States and Processes for Mental Health

Advancing Psychotherapy Effectiveness

States and Processes for Mental Health

Advancing Psychotherapy Effectiveness

Brad Bowins
Psychiatrist, Researcher,
and Founder of the Centre
for Theoretical Research in
Psychiatry and Clinical Psychology,
Toronto, Canada

ELSEVIER

ACADEMIC PRESS
An imprint of Elsevier
elsevier.com/books-and-journals

Academic Press is an imprint of Elsevier
125 London Wall, London EC2Y 5AS, United Kingdom
525 B Street, Suite 1650, San Diego, CA 92101, United States
50 Hampshire Street, 5th Floor, Cambridge, MA 02139, United States
The Boulevard, Langford Lane, Kidlington, Oxford OX5 1GB, United Kingdom

British Library Cataloguing-in-Publication Data
A catalogue record for this book is available from the British Library

Library of Congress Cataloging-in-Publication Data
A catalog record for this book is available from the Library of Congress

ISBN: 978-0-323-85049-0

For Information on all Academic Press publications visit our website at https://www.elsevier.com/books-and-journals

Publisher: Nikki Levy
Acquisition Editor: Joslyn Chaiprasert-Paguio
Editorial Project Manager: Sam W. Young
Production Project Manager: Niranjan Bhaskaran
Cover Designer: Greg Harris

Typeset by Aptara, New Delhi, India

To my children, Emma, Mark, and Breanna,
and my wife Lynne.

Contents

Section II
Forms of psychotherapy and non-specific factors proof of concept

Preface

Psychotherapy constitutes the most prominent mental health intervention given the diversity of issues it is applied to. However, despite its prominence the mechanism of action is still unknown, and surprisingly or even shockingly, little attention is paid to this crucial topic relative to efficacy and process research. An accurate understanding of how psychotherapy works will place it on a more solid scientific foundation, and guide highly targeted and effective interventions. The current discrete approach to psychotherapy informs regarding how this treatment modality is commonly perceived to work: distinct types designed to remedy psychopathology. For example, cognitive therapy altering negative cognitions and interpersonal psychotherapy correcting defective relationship patterns. Mental health is then indirectly advanced by remedying psychopathology. While at a surface level the rational appears to have merit, a closer look reveals profound conceptual and practical problems. Three major conceptual concerns stand out. First, there are far too many discrete forms of psychotherapy directed at a given type of mental illness such as depression, an unlikely occurrence due to how problems require specific solutions and rarely respond to countless interventions. For instance, physical health issues such as heart disease require precise interventions. Second, virtually every form of psychotherapy is applied to remedy numerous types of mental illness, equivalent to heart treatments directed to multiple organ systems, a scenario that is absurd in the physical health domain. Third, how nonspecific factors are inexplicable, if it is indeed the special sauce of a given form of psychotherapy that is instrumental in remedying psychopathology to improve mental health. Nonspecific factors, such as hope, the therapeutic alliance, and placebo effect, are very robust, but in the context of specific interventions to remedy psychopathology this impact is impossible to understand, or tortuous at best.

In terms of practical problems, three further issues stand out, the first being the sheer number of psychotherapy types. Presently there are numerous forms of psychotherapy, with the numbers increased by subtypes, applications specific to individual, family, and couple therapy, and also how each of these is often combined with other forms of psychotherapy, such as mindfulness and cognitive therapy. Hundreds of specific types of psychotherapy currently exist, and as the expansion trend continues it is inevitable that in 50–100 years the number will easily exceed 1000! The overwhelming array of psychotherapy types both now and in the future creates confusion, stress, and cost for consumers, providers, educators, and funders. Efficacy research is focused on to ensure adequate funding for the given form of psychotherapy, bringing into play the second practical problem—research bias. Whenever a product such as psychotherapy is involved there is a high potential for research bias, and the literature is saturated with poorly controlled studies typically conducted by the originator or students of the psychotherapy type, as opposed to truly independent and objective evaluations. Fads and fades comprise the third practical problem: history reveals that heavy promotion of a psychotherapy type produces fads (popularity substantially outstripping robust evidence) that fade once the originator and a generation or two of students fade away. For example, Rational-Emotive Therapy and Person-Centered Therapy were once extremely popular with their application outstripping solid evidence, but now are rarely practiced. These very profound conceptual and practical problems even individually, but certainly in combination, result in a very weak foundation for psychotherapy. Consequently, a new approach to psychotherapy is required that resolves the conceptual and practical problems associated with the current understanding.

States and Processes for Mental Health: Advancing Psychotherapy Effectiveness presents a novel mechanism of action for psychotherapy. Mental health is characterized by key states and processes—activity, psychological defense mechanisms, social connectedness, regulation, human-specific cognition, self-acceptance, and adaptability—with positive affectivity over negative affectivity following from them if it is to be sustainable. Intact functioning on these states and processes fosters mental health, and impairments to each of them produce mental illness. Psychotherapy directly enhances these key states and processes for mental health through both factors specific to a given form of therapy and nonspecific factors. Mental illness is remedied and overall mental health improved. By emphasizing the most robust specific and nonspecific factors enhancing the states and processes for mental health, the effectiveness of psychotherapy is advanced.

The approach to psychotherapy based on states and processes for mental health resolves the conceptual and practical problems arising from the current discrete psychotherapy approach. Pertaining to the conceptual issues, excessive generalizability in terms of too many forms of psychotherapy directed to a specific form of mental illness such as depression, and most forms of psychotherapy applied to many mental illnesses, will no longer transpire. The most robust specific and nonspecific strategies will be applied to directly enhance states and processes for mental health, an approach that resolves mental illness. For example, improving emotion regulation enhances the regulation state and process for mental health remedying depression, anxiety, and other mental health problems ensuing from emotional dysregulation. Likewise, behavioral activation advances another key state and process for mental health—activity—remedying mental illnesses that arise from impaired activity and excessive inhibition. As these examples suggest, the approach is both transdiagnostic and transtherapy: the states and processes characterizing mental health span diagnoses and forms of psychotherapy, and the strategies for advancing these states and processes apply to various forms of mental illness and follow from several specific forms of psychotherapy. The perplexing divide between specific and nonspecific psychotherapy factors is resolved, because both advance the states and processes for mental health.

In regards to practical problems, instead of hundreds and potentially over a thousand forms of psychotherapy, states and processes for mental health are directly enhanced by applying robust specific and nonspecific strategies. Research to establish efficacy for a given form of psychotherapy is no longer required, reducing research bias. Solid strategies derived from specific forms of psychotherapy will be preserved, ending the fad and fade scenario that history reveals. This new understanding of how psychotherapy actually works is presented in three sections:

Section 1 identifies the key states and processes for mental health: activity, psychological defense mechanisms, social connectedness, regulation, human-specific cognition, self-acceptance, and adaptability. The role of each in mental health and illness will be described, as well as how they contribute to positive emotions exceeding negative emotions in a stable fashion.

Section 2 examines 15 major forms of psychotherapy (Acceptance & Commitment Therapy, Behavioral Therapy, Cognitive Therapy, Compassion-Focused Therapy, Emotion-Focused Therapy, Existential Psychotherapy, Gestalt Therapy, Interpersonal Psychotherapy, Mindfulness-Based Therapy, Narrative Therapy, Person-Centered Therapy, Positive Psychotherapy, Problem-Solving Therapy, Psychoanalytic Therapy, Rational-Emotive Therapy) and nonspecific factors, providing a comprehensive overview of what distinguishes each, with an empirical and theoretical proof of concept showing how they do indeed enhance the states and processes for mental health.

Section 3 first takes a close look at the conceptual and practical problems inherent in the current discrete psychotherapy approach, whereby various forms of psychotherapy are oriented to remedying psychopathology. The new approach to psychotherapy is then presented, applying general strategies and those derived from existing forms of psychotherapy to advance each of the states and processes for mental health. The most robust strategies derived from those detailed in Section 2 are clearly identified.

This transdiagnostic and transtherapy model of psychotherapy emphasizing states and processes for mental health, advances psychotherapy effectiveness by placing it on a solid scientific foundation, resolving the conceptual and practical problems inherent in the current discrete approach to psychotherapy, aligning specific and nonspecific factors, and providing robust therapeutic strategies. Psychotherapists, students of psychotherapy, educators, payers, and consumers will all benefit. Change is always a challenge, but given that the only constant is change it is inevitable, and with the insurmountable problems inherent in the psychopathology-based understanding of psychotherapy, that change necessitates a different understanding of how psychotherapy actually works, and a new approach based on this reformulation.

Section I

States and processes for mental health

Chapter 1

Introduction

For many psychotherapists, the notion of focusing on what constitutes mental health might ironically seem unusual, given how we are so focused on mental illness. However, everything considered we are ultimately restoring mental health. It is interesting that despite helping people achieve good mental health, psychotherapists are often at a loss regarding what states and processes actually characterize it. Prior to writing this section, I informally asked several psychotherapists what they believe characterizes mental health. Both the nonverbal and verbal responses were very informative and telling of how alien the mental health focus is. In contrast to being asked what mental illness involves, with terms such as depression, anxiety, trauma, psychological conflict, flowing without hesitation, there was a lag in responding indicating that conscious, nonautomatic processing was being engaged. The responses frequently being of the form, "Not being depressed or anxious," which is really just negating psychopathology as the focus, or some generic response such as "Happiness and contentment," which pops out from pop psychology. Equally telling, I often had more luck asking lay people who had never conducted psychotherapy, with responses such as, "Regulation of emotions," "Self-improvement," "Being yourself." Lay people are often more focused on what good mental health entails than psychotherapists!

One of my initial purposes in asking psychotherapists what characterizes mental health was to get a diverse perspective on the topic. Considering several of my own peer-reviewed publications, I realized that although my focus was more on psychopathology, I had inadvertently addressed what constitutes mental health by uncovering and describing various states and processes that suffer with mental illness such as activity, regulation, human specific cognition, and psychological defenses. These and others revealed through further research yielded the following states and processes for mental health:

Activity
Psychological Defense Mechanisms
Social Connectedness
Regulation
Human-Specific Cognition
Self-Acceptance
Adaptability

States and Processes for Mental Health. DOI: 10.1016/C2020-0-00574-8

Given that there are numerous aspects to mental health, as there are to mental illness, this set is not necessarily exhaustive and future research might address additional states and processes characterizing it. However, I strongly recommend not diffusing options to the point where they become unworkable or meaningless, and instead adhering to core characteristics. Some readers might be surprised at the omission of a happiness theme, but as we will see the positive emotions of happiness and interest really only transpire under special circumstances as brief responses. The quest for this state being ever present ends up being misguided and futile as revealed in the Adaptability chapter. More reasonable is a scenario whereby positive emotions exceed negative emotions, or in other words, positive affectivity over negative affectivity. This scenario aligns with mental health, but for reasons that we will get to it follows from activity, psychological defense mechanisms, social connectedness, regulation, human-specific cognition, self-acceptance, and adaptability if it is to be sustainable.

The core states and processes for mental health are compromised with mental illness, both formal variants such as depression, anxiety, psychosis, schizophrenia, mania, posttraumatic stress disorder, eating disorders, addictions, and more informal scenarios that often lead people to seek psychotherapy. These latter presentations encompass a diverse array of issues, including self-concept and self-esteem deficits, loneliness and social isolation, recurrent maladaptive behavior, failure to progress in life, and countless more. Indeed, if functioning on all of the core states and processes is robust the person has no need for psychotherapy or any form of mental health intervention, but when functioning is impaired psychotherapy is required. We will now see how activity, psychological defense mechanisms, social connectedness, regulation, human-specific cognition, self-acceptance, and adaptability enhance mental health, and when impaired produce mental illness.

Chapter 2

Activity

During our evolution in hunting–gathering groups, being active was crucial. There were no grocery stores, houses, and security from predators. Food had to be gathered and hunted, warm and secure sleeping sites sought out wherever the group moved to in search of resources, and although our ancestors were not the meatiest animal they were on the menu of various predators. Doing as little as "humanly" possible probably would not have worked out so well under the vast majority of circumstances. Evolutionary research reveals how we evolved to be physically active related to a hunting–gathering way of life, and how inactivity, although fine for our more sedentary Great Ape relatives, is very detrimental for humans (Pontzer, 2017; Raichlen and Alexander, 2017). Hence, activity is consistent with human evolutionary success (fitness) and health, while inactivity hinders both. Success in finding good food, safe sleeping and resting sites, and other valuable resources contributed to physical and mental wellbeing.

Backing up the assertion that activity characterizes good mental health are the profiles on two ancient motivational systems: behavioral approach/activation system (BAS) and behavioral inhibition system (BIS). As is evident from the names BAS is approach and activation focused generating reinforcement, whereas the BIS system emphasizes withdrawal and inhibited behavior more consistent with a lack of reinforcement and punishment (Fowles, 1988; Gray, 1987). Levels on both occur on a continuum, but we will consider low and high points. Low behavioral activation and high behavioral inhibition is the profile found with depression. For instance, Kasch et al. (2002) compared 62 patients with major depressive disorder (High Hamilton Depression Inventory Scores and Low Global Assessment of Functioning Scale Scores) to 27 matched nondepressive controls, finding that the depressed subjects scored significantly lower on BAS than did the nondepressed controls. They also found that the depressed subjects had high behavioral inhibition (BIS). Anxiety involves high behavioral inhibition (Bowins, 2012a; Fowles, 1988; Gray, 1987; Kasch et al., 2002; Schneier et al., 2002; Scholten et al., 2006). Consistent with these outcomes for depression and anxiety, BIS and negative affectivity are related concepts, sometimes used interchangeably, as are BAS and positive affectivity (Gray, 1987; Kasch et al., 2002). Positive and negative affectivity can be viewed as expressions of BAS and BIS, respectively (Kasch et al., 2002). Hence, by altering BAS and BIS changes in affectivity transpire.

States and Processes for Mental Health. DOI: 10.1016/C2020-0-00574-8

High behavioral inhibition blocks or limits actions and is consistent with anxiety and the root emotion, fear. Emotions are brief responses to external and internal stimuli, typically lasting seconds to minutes, or at most hours to days as an extended mood state. Fear, sadness, anger, disgust, shame, happiness, interest, and surprise appear to be universal, based on research focusing on preliterate societies having little contact with the larger world (Ekman, 1972, 1994; Ekman and Friesen, 1971; Izard, 1977; Tomkins, 1962, 1963). These societies have mostly vanished and so it is very important that we have this earlier research to go by. For example, Ekman and Friesen (1971) gave isolated New Guinea tribal people photographs each containing facial expressions of either happiness, sadness, anger, disgust, surprise, and fear, and told them a story that involved one emotion. These people were able to match stories to facial expressions for the six emotions beyond that predicted by chance. The researchers went one step further and had nine New Guineans show how their face would appear if they were the person in the story. The unedited videotapes were shown to college students in the United States who quite accurately recognized the displayed emotion (Ekman, 1972).

If based on this evidence we accept that certain emotions that we are all very familiar with are universal, even in those having little contact with the larger world, then it is logical to conclude that they are genetically based, and from this must have served an evolutionary function. Indeed, further research has identified the so-called "deep structures," or in other words core themes, intrinsic to each universal emotion (Beck, 1991; Boucher and Carlson, 1980; Eley and Stevenson, 2000; Finlay-Jones and Brown, 1981; Izard, 1991; Keltner and Buswell, 1997; Rozin et al., 1999; Shaver et al., 1987; Vrana, 1993):

- Fear—threat or danger.
- Sadness—loss.
- Anger—violation or damage.
- Disgust—physically or morally repulsive stimuli.
- Shame—social or perhaps moral transgression.
- Happiness—gain.
- Interest—potential reward.
- Surprise—unanticipated occurrences either positive or negative.

A quick consideration of these core themes suggests that they cover a wide range of occurrences, and also that how we respond to these circumstances impacts success and failure outcomes. For example, failure to respond to threat or danger results in negative consequences, in some cases tragic. Managing loss can stem the depletion and either restore the resources or compensate. Violation and damage needs to be challenged. Social, and possible moral, transgression requires alterations in behavior often appeasement oriented. Gain indicates success, and maintaining behavior producing this outcome often leads to further gains. Potential reward motivates actions directed toward it. Positive surprise motivates efforts to capitalize on the unexpected scenario, while negative surprise encourages withdrawal.

I have proposed that the evolution of human intelligence amplified emotional states—the amplification effect—by making the conscious and unconscious cognitive activating appraisals that trigger emotions more intensive, extensive, and adding a temporal dimension (Bowins, 2004, 2006). For example, a person processes negative feedback from a boss as a threat, triggering fear. This person then thinks of all the implications for the job intensifying the threat. Repercussions in other areas are also dwelled on, such as how the identified negative characteristic or behavior impacts social relationships outside of work, thereby extending the threat. These various threat-oriented scenarios are replayed adding a temporal dimension. Consequently, the threat and emotional reaction of fear is amplified. Amplified fear produces anxiety, while amplified sadness contributes to depression (Bowins, 2004, 2006). Likewise, amplified anger results in excessive aggression.

The amplification effect also plays out with behavioral inhibition and behavioral activation, given that cognitive activating appraisals play a role (Bowins, 2004, 2006). For example, a thought such as, "I know this is going to result in a bad outcome," will intensify inhibition, while the thought, "Although it will be challenging, there is little risk," greatly diminishes inhibition. Likewise, the thought, "This setback is just too much, I've had enough," diminishes behavioral activation, while the thought, "I've learned from this experience and now know how to succeed," intensifies behavioral activation.

Amplified fear and intensified cognitive activating appraisals for behavioral inhibition ensure that BIS is high in anxiety states. Amplified sadness involves high BIS and also intensified cognitive activating appraisals favoring low behavioral activation (low BAS), hence it is not surprising that depression is also characterized by behavioral inhibition and withdrawal. The opposite BAS and BIS profile—high BAS and low BIS—is consistent with mental health in terms of an absence of anxiety and depression, with behavioral activation > behavioral inhibition, or even behavioral activation >> behavioral inhibition, contributing to reinforcing experiences and elevated mental wellbeing. During the 95% or so of our evolution in hunting-gathering groups this BAS and BIS profile would likely have increased evolutionary fitness.

Hence, based on the ancient motivational systems of BAS and BIS, activity is good for mental health. Most people tend to feel better when they are active, so long as the activity is not inherently negative to them. For example, a person who does not have good muscle strength and fears heights, will probably feel worse with mountain climbing, although if determined to overcome their fear, positive mental health outcomes might ensue. Consistent with this suggestion, research has revealed that physical, nature, social, art/hobby, and music activity advance mental health, both in terms of lower mental illness and enhanced mental wellbeing in the general population (Bowins, 2020). Cognitive activity likely does so as well, but research is almost exclusively focused on cognitive activity and cognitive, not emotional, functioning. We will now look at how physical, nature, art/hobby, and music forms of activity benefit mental health, leaving social activity to the Social connectedness chapter. Since this book is proposing an alternative model for understanding psychotherapy, and such therapies are oriented to mental health, we will not be examining physical health outcomes, although better physical health frequently translates into improved mental health.

Physical activity

Body and mind are connected, and from this alone it follows that physical activity can improve mental health, given that physical activity is very good for physical health. Beyond the body and mind relationship there is a great deal of evidence supporting the mental health benefits of physical activity (Bowins, 2020). We will now look at why physical activity has such a benefit by presenting research that backs up the assertion. Perhaps the most obvious way that such activity advances mental health is by making people feel better emotionally. Investigating this possibility, Hyde and fellow researchers (Hyde et al., 2011) assessed 190 university students for varying feeling states potentially following from physical activity. The Leisure Score Index of the Godin Leisure Time Exercise Questionnaire was applied to assess physical activity, and questions evaluated feeling states. Pleasant-activated feelings were associated with physical activity, and the level of such feelings increased with more physical activity, even on a given day. This outcome might occur, at least in part, due to enhanced synaptic (between nerve cells) transmission of chemical messengers known as monoamines in the brain, including dopamine, norepinephrine, and serotonin: the monoamine enhancement theory (Lubans et al., 2016). However, even though exercise does increase neurotransmitters in the peripheral nervous system, this does not directly impact the brain, given that these neurotransmitters cannot cross the blood-brain barrier (Lubans et al., 2016). Hence, the way that neurotransmitters might mediate this influence of physical activity on emotions is not clear.

Bolstering positive feelings aligns with physical activity reducing negative feelings and stress. Puterman et al. (2017) studied this option as part of the National Study of Daily Experiences, assessing 2,022 adults aged 33–84, questioning them on 8 consecutive nights regarding their general affect and affective responses to stressful events, as well as their engagement in physical activities. Their results revealed that negative affect was significantly elevated on days with stressful events compared to days free of such events, and physical activity reduced the impact. In addition, the closer the time frame between the stressor and physical activity, the less impact in terms of negative mood, and in active participants, negative affect in response to stressors remained low if they were active that day (Puterman et al., 2017). So, physical activity enhances positive affect and also diminishes negative affect and stress responses! The combination certainly underscores the emotional benefits of physical activity.

The question arises as to how physical activity might favor positive over negative emotions? The answer appears to reside in absorption in the physical activity, which is typically positive to the individual, hence absorption in a positive activity. In line with this possibility is the response style theory proposing that physical activity acts as a distraction from negative thoughts, and as an ongoing response style is an effective way to counter negativity (Nolen-Hoeksema et al., 2008). In the case of depression there is a negative focus mostly on loss-related real or potential occurrences, and anxiety threat relevant thoughts. Physical activity potentially distracts a person from such negative thoughts, promoting better mental health as an ongoing response pattern. Flow theory proposed by Csikszentmihalyi (1990) indicates that when a person becomes engaged in an activity, detrimental thoughts and feelings are pushed aside.

Various psychosocial influences have been suggested including self-efficacy, mastery, self-acceptance, self-esteem, self-concept, physical self-perceptions, purpose in life, and motivation. These potential mechanisms have varying levels of support and confusion arises from an overlap in terms, such as self-concept, physical self-perceptions, and self-esteem. None stands out as being fully relevant to most or all people who engage in physical activity, but improved and diversified motivation appears quite robust. Combining cross-sectional and longitudinal research designs Aaltonen et al. (2014) assessed the motives for leisure time physical activity, among 2,308 active and inactive participants. Motives for physical activity were based on responses to the Recreational Exercise Motivation Measure. The active participants scored higher on mastery, physical fitness, social aspects of physical activity, psychological state, enjoyment, willingness to be fitter/look better than others, and appearance than inactive participants, and this outcome was consistent for a decade of results, suggesting that these benefits align with ongoing physical activity. Inactive participants only scored higher on the conforming to expectations motivation.

One good thing often leads to another, due to enhanced motivation and reinforcement. For example, with enhanced positive motivations like participants in the Aaltonen et al. (2014) study experienced, physically active people might feel better about themselves with improved confidence and self-efficacy, then engage in more positive activity. Consistent with this possibility, Dinger et al. (2014) examined physical activity and health-related behaviors among 67,861 US college students who completed the National College Health Assessment II during the 2008–2009 academic year. Those who met moderate to vigorous physical activity recommendations also tended to have adequate daily fruit and vegetable consumption, positive perception of general health, healthy body mass index, consistent seatbelt use, not smoking cigarettes, less perceived depression, and adequate sleep. Physical activity and the enhanced motivation then lead to additional healthy behaviors with reinforcing effects.

Returning to neurological explanations, beyond neurotransmitters that tend to act in shorter time frames, there is evidence for longer term changes induced by physical activity. For example, Lubans et al. (2016) indicate how exercise appears to increase the growth of new blood vessels in the brain, aiding the transportation of nutrients to neurons which enhances their growth and survival. Deslandes et al. (2009) provide evidence for exercise increasing blood flow in several cortical and subcortical areas, thereby promoting neurogenesis. Presumably, by enhancing blood flow and neurogenesis there could be some downstream benefits to mental health, and resilience to mental illness.

Acting through several pathways physical activity promotes mental health. Such activity tends to increase positive feelings and reduce negative feelings, likely due to absorption in the positive pursuit that can even generate a "flow" experience. As an ongoing response style this absorptive benefit derived from physical activity helps maintain good mental health, and blocks or counters the negativity inherent in depression and anxiety. Psychosocial advantages can follow from physical activity, with enhanced positive motivation likely a key one leading to further healthy behavior and reinforcing effects. Longer range neurological changes pertaining to enhanced blood flow and neurogenesis might also help explain the mental health benefits of physical activity.

Nature activity

Being in nature does tend to make most people feel calmer, and consistent with this occurrence a major research outcome is how nature activity increases nervous system relaxation responses while diminishing stress responses (Bowins, 2020). The autonomic nervous system generally divides into parasympathetic and sympathetic, the former is active with relaxation responses and the latter is active when stress responses occur. Eating and romance typically activates the parasympathetic autonomic nervous system, while running from a predator, if any still exist for most people, activates the sympathetic autonomic nervous system. One of these systems usually dominates at a given point, although the time frame can be short. For instance, while running from a predator you are unlikely to be thinking about eating (maybe being eaten) or romance until the threat is over. By enhancing relaxation responses and diminishing stress responses, nature activity can advance mental health in the moment, and also ongoing if a person engages in such activity on a frequent basis.

Regarding research supporting the notion of increased relaxation parasympathetic autonomic nervous system activity and reduced stress-related sympathetic autonomic nervous system activity, there are some interesting field experiments. One of these is by Song et al. (2014) who had 17 males in their early twenties walk a predetermined course in an urban park and also nearby city area during the spring season. Physiological measures consisted of heart rate and heart rate variability, and the Profiles of Mood States and State-Trait Anxiety Inventory assessed mental health parameters. Heart rate was lower while walking in the urban park compared to the city area indicating relaxation responses. Heart rate variability is a measure of autonomic control of the heart, particularly vagal activity, with lower variability linked to cardiovascular disease. Based on this measure the urban park walk produced higher healthy parasympathetic nervous system activity and the city street walk elevated sympathetic nervous system activity. Subjective responses were in line with the physiological results, the urban park walk producing higher indications of comfortable, natural, and relaxed. On the Profiles of Mood States, tension-anxiety and fatigue scores were lower and the vigor scores higher for the urban park walk. Another research study using heart rate variability as a measure is that by Gladwell et al. (2016), assessing it during sleep for 13 adult participants after lunchtime walks in nature and built-up areas. The walks were over 1.8 km distances and the speed was the same in both settings. Heart rate variability was greater during sleep after the nature walk, suggesting enhanced relaxation responses to this form of activity compared to similar walks in built-up areas.

Nature can be so relaxing that the citizens of Japan embrace "forest bathing" or Shinrin-yoku, meaning taking in the forest. People partake in forest bathing excursions to relieve stress. Investigating the benefit, Park et al. (2010) conducted field experiments in 24 forests and city areas across Japan. Each area had 12 participants with 6 walking in the given forest area and 6 in the nearby urban area on the first day, reversing the area on the second day. Each participant also viewed scenes from the given setting without walking. Physiological measurements including salivary cortisol, blood pressure, pulse, and heart rate variability were conducted in the morning and before and after each walk and viewing. Physiological results were compatible with increased parasympathetic and reduced sympathetic autonomic nervous system activity in response to the forest walks, but not the urban walks. Even just viewing the forest setting produced the same relaxation pattern.

Forest bathing has even been found to reduce inflammation that might be associated with mental illness. Mao et al. (2012) recruited 20 healthy male university students and randomly sent 10 to stay 2 nights in a broad-leaved evergreen forest, and the other 10 to stay 2 nights in a city area. Markers of inflammation including cortisol, plasma endothelin-1, interleukin-6, and tumor necrosis factor were measured before and after the stays. The Profile of Mood States assessed emotional changes. Levels of the inflammatory markers were the same for both groups at the start, but dropped in the forest group, as did negative moods, while vigor scores increased. Instead of participants just going to city settings, Li (2010) had female and male "controls" conduct their normal work routines in urban areas, while other participants engaged in "forest bathing." Tests for inflammation took place before the outings, at the end, as well as 7 and 30 days after. Indicators of inflammation were reduced in the forest participants, and natural killer cells that perform a very important function in destroying foreign organisms entering the body were still elevated 30 days after the forest stay! To the extent that inflammation impacts mental illness, there might conceivably be a benefit to mental health via reduced inflammation from nature activity.

Enhanced parasympathetic relaxation responses and diminished sympathetic stress responses do seem to arise from nature activity, consistent with what is known as the Stress Reduction Theory by Ulrich et al. (1991), but why does this occur? In some instance, nature can be stressful such as when there are mosquitos or settings that might be hiding a dangerous animal or person. Indeed, Gatersleben and Andrews (2013) have found that nature settings low in prospect (clear field of vision) and high in refuge (places to hide) can actually induce stress responses. The initial part of their study involved an online survey of 269 participants, with them rating perceived restorativeness of environments presented in slides that varied in prospect and refuge. They then had 17 of the participants engage in walks and watch videos of the walks, varying prospect and refuge features. Natural environments low in prospect and high in refuge were not rated as restorative and appeared to increase stress and attentional fatigue, both with online viewing and actual walks. However, assuming that the natural setting is perceived to be safe, such as with high prospect and low refuge, and generally in a safe area, relaxation responses ensue.

To explain the benefits of nature activity, E.O. Wilson (Wilson, 1984) proposed the Biophilia Hypothesis, stating that based on our evolution in natural settings humans have an innate tendency to seek contact with nature and other life forms, resulting in positive feelings from such contact. Due to this evolutionary influence, the human brain might synchronize with features of nature. Florence Williams (Williams, 2017) indicates how aspects of natural environments including fractal patterns, color saturation, rounded and smooth contours, and spatial frequency are pleasing to us generating positive feelings, because they align with how the brain evolved. Fractal patterns are those that repeat from larger to smaller, such as a tree branching from trunk to limbs to smaller extensions. Spatial frequency refers to amount of detail per degree of spatial angle; we prefer moderate levels of spatial frequency characterizing nature to limit information processing demands. This alignment of natural features and evolution of the human brain helps explain why nature activity induces relaxation responses.

A more specific way that nature might advance relaxation responses is by shifting negative thought processes consistent with depression and anxiety to positive ones. A negative process everyone has experienced is worry, greatly heightened in depression, anxiety, and stress (Olatunji et al., 2010), and referred to as ruminations in the case of depression. Bratman et al. (2015) found that nature walks reduce rumination, in a study where 38 adult participants underwent regional cerebral blood flow measurements and filled out the Reflection Rumination Questionnaire, before and after a 90-min walk in either a natural or urban setting with random assignment to each. Only the nature walk reduced rumination scores and also activity in a brain region known as the subgenual prefrontal cortex that shows increased activity during sadness, behavioral withdrawal, and negative self-reflection, all linked to rumination. People tend to seek out environments that transform negative psychological states to positive ones, and these environments are typically natural with pleasing aesthetic qualities, such as open spaces and quiet (Bratman et al., 2015). Much like with physical activity, nature activity shifts negative thought processes into positive ones, producing an absorption in a positive focus.

Nature activity advances mental health largely by enhancing relaxation inducing parasympathetic autonomic nervous system activity, and diminishing stress-related sympathetic nervous system activity. By enhancing the former, the latter is diminished as these systems counter one another. The synchronicity of our brain structure to core features of nature, such as fractal patterns, color saturation, rounded and smooth contours, and spatial frequency, based on evolution in natural settings, appears to play a key role in the relaxation response with nature activity. A shift of negative thoughts to positive ones consistent with the relaxation response generates absorption in a positive experience further advancing mental health.

Art/hobby activity

Drawings by early humans etched into cave walls and colored with pigments suggest that creativity has been part of human nature for a long time. With the stresses that modern humans face working long hours and raising children, commonly without the support of a larger group or community, creative pursuits are often sacrificed. However, when people take the time they usually feel better from engaging in art and hobby activities. Research focused on arts and mental health tends to be qualitative yielding narrative outcomes, and while this is a limitation in a sense given it does not provide objective results, it is strength in many ways by generating very personally meaningful information (Bowins, 2020). Reviewing these qualitative studies (Davies et al., 2016; Lawson et al., 2014; Makin and Gask, 2012; Margrove et al., 2013; Stickley and Eades, 2013; Van Lith et al., 2011; Zarobe and Bungay, 2017) several core ways that art and hobby activity benefits mental health emerge consisting of the following (Bowins, 2020):

- Empowerment: Enhancement of self-confidence, self-esteem, self-worth, competency, self-expression, and a greater sense of control in life, with the overriding theme empowerment.
- Absorption: Shifting away from negative foci and immersion in positive experiences, based on heightened concentration providing a flow experience, distraction from negative emotions, and absorption in an activity.
- Self-actualization: Maslow's (1934) hierarchy of needs pyramid is relevant, with self-actualization possible once more basic needs including physiological, safety, love/belonging, and self-esteem are satisfied. Narrative themes indicating self-actualization from art/hobby activity consist of practical and aspirational achievement, broadened horizons, accessing new worlds, assuming and sustaining identities, acquisition of valued skills, greater knowledge, personal achievement, heightened creativity, and transformative.
- Social connectedness: This only applies when art and hobby activity is done in a social context which is common for research studies. Sense of belonging, improved social and communication skills, peer support, sense of community, and connection to the larger community indicate that social connectedness is a way that art/hobby activity benefits mental health.

- Motivation: Enhancement of general motivation from having a purposeful activity, cognitive and creative challenge, setting goals, intrinsic motivation, and meaningful pursuits.

These benefits individually or in combination can clearly improve mental illness and advance mental health in the general population. An example of a research study demonstrating that art and hobby activity can improve mental illness is that by Makin and Gask (2012), who investigated benefits of the United Kingdom Arts on Prescription Program for people with chronic mental health issues. Qualitative in-depth interviews were applied to 15 participants with persistent anxiety and depression. Key benefits consisted of the therapeutic effect of absorption in an activity, the creative potential of art, and the social aspect of attendance. Another analysis of the Arts on Prescription program conducted by Stickley and Eades (2013) revealed narrative themes of education, practical and aspirational achievements, broadened horizons, accessing new worlds, assuming and sustaining identities, and social and relational perceptions. Shifting to Australia, Van Lith et al. (2011) interviewed 18 participants who attended an arts program in Australia for people with mental illness. The participants described the experience as transformative, enabling them to take more control of their life, and this in turn generated a feeling of strength, confidence, and sense of playing a role in their recovery, each of these contributing to a sense of empowerment.

Beyond the qualitative research, there are some experimental studies looking at the mental health benefits of art and hobby activity. One such study conducted in England and applying a very naturalistic experimental design is that by Margrove et al. (2013) who compared 26 people completing a 12-week course in Open Arts to 32 individuals on the wait list, the latter providing a control condition. Mental health was measured at baseline and after the 12 weeks via the Warwick Edinburgh Mental Well-Being Scale. The baseline measurements did not reveal any significant differences between the two groups, but after the Open Arts course participants scored significantly higher than the wait list people. Course participants reported enjoying the activities (96%), improved confidence (81%), and enhanced motivation (88%).

Art and hobby activity does counter mental illness and advance mental health in the general population. This is not surprising given the psychosocial benefits including empowerment, absorption, self-actualization, social connectedness (when in a group setting), and motivation. The benefits once experienced often lead to further creative activities providing an additive advantage. I often say that everyone needs a hobby (while few seem to have one), and the research backs up my assertion.

Music activity

Everyone seems to like music, mostly listening but frequently singing, dancing, or playing an instrument. However, just because we like it does not necessarily mean that it is good for mental health. Fortunately, quite an extensive body of research demonstrates that music activity improves mental illness and advances mental wellbeing in the general population (Bowins, 2020). Regarding mental illness, Pylvanainen et al. (2015) compared dance therapy to treatment as usual for adults with moderate to severe depression. Dance therapy consisted of 12 weeks of group dance intervention with assessment before, just after, and 3 months later for depressive symptoms. Dance therapy participants improved more than those in treatment as usual which included antidepressant medication. Studying depressed elderly people living in the community within Hong Kong, Chan et al. (2009) conducted a randomized controlled study of 47 people with 23 assigned to a music group and 24 to a no music control condition. Music listening was the focus, with depression levels, blood pressure, heart rate, respiratory rate, assessed. After a month depression levels and blood pressure were significantly lower for those in the music group than in the no music group.

An interesting study conducted in Norway, Austria, and Australia by Gold et al. (2013) randomly assigned 144 people with various mental health issues—schizophrenia, depression, and substance abuse—and low therapy motivation to music therapy plus treatment as usual or just treatment as usual. Music therapy was superior to treatment as usual, which included medications, for total negative symptoms, functioning, clinical global impressions, social avoidance, and vitality. Low motivation frequently translates into limited benefits for any psychological intervention, hence these results for music therapy are particularly impressive.

Regarding mental health for those in the general population, a comprehensive review by Daykin et al. (2017) involved 61 relevant studies, with music activity consisting of listening or regular group singing. Their results provide solid support for the notion that music activity improves, or at least is associated with, mental wellbeing. A study by Coulton et al. (2015) of elderly people in the general population randomly assigned 258 participants to either a community singing activity or usual activities group. By 3 months, mental health quality of life was superior in the singing condition, and anxiety and depression were also lower.

How might music activity benefit mental health? A major way that this appears to transpire is in the processing of emotions, that can involve regulating responses, such as when feeling sad listening to upbeat music, or expressing emotions as with listening to a sad song when feeling sad. Carlson et al. (2015) demonstrated how music processes emotions by applying the Music in Mood Regulation scale and assessing depression, anxiety, and neuroticism with the young participants also undergoing magnetic resonance imaging (MRI) to measure responses to musical scores designed to elicit both positive and negative emotions. Music eliciting negative emotions produced regulation responses for females with high diversion scores on the Music in Mood Regulation scale, indicated by increased activity of the medial prefrontal cortex (mPFC). Males and particularly those higher in anxiety and neuroticism showed reduced mPFC activity in response to negative emotion eliciting music, which aligned with high discharge responses. The emotion processing induced by music can then entail regulation and expression (discharge) responses.

Music production in the younger years of life appears to advance brain maturation, which might have upstream benefits for mental health. Hudziak et al. (2014) conducted a project as part of the United States National Institutes of Health Magnetic Resonance Imaging Study of Normal Brain Development, applying MRI and behavioral testing to 232 youths from 6 to 18 years of age, with up to three separate visits 2 years apart. The music training of participants was included in the analysis. They found that playing an instrument produced more rapid cortical thickening (maturation) in several brain regions including motor, premotor, and supplementary motor cortices, as well as prefrontal and parietal cortices; areas involved in motor planning and coordination, visuospatial ability, and emotion and impulse regulation. The emotion results backup the emotional processing role of music activity (Hudziak et al., 2014).

Music activity also appears to have a beneficial impact on immune system mediators of stress responses, as found by Fancourt et al. (2016) who investigated those with cancer (55), bereaved caregivers (66), and caregivers still dealing with a person suffering from cancer (72). Group singing comprised the intervention, and measures of mood, stress, and immune system status were conducted before and after singing sessions. Singing was associated with a reduction in negative emotions and increase in positive emotions, and biological immune system mediators improved with increases in cytokines and reductions in cortisol, beta-endorphin, and oxytocin for all three groups (Fancourt et al., 2016). Music then assists with stress responses even at an immune system level.

Qualitative research yielding narrative themes suggests additional ways that music activity can benefit mental health (Orjasaeter et al., 2017; Perkins et al., 2016; Solli et al., 2013). These themes include the development of strengths and resources contributing to a positive identity, becoming a whole person with multiple identities, connection with life through rhythm, and sense of purpose via progression and creative expression. They each involve immersion in positive experiences and a disconnect from negativity.

Music activity does seem to improve mental illness and advance mental health in the general population. A key way that this transpires is the processing of emotions in terms of regulation and expression. Almost everyone has listened to a happy song to regulate sadness, and a sad song to express sadness. Additional biological and psychosocial benefits consistent with good mental health also seem to follow from music activity. Of "note," given that people listen to or produce music that resonates with them, there is also a shift from negativity to absorption in a positive focus countering depression and anxiety and advancing mental wellbeing.

How activity in general benefits mental health

The ways that activity of specific types advances mental health inform regarding how activity in general counters mental illness and advances mental health in the larger population. A theme for specific types of activity is a disconnect from negativity and absorption in positive experiences (Bowins, 2020). Absorption is a milder constructive form of dissociation, and as such represents a psychological defense—adaptive (therapeutic) dissociation (Bowins, 2012b) (see the Psychological defense mechanisms chapter for further information). Immersion in the positive focus of activity then entails dissociative absorption. Activity of the types described also fosters balance, which acts defensively by helping assure that some positivity will transpire: if a person places all their eggs in the proverbial one basket and that area suffers, then great negativity ensues, but with diverse activities good outcomes are always likely in one or more areas helping to preserve mental health.

The narrative studies reviewed inform regarding various psychosocial benefits that likely follow from absorption in positive activities, including empowerment from enhanced competence and confidence, social connectedness, greater motivation, self-actualization, positive identity, sense of purpose, and hope (Bowins, 2020). These benefits help resolve and prevent mental illness, and advance mental wellbeing and other aspects of mental health in the general population. One thing frequently leads to another, and this applies well to the psychosocial gains from activity. For example, with greater motivation a person becomes more active, and this brings into play other benefits and further motivation. People who are active often progress to a healthier lifestyle generally, such as better eating, less alcohol and drug consumption, and engagement in additional constructive pursuits. Hence, mutually reinforcing effects amplify the psychosocial benefits of activity.

Ultimately, activity aligns with the behavioral activation/approach (BAS) and behavioral inhibition (BIS) requirements of our evolution covered at the start of the chapter. The approach over avoidance behavior consistent with activity, equates with higher BAS and lower BIS, affording the capacity to seek out valuable resources while responding to objective threats. This combination optimizes reinforcement, which in turn enhances motivation, contributing to further constructive actions, more reinforcement, additional motivation, thereby generating a mutually reinforcing positive cycle linking constructive actions, reinforcement, and enhanced motivation. Of relevance, hypomanic also consists of high BAS and low BIS (Akiskal and Pinto, 1999; Bowins, 2008; Meyer et al., 1999). Unfortunately, there is a tendency within mental health disciplines to view hypomania as simply a prelude to mania requiring medication, instead of a defensive response to depression (and anxiety). However, hypomania in its modal duration of 1–3 days rarely progresses to mania even in people with a history of this condition, being approximately equivalent in frequency of occurrence to depression as would be expected if it is acting as a defense (Akiskal, 1996; Benazzi and Akiskal, 2001; Cassano et al., 1992; Coryell et al., 1989; Klein et al., 1996). The conversion of mostly adaptive hypomania to largely maladaptive mania appears to involve deficient regulation, often induced by psychoactive substances and negative symptoms (Bowins, 2008, 2016), a topic we will revisit in the Regulation and Human-specific cognition chapters. A personality variant of hypomania—hyperthymia or hyperthymic personality—confers success across the lifespan and resilience to depression (Akiskal and Pinto, 1999). Hence, activity with high BAS and low BIS aligns with evolutionary success, and the activity requirements for mental health reflect this occurrence.

References

Aaltonen, S., Rottensteiner, M., Kaprio, Jaakko, K., Kujala, U.M., 2014. Motives for physical activity among active and inactive persons in their mid-thirties. Scand. J. Med. Sci. Sports 24 (4), 727–735.

Akiskal, H.S., 1996. The prevalent clinical spectrum of bipolar disorders: beyond DSM-IV. J. Clin. Psychopharmacol. 16, 4S–15S.

Akiskal, H.S., Pinto, O., 1999. The evolving bipolar spectrum: prototypes I, II, III, and IV. Psychiatr. Clin. North Am. 22, 517–534.

Beck, A., 1991. Cognitive therapy: a 30-Year retrospective. Am. Psychol. 46 (4), 368–375.

Benazzi, F., Akiskal, H.S., 2001. Delineating bipolar II mixed states in the Ravenna-San Diego collaborative study: the relative prevalence and diagnostic significance of hypomanic features during major depressive episodes. J. Affect. Disord. 67, 115–122.

Boucher, J., Carlson, G., 1980. Recognition of facial expression in three cultures. J. Cross Cult. Psychol. 11, 263–280.

Bowins, B.E., 2004. Psychological defense mechanisms: a new perspective. Am. J. Psychoanal. 64, 1–26.

Bowins, B.E., 2006. How psychiatric treatments can enhance psychological defense mechanisms. Am. J. Psychoanal. 66, 173–194.

Bowins, B., 2008. Hypomania: a depressive inhibition override defense mechanism. J. Affect. Disord. 109, 221–232.

Bowins, B.E., 2012a. Augmenting behavioural activation treatment with the behavioural activation and inhibition scales. Behav. Cogn. Psychother. 40, 233–237.

Bowins, B.E., 2012b. Therapeutic dissociation: compartmentalization & absorption. Couns. Psychol. Q. 25 (1), 307–317.

Bowins, B., 2016. Defining Mental Illness: Continuums, Regulation, and Defense. Routledge, London.

Bowins, B., 2020. Activity for Mental Health. Academic Press, Cambridge, Massachusetts.

Bratman, G.N., Hamilton, J.P., Hahn, K.S., Daily, G.C., Gross, J.J., 2015. Nature experience reduces rumination and subgenual prefrontal cortex activation. Proc. Natl. Acad. Sci. USA. 112 (28), 8567–8572.

Carlson, E., Saarikallio, S., Toiviainen, P., Bogert, B., Kliuchko, M., Brattico, R., 2015. Maladaptive and adaptive emotion regulation through music: a behavioral and neuroimaging study of males and females. Front. Hum. Neurosci. 9, 466–488.

Cassano, G.B., Akiskal, H.S., Savino, M., Musetti, L., Perugi, G., 1992. Proposed subtypes of bipolar II and related disorders: with hypomanic episodes (or cyclothymia) and with hyperthymic temperament. J. Affect. Disord. 26, 127–140.

Chan, M.F., Chan, E.A., Mok, E., Kwan-Tse, F.Y., 2009. Effect of music on depression levels and physiological responses in community-based older adults. Int. J. Ment. Health Nurs. 18 (4), 285–294.

Coryell, W., Endicott, J., Keller, M., Andreasen, N., Grove, W., Hirshfeld, R.M., et al., 1989. Bipolar affective disorder and high achievement: a familial association. Am. J. Psychiatry 146, 983–988.

Coulton, S., Clift, S., Skingley, A., Rodriquez, J., 2015. Effectiveness and cost-effectiveness of community singing on mental health-related quality of life of older people: randomised controlled trial. Br. J. Psychiatry 207 (3), 250–255.
Csikszentmihalyi, M., 1990. Flow: The Psychology of Optimal Experience. Harper Collins, New York.
Davies, C., Knuiman, M., Rosenberg, M., 2016. The art of being mentally healthy: a study to quantify the relationship between recreational arts engagement and mental well-being in the general population. BMC Public Health. doi:10.1186/s12889-015-2672-7.
Daykin, N., Mansfield, L., Meads, C., Julier, G., Tomlinson, A., Payne, A., et al., 2017. What works for wellbeing? A systematic review of wellbeing outcomes for music and singing in adults. Pers. Public Health. doi:10.1177/1757913917740391.
Deslandes, A., Moraes, H., Ferreira, C., Veiga, H., Silveira, H., Mouta, R., et al., 2009. Exercise and mental health: many reasons to move. Neuropsychobiology 59, 191–198.
Dinger, M.K., Brittain, D.R., Hutchinson, S.R., 2014. Associations between physical activity and health-related factors in a national sample of college students. Am. Coll. Health 62 (1), 67–74.
Ekman, P., 1972. Emotions in the Human Face. Cambridge University Press, New York.
Ekman, P., 1994. Antecedent events and emotion metaphors. Nature of Emotions. Oxford University Press, Oxford.
Ekman, P., Friesen, W., 1971. Constants across cultures in the face and emotion. J. Pers. Soc. Psychol. 17, 124–129.
Eley, T., Stevenson, J., 2000. Specific life events and chronic experiences differentially associated with depression and anxiety in young twins. J. Abnorm. Child Psychol. 28 (4), 383–394.
Fancourt, D., Williamon, A., Carvalho, L.A., Steptoe, A., Dow, R., Lewis, I., 2016. Singing modulates mood, stress, cortisol, cytokine and neuropeptide activity in cancer patients and carers. Ecancermedicalscience. doi:10.3332/ecancer.2016.631.
Finlay-Jones, R., Brown, G., 1981. Types of stressful life event and the onset of anxiety and depressive disorders. Psychol. Med. 11, 803–815.
Fowles, D.C., 1988. Psychophysiology and psychopathology: a motivational approach. Psychophysiology 25, 373–391.
Gatersleben, B., Andrews, M., 2013. When walking in nature is not restorative-the role of prospect and refuge. Health Place 20, 91–101.
Gladwell, V.F., Kuoppa, P., Tarvainen, M.P., Rogerson, M., 2016. A lunchtime walk in nature enhances restoration of autonomic control during night-time sleep: results from a preliminary study. Int. J. Environ. Res. Public Health 13 (3), E280. doi:10.3390/ijerph.
Gold, C., Mossler, K., Grocke, D., Heldal, T.O., Tjemsland, L., Aarre, T., et al., 2013. Individual music therapy for mental health care clients with low therapy motivation: multicentre randomised controlled trial. Psychother. Psychosom. 82 (5), 319–331.
Gray, J.A., 1987. Perspectives on anxiety and impulsivity: a commentary. J. Res. Per. 21, 493–509.
Hudziak, J.J., Albaugh, M.D., Ducharme, S., Karama, S., Spottswood, M., Crehan, E., et al., 2014. Cortical thickening maturation and duration of music training: health-promoting activities shape brain development. J. Am. Acad. Child Adolesc. Psychiatry 53 (11), 1153–1161.
Hyde, A.L., Conroy, D.E., Pincus, A.L., Ram, N., 2011. Unpacking the feel good effect of free-tine physical activity: between- and within-person associations with pleasant-activated feelings states. J. Sport. Exerc. Psychol. 33 (6), 884–902.
Izard, C., 1977. Human Emotions. Plenum, New York.
Izard, C., 1991. The Psychology of Emotions. New York, Plenum Press.
Kasch, K.L., Rottenberg, J., Arnow, B.A., Gotlib, I.H., 2002. Behavioral activation and inhibition systems and the severity and course of depression. J. Abnorm. Psychol. 111, 589–597.

Keltner, D., Buswell, B., 1997. Embarrassment: its distinct form and appeasement functions. Psychol. Bull. 122 (3), 250–270.

Klein, D.N., Lewinsohn, P.M., Seeley, J.R., 1996. Hypomanic personality traits in a community sample of adolescents. J. Affect. Disord. 38, 135–143.

Lawson, J., Reynolds, F., Bryant, W., Wilson, L., 2014. 'It's like having a day of freedom, a day off from being ill': exploring the experiences of people living with mental health problems who attend a community-based arts project, using interpretative phenomenological analysis. J. Health Psychol. 19 (6), 765–777.

Li, Q., 2010. Effect of forest bathing trips on human immune function. Environ. Health Preven. Med. 15, 9–17.

Lubans, D., Richards, J., Hillman, C., Faulkner, G., Beauchamp, M., Nilsson, M., et al., 2016. Physical activity for cognitive and mental health in youth: a systematic review of mechanisms. Pediatrics 138 (3), 1–27.

Makin, S., Gask, L., 2012. 'Getting back to normal': the added value of an art-based programme in promoting 'recovery' for common but chronic mental health problems. Chronic Illn. 8 (1), 64–75.

Mao, G.X., Lan, X.G., Cao, Y.B., Chen, Z.M., He, Z.H., Lv, Y.D., 2012. Effects of short-term forest bathing on human health in a broad-leaved evergreen forest in Zhejiang Province. China Biomed. Environ. Sci. 25 (3), 317–324.

Margrove, K.L., Se-Surg (South Essex Service User Research Group), Heydinrych, K., Secker, J., 2013. Waiting list-controlled evaluation of a participatory arts course for people experiencing mental health problems. Perspect. Public Health 133 (1), 28–35.

Maslow, A., 1934. A theory of human motivation. Psychol. Rev. 50 (4), 370–396.

Meyer, B., Johnson, S.L., Carver, C.S., 1999. Exploring behavioral activation and inhibition sensitivities among college students at risk for bipolar spectrum symptomatology. J. Psychopathol. Behav. Assess. 21, 275–292.

Nolen-Hoeksema, S., Wisco, B.E., Lyubomirsky, S., 2008. Rethinking rumination. Perspect. Psychol. Sci. 3 (5), 400–424.

Olatunji, B.O., Broman-Fulks, J.J., Bergman, S.M., Green, B.A., Zlomke, K.R., 2010. A taxometric investigation of the latent structure of worry: dimensionality and associations with depression, anxiety, and stress. Behav. Ther. 41 (2), 212–228.

Orjasaeter, K.B., Stickley, T., Hedlund, M., Ness, O., 2017. Transforming identity through participation in music and theatre: exploring narratives of people with mental health problems. Int. J. Qual. Stud. Health Well-being 12 (sup 2), 17–24.

Park, B., Tsunetsugu, Y., Kasetani, T., Kagawa, T., Miyazaki, Y., 2010. The physiological effects of Shrinrinyoku (taking in the forest or forest bathing): evidence from field experiments in 24 forests across Japan. Environ. Health Prev. Med. 15 (1), 18–26.

Perkins, R., Ascenso, S., Atkins, L., Fancourt, D., Williamson, A., 2016. Making music for mental health: how group drumming mediates recovery. PWB 6 (1), 11–17.

Pontzer, H., 2017. The crown joules: energetics, ecology, and evolution in humans and other primates. Evol. Anthropol. 26 (1), 12–24.

Puterman, E., Weiss, J., Beauchamp, M.R., Mogle, J., Almeida, D.M., 2017. Physical activity and negative affective reactivity in daily life. Health Psychol. doi:10.1037/hea0000532.

Pylvanainen, P.M., Muotka, J.S., Lappalainen, R., 2015. A dance movement therapy group for depressed adult patients in a psychiatric outpatient clinic: effects of the treatment. Front Psychol. doi:10.3389/fpsyg.2015.00980.

Raichlen, D.A., Alexander, G.E., 2017. Adaptive capacity: an evolutionary neuroscience model linking exercise, cognition, and brain health. Trends Neurosci. 40 (7), 408–421.

Rozin, P., Lowery, L., Imada, S., Haidt, J., 1999. The CAD triad hypothesis: a mapping between three moral emotions (contempt, anger, disgust) and three moral codes (community, autonomy, divinity). J. Pers. Soc. Psychol. 76 (4), 574–586.

Schneier, F.R., Blanco, C., Antia, S.X., Liebowitz, M.R., 2002. The social anxiety spectrum. Psychiatr. Clin. North Am. 25, 757–774.

Scholten, M.R., van Honk, J., Aleman, A., Kahn, R.S., 2006. Behavioral Inhibition system (BIS) and the behavioral activation System (BAS) and schizophrenia: relationship with psychopathology and physiology. J. Psychiatr. Res. 40, 638–645.

Shaver, P., Schwartz, J., Kirson, D., O'Connor, C., 1987. Emotion knowledge: further exploration of a prototype approach. J. Pers. Soc. Psychol. 52 (6), 1086–1091.

Solli, H.P., Rolvsjord, R., Borg, M., 2013. Toward understanding music therapy as a recovery-oriented practice within mental health care: a meta-synthesis of service users' experiences. J. Music Ther. 50 (4), 244–273.

Song, C., Ikei, H., Igarashi, M., Miwa, M., Takagaki, M., Miyazaki, Y., 2014. Physiological and psychological responses of young males during spring-time walks in urban parks. J. Phys. Anthropol. 33 (8). doi:10.1186/1880-6805-33-8.

Stickley, T., Eades, M., 2013. Arts on prescription: a qualitative outcomes study. Public Health 127 (8), 727–734.

Tomkins, S., 1962. Affect, Imagery, Consciousness: The Positive Effects (Volume 1). Springer, New York.

Tomkins, S., 1963. Affect, Imagery, Consciousness: The Negative Effects (Volume 2). Springer, New York.

Ulrich, R.S., Simons, R.F., Losito, B.D., Fiorito, E., Miles, M.A., Zelson, M., 1991. Stress recovery during exposure to natural and urban environments. J. Environ. Psychol. 11 (3), 201–230.

Van Lith, T., Fenner, P., Schofield, M., 2011. The lived experience of art making as a companion to the mental health recovery process. Disabil. Rehabil. 33 (8), 652–650.

Vrana, S., 1993. The psychophysiology of disgust: differentiating negative emotional contexts with facial EMG. Psychophysiology 30, 279–286.

Williams, F., 2017. The Nature Fix: Why Nature Makes Us Happier, Healthier, and More Creative. W. W. Norton & Company, New York.

Wilson, E.O., 1984. Biophilia. Harvard University Press, Cambridge.

Zarobe, L., Bungay, H., 2017. The role of arts activities in developing resilience and mental wellbeing in children and young people a rapid review of the literature. Perspect. Public Health 137 (6), 337–347.

Chapter 3

Psychological defense mechanisms

Much as there are ongoing challenges to the integrity of the biological system from pathogens, emotional stressors are ever present. Biological defense takes the form of the immune system, while psychological defense mechanisms protect against emotional stress. Defense, both biological and psychological, is necessary for physical and emotional wellbeing. Psychological defense mechanisms originated with Sigmund Freud who commented, "I have the distinct feeling that I have touched on one of the greatest secrets of nature" (Personal communication to his friend Wilhelm Fliess, cited in Masson (1985). Sigmund Freud, along with his daughter, Anna Freud, described psychological defense mechanisms and identified five of their important properties (Freud, 1964; Vaillant, 1994):

- Major means of managing conflict and disturbing affect.
- Relatively unconscious.
- Discrete from one another.
- Reversible despite being the hallmark of major psychiatric syndromes.
- Adaptive as well as pathological.

The notion of adaptive and pathological manifestations relates to the maturity level of psychological defense mechanisms, described largely by Vaillant (1977, 1994). Maturity level refers to both the adaptive value of the defense and the age when it is most likely to be expressed (Vaillant, 1977). For instance, mature defenses are highly adaptive and typically expressed in adults, while immature defenses are commonly expressed in childhood-adolescence and are less adaptive, particularly when a person is older. However, immature psychological defenses are adaptive relative to no defenses in very young people. We will now look at what psychological defenses fall under mature, intermediate/neurotic, and immature (Trijsburg et al., 2000; Vaillant, 1977, 1994; Wastell, 1999).

Classical psychological defense mechanisms:

Immature psychological defense mechanisms

Immature psychological defense mechanisms include splitting, idealization and devaluation, projection, hypochondriasis and somatization, undoing,

States and Processes for Mental Health. DOI: 10.1016/C2020-0-00574-8

acting out, schizoid fantasy, and denial (Kaplan et al., 1994; Vaillant, 1994; Weinberger, 1990).

- Splitting: Division of external objects, namely people, into all good and all bad, with shifts of an object from one extreme to the other.
- Idealization and devaluation: Endow "all good" and "all bad" objects with great power resulting in the former being seen as ideal and the latter devalued.
- Projection: Alters experience such that it is believed that unacceptable impulses and attitudes arise not from the self but from another object. Hence, aggressive urges are perceived and reacted to as coming from someone else when they are really your own.
- Hypochondriasis: Transforms reproach toward others into self-reproach and complaints of illness.
- Somatization: Psychic derivatives are converted into bodily symptoms.
- Undoing: Symbolic negating of an unacceptable behavior by acting in reverse.
- Acting out: Translates disturbing impulses into action so fast that the person escapes feeling or thinking.
- Schizoid fantasy: Retreat into a fantasy world and avoidance of intimacy.
- Denial: Negates awareness of some disturbing aspect of experience, however, when denial only involves an isolation of affect it is significantly more adaptive than when a near-psychotic distortion of reality transpires (Steiner et al., 2001).

Intermediate/neurotic psychological defense mechanisms

Intermediate/neurotic defenses including intellectualization, rationalization, repression, isolation, reaction formation, and displacement are expressed by everyone, particularly during difficult periods of life (Freud, 1915, 1915; Kaplan et al., 1994; Vaillant, 1977, 1994; Weinberger, 1990).

- Intellectualization: Transforms events into a nonemotional experience through the overuse of conscious thought processes.
- Rationalization: Makes unacceptable attitudes, beliefs, and behaviors more palatable by providing a socially acceptable meaning.
- Repression: Expulsion or withholding of a distressing idea from consciousness while allowing affect to remain, in contrast to isolation, thereby attenuating conscious realization of what object or situation is related to the affect.
- Isolation: Spares the idea but modifies awareness of affect, opposite to repression.
- Reaction formation: Transforms an unacceptable impulse into its opposite, for example, instead of accepting a desire to have sex with multiple partners a person preaches the virtues of celibacy.
- Displacement: Shifts affect and the focus of attention from an object that is unacceptable to a safer one.

- Dissociation: While it is usually included in the neurotic defenses, the definition in this regard is restricted to a severe form involving a breakdown of psychological functions, and a drastic modification of one's own character (Trijsburg et al., 2000; Vaillant, 1977).

Mature psychological defense mechanisms

Mature defenses including humor, sublimation, anticipation, altruism, and suppression represent well-orchestrated composites of less mature defenses (Kaplan et al., 1994; Vaillant, 1977, 1994).

- Humor: Alters the content of a potentially disturbing scenario so that it becomes lighter and more tolerable.
- Sublimation: Transforms disturbing impulses and feelings by channeling them into acceptable pursuits, and in the process, modifies awareness of negative states.
- Anticipation: Shifts attention away from current experience to prepare for some perceived outcome.
- Altruism: Involves giving to others what you would actually like to receive allowing personal needs to be satisfied vicariously, and can entail the not always realistic assumption that if you help someone or something then you will receive assistance yourself.
- Suppression: Reduces the focus on disturbing intrapsychic states, shifting attention away from them while maintaining some awareness.

Even a quick review of these diverse psychological defense mechanisms reveals how maturity level is relevant, in that the mature ones do seem to equate with good mental health. Shifting negative content to something lighter and more positive via humor replaces negative feelings with positive ones. Channeling negative energy into constructive pursuits with sublimation transforms negativity into success, a defense that likely characterizes people who excel—it is impossible to avoid negativity, but harnessing the energy for positivity is powerful. Instead of worrying about potential negative scenarios, anticipating issues and proactively preparing for them improves outcomes without the emotional drain of worry. Negative treatment by others can often trigger more negative behavior, generating enormous stress, but by acting altruistically both hope and the possibility of reciprocation is generated. Successful people are usually able to suppress disturbing emotional states in the moment to remain productive.

Contrast the adaptive functioning conferred by mature psychological defense mechanisms to that provided by immature defenses. Splitting for example can alienate people who the person interacts with, although to a child this defense provides a simple good and bad template for understanding what to expect from others. Idealization and devaluation creates a rollercoaster of emotions, but as with splitting provides a simple good/bad template applied to a single person and can help in the acquisition of resources. Acting out is grossly inadequate for coping as an adult, although it does help young children gain attention, and parents often desperate to end the display give into to what is wanted. Adults who throw themselves down on the floor and have temper tantrums are much less likely to get what they want. Retreating into a fantasy world can work for children under severe stress, but represents psychosis in adults. Hence, mature psychological defenses advance functioning and mental health outcomes, while immature defenses greatly limit success and impair mental health, at least in adulthood.

The categorization of psychological defense mechanisms covered so far represents a discrete model with mature, intermediate/neurotic, and immature. To simplify information processing, we have a preference for discreteness while psychological, and natural processes generally, occur on continuums (Bowins, 2016). Psychological defense mechanisms actually are continuous ranging from immature to mature, as revealed by the work of Trijsburg et al. (2000) who had experienced psychoanalysts rate the maturity level of psychological defense mechanisms, and then applied various statistical analyses to the data including factor analysis. Support was found for a unidimensional representation from least to most mature: splitting, dissociation, autistic (schizoid) fantasy, somatization, acting out, projection, devaluation, denial, passive aggressive behavior, idealization, isolation, undoing, reaction formation, displacement, repression, rationalization, suppression, altruism, humor, anticipation, and sublimation. They stressed that dissociation was rated toward the immature end of the spectrum because of the definition applied—a breakdown of functioning. So instead of the discrete framework proposed by Vaillant (1977), psychological defense mechanism occur on a continuum from least to most mature.

Beyond classical psychological defense mechanisms:

At this point, my research pertaining to psychological defense mechanisms is relevant as it emphasizes continuums and natural valid divisions. In the Activity chapter, we looked at the Amplification Effect whereby the evolution of human intelligence has amplified emotional states by making the cognitive activating appraisals that underlie emotions more intensive, extensive, and adding a temporal dimension (Bowins, 2004). On the positive side with happiness and interest this produces a very good experience, but amplified negative emotions detract from mental health and foster depression and anxiety via excessive and extensive sadness and fear, respectively. This outcome likely reduced adaptive capacity, thereby diminishing evolutionary fitness during our evolution (Bowins, 2004). To counter the evolutionary fitness reducing impact of excessive negative emotions, psychological defense mechanisms evolved (Bowins, 2004). They operate ongoing largely unconsciously to protect our psychological integrity and foster emotional resilience. Given that natural events are organized continuously, as opposed to numerous discrete entities, psychological defense mechanism templates occur, namely positive cognitive distortions and dissociation, with a continuous organization of defenses within each.

Positive cognitive distortions

A spectrum from mild to extensive transpires with cognitive distortions. The term "distortion" fits because first, reality is extremely difficult to accurately characterize even by scientists devoting careers to this pursuit, and with life in motion a person can at best hope to have a perspective on what is transpiring; second, when thoughts link to emotions there is a negative or positive distortion because neutral does not apply to emotional states and reactions: +1 and -1 do not = 0, but both coexist. Milder positive cognitive distortion variants consist of seeing events through the proverbial rose-colored glasses, self-enhancing spins on events, being excessively optimistic about the future, and remembering the past in a selective fashion favoring the positive side of experiences (Bowins, 2004; Nelson and Craighead, 1977; Tiger, 1979). Attribution biases are often involved whereby unfavorable events are attributed to external, unstable, and specific factors, and good events are attributed to internal, stable, and global factors (Cohen, 1989). Good mental health is distorting experience to enhance the self and provide a positivity bias, while diminishing negativity (Beck, 1991; Beck and Clark, 1997). Mild cognitive distortions enable people to slightly alter their perceptions of various experiences by placing a positive, self-enhancing spin on them so that they are less negative and threatening. Perhaps one of the most powerful is having hope that good outcomes will ensue. More moderate-level positive cognitive distortions entail occurrences such as excessive fantasy involvement, magical thinking, and over-valued ideas. Examples of magical thinking include superstitious thoughts, a belief in fortune-telling and horoscopes, and acceptance of mystical modes of healing. Belief in paranormal type events can also be included, and it has been found that such beliefs are not uncommon (Ross & Joshi, 1992). Progressing to extensive cognitive distortions, delusions not at all consistent with reality occur. Psychotic cognitions are then at the extreme end of a cognitive distortion continuum (Kingdon and Turkington, 1994; Landa et al., 2006).

Classical psychological defense mechanisms involve cognitive distortions (Steiner et al., 2001), and can largely be subsumed under this psychological defense mechanism template, with some having strong elements of dissociation (Bowins, 2004). I proposed that there is an inverse relationship between the level of defense maturity and the degree of cognitive distortion: as the maturity level increases, the degree of cognitive distortion decreases (Bowins, 2004). Immature defenses such as schizoid fantasy and projection involve extensive cognitive distortions; in the case of schizoid fantasy a person retreats into a fantasy world, and with projection negative qualities of the self are seen as being part of another person. Intermediate/neurotic defenses involve a lesser degree of cognitive distortion but still quite significant. For example, intellectualization transforms events into a nonemotional experience through the overuse of conscious thought processes. Repression removes ideation allowing affect to remain, thereby attenuating conscious realization of what object or situation is related to the affect, while isolation spares the idea but modifies awareness of affect. Mature classical psychological defenses entail milder cognitive distortions attenuating awareness of negative events. For instance, humor places a lighter spin on stressful occurrences, and sublimation channels disturbing impulses and feelings into positive pursuits.

As a general rule, the greater the degree of cognitive distortion, the less adaptive the defense, except under extreme circumstances (Bowins, 2004). For example, while schizoid fantasy greatly impedes adaptive functioning under the vast majority of circumstances, it might be very helpful if captured by terrorists and facing certain torture and/or execution. Mature defenses such as humor, sublimation, and suppression might not cut it under such extreme circumstances. Meanwhile, more common stressors such as a challenging political situation at work respond far better to mature defenses involving milder cognitive distortions; immature defenses entailing much more extensive cognitive distortions invariably worsen a person's capacity to cope effectively under these circumstances. Hence, beyond extreme circumstances psychological defense mechanisms involving milder positive cognitive distortion (more mature) are the most adaptive, countering sadness and fear, and the amplification to depression and anxiety, respectively. They also augment positive emotional states advancing mental health.

Dissociation

Psychological dissociation has drawn the attention of theorists and researchers over many years. One of the first was Janet who viewed dissociation as the division of mental functions resulting from the failure of integrative processes (in Van Der Hart and Friedman (1989)). Aligning with Janet's view, some later researchers conceptualize dissociation as simply a breakdown or disruption in the usually integrated functions of consciousness (Marmar et al., 1994; Putman, 1985; Trijsburg et al., 2000). This disruption is typically seen as arising from traumatic experiences (Marmar et al., 1994). Emphasizing the positive aspects, Watkins and Watkins (1997) see it as a natural organizing principle of the psyche giving humans the ability to adapt, think, act, and respond. Dissociative states have also been separated into negative involving a loss such as amnesia, and positive consisting of added activity as with absorption (Nijenhuis et al., 1996). Appreciating the defensive value, Freud (1894, 1895) indicated that dissociation can dislocate affect from ideas, while Vaillant (1977) suggests that dissociation permits the ego to so alter the internal state that the pain of conflict seems irrelevant. Dissociation essentially provides the ability to detach from adverse emotional states and circumstances, and represents a key psychological defense mechanism template (Bowins, 2004, 2012).

In line with dissociation being listed as an intermediate/neurotic or immature classical psychological defense negating awareness (see above), many clinicians view it as largely or entirely dysfunctional. However, dissociation actually encompasses a spectrum of manifestations from mild to extensive, with the milder ones generally highly adaptive, and the more extensive less adaptive and usually only functional in extreme circumstances, such as abuse (Bowins, 2004). The dissociation continuum from mild to more extensive includes emotional numbing, absorption with or without imaginative involvement, compartmentalization, depersonalization and derealization, amnesia, and identity fragmentation (Allen and Lolafaye, 1995; Ross et al., 1990, 1991).

Emotional numbing: Occurs when feelings that can interfere with functioning are unconsciously diminished or blocked. For instance, when dealing in the moment with a traumatic situation responders often feel somewhat numb and emotionally detached.

Absorption with or without imaginative involvement: Absorption is arguably the most common dissociative psychological defense, consisting of immersion in a positive focus producing a detachment from negativity. For example, immersion in a hobby to remove oneself from work stress, and becoming absorbed in a video on a cell phone to detach from negative thoughts. In some instances, imaginative involvement (fantasy) occurs adding a very positive component. For instance, while at a very boring work meeting your eyes glaze over (detachment) and you fantasize about the upcoming sailing season. Nowadays online videos seem to have replaced fantasy for many individuals, but it still transpires with absorption. When the source of an adverse emotion does not have to be consciously attended to absorption can occur; if conscious attention is required emotional numbing is more likely to transpire. There are actually various forms of absorption identified by Ross et al. (1991) including missing part of a conversation, remembering past events so vividly one seems to be reliving it, not sure if a remembered event happened or was a dream, absorption in a television program or a movie, so involved in a fantasy that it seemed real, able to ignore pain, staring into space, talking out loud to oneself when alone, not sure whether one has done something or only thought about it, finding evidence off having done things one cannot remember doing.

Demonstrating how common dissociative absorption is, Ross et al. (1991) applied the Dissociative Experiences Scale to a stratified sample of 1,055 Winnipeg, Manitoba residents. Results for various types of absorption are as follows: the first number is the percentage experiencing it on some occasions and the second number is those experiencing it 30% of the time or more:

- Missing part of a conversation (83, 29).
- Remembering past events so vividly one seems to be reliving it (60.4, 19.2).
- Not sure if a remembered event happened or was a dream (54.6, 12.5).
- Absorption in a television program or a movie (63.9, 24.2).
- So involved in a fantasy that it seemed real (44.5, 10.9).
- Able to ignore pain (74.7, 33.4).
- Staring into space (62.6, 25.7).
- Talking out loud to oneself when alone (55.6, 17.7).

- Not sure whether one has done something or only thought about it (73.1, 24.7).
- Finding evidence off having done things one cannot remember doing (58.4, 14.3).

When informed that these familiar experiences are actually a mild form of dissociation—absorption—many people feel relieved, as they assume they are losing their memory or mind, or both. For instance, virtually everyone has missed part of a conversation, and many people are not sure whether they did something or only thought about it. Is this memory loss? No, typically it is dissociative absorption unconsciously activated when a person is stressed to give the mind a rest. Over half of people talk out loud to themselves when alone, commonly attributed to "insanity," even though it is just a milder psychological defense! I like to say that it does not indicate insanity but a defense to help prevent insanity. Psychological pain control techniques rely on diverting attention from the source of pain to a neutral or pleasing focus, in line with about 75% of people being able to ignore pain at some point and 33% a third or more of the time. Highway hypnosis is a common variant of dissociative absorption, whereby a driver shifts conscious attention away from a monotonous stretch of road to some thought or fantasy, but still manages to drive. An interesting experience I have had several times while explaining absorption to those who only see dissociation as a severe problem, is to watch their eyes glaze over and mind drift off. When I express that I just induced dissociative absorption (with or without imaginative involvement) they typically deny that it occurred, but yet cannot repeat what I just explained. None of these individuals suffered from memory loss. The various forms of absorption are healthy protecting the mind when stress and negativity arises. Kihlstrom et al. (1994) indicate that there is nothing inherently pathological about these experiences, even when displayed at high levels, and people displaying them are well adjusted. In addition, those who score high on fantasy proneness (the imaginative involvement component) tend to have a positive response bias (Merckelbach et al., 2000).

Meditation is likely a form of dissociative absorption, or at the very least largely works via this form of dissociation. With meditation, and also Yoga, there is absorption in a pleasing or neutral focus, and mental detachment from disturbing thoughts and emotional occurrences (Bowins, 2004, 2012; Castillo, 2003; Waelde, 2004). Absorption in repeated vocalizations, breathing, other bodily sensations, peaceful thoughts, images, or external stimuli produce a trance-like state that dissociates the person from distressing reality allowing pleasing mental images or fantasies to dominate conscious awareness (Castillo, 2003). Active instruction in how to redirect attention away from distressing cognitions, emotions, and memories, maximizing the more positive or neutral stimulus focus consistent with the particular form of meditation, is provided (Waelde, 2004). Despite the various types, meditation might be separable into concentrative and mindful types (Waelde, 2004). Concentrative meditation focuses on an object of meditation, whereas mindfulness meditation maintains awareness of the present moment (Waelde, 2004). Both involve the absorption form of dissociation with or without imaginative involvement, in that a person becomes absorbed in the focus of meditation in the concentrative form, and in the safe, positive, or neutral present in the mindfulness variety. Yoga involves absorption in the various movements and breathing exercises, with aerobic variants having the added advantage of releasing endogenous opioids that likely enhance the dissociative state.

Compartmentalization: Consists of learning to place simultaneous experiences in separate psychological spaces to aid in coping. People who cope well despite enormous stress typically place various aspects of their overall experience in separate psychological compartments. Imagination can be used to enhance the compartments, such as picturing a tool box with separate drawers and even larger compartments subdivided into smaller spaces. Work and social life might occupy the larger compartments, and the subdivisions various components of each, such as general meetings, client appointments, interactions with managers, and individual work. Negative experiences in one compartment are then contained, not compromising performance in others.

Depersonalization and derealization: These related moderate-level dissociative experiences involve a disconnection from some aspect of experience; in the former one's own identity, and in the latter the surrounding environment. Based on the work of Ross et al. (1991) various forms occurring are listed here: with the first number the percentage experiencing it on some occasions and the second number those experiencing it 30% of the time or more:

- Not recognizing one's reflection in a mirror (13.6, 1.2).
- Other people and objects do not seem real (26.3, 4.1).
- Feeling as though one's body is not one's own (22.7, 3.6).
- Hearing voices inside one's head (26, 7.3).
- Looking at the world through a fog (26.3, 4.0).

While much less familiar than the absorption forms of dissociation, many people have experienced one or more of these, at least on some occasions. Supporting the relative commonalty of these moderate level forms of dissociation, it has been found that up 46% of college students experience depersonalization (Simeon, 1997). Depersonalization and derealization often arise when a person is tired and stressed, and although this might appear to be completely dysfunctional, these dissociative experiences defensively detach the mind from very stressful and overwhelming experiences in the moment. For example, if a person has a highly embarrassing and humiliating experience he or she might feel disconnected from oneself (depersonalization) as a way of coping with the emotional distress.

Amnesia: An extensive form of dissociation consisting of a complete detachment of memory and cognitive processes from an emotionally disturbing event. Interestingly, even this type of dissociative experience is not all that rare. Different forms of amnestic states are as follows: with the first number listing the percentage experiencing it on some occasions and the second those experiencing it 30% of the time or more (Ross et al., 1991):

- Finding oneself in a place but unaware of how one got there (18.8, 2).
- Finding oneself dressed in clothes one cannot remember putting on (14.6, 1.4).
- Finding unfamiliar things among one's belongings (22.1, 4.1).
- Not recognizing friends or family member (25.8, 4.6).

Amnesia often occurs in response to horrific occurrences as a way of protecting the psyche. Although most traumatic experiences are remembered, some are not. However, it is not a memory problem as they often resurface at some point such as during psychotherapy. In the field of Post-Traumatic Stress Disorder, there are even attempts to induce amnesia right after trauma either chemically or with sleep deprivation.

Identity fragmentation: This is the most extensive form of dissociation that typically occurs within the context of severe physical and/or sexual abuse during the early years of life. Personality fragments into different states, some of which usually remain sheltered from the damaging effects of the trauma. Identity fragmentation characterizes dissociative identity disorder. Although this condition is quite rare, the substrate is present in the population based on the finding that 11.8% of people have felt "almost as if they were two different people" more than 30% of the time (Ross et al., 1991).

Dissociation routinely occurs with stress and in healthy individuals, as revealed in a study by Morgan (2001) who investigated dissociative responses of general infantry and Special Forces soldiers with survival training, the 19 days involving semistarvation, sleep deprivation, lack of control over personal hygiene, and external control over movement, social contact, and communication. The Clinician-Administered Dissociative States Scale assessed dissociative symptoms before and after training. From before to just after survival training the following dissociative symptoms increased:

- Things seemed to take much longer than you would have expected.
- Things seemed very real, as if there were a special sense of clarity.
- Things happened that you were unable to account for later.
- Things seemed unreal, as if in a dream.
- You spaced out or lost track of what was going on.
- You had a feeling of separation from what was happening, as if you were watching a movie or a play or as if you were an automaton.

Given the excellent physical, and likely mental, health of participants in the Morgan (2001) study, defensive psychological dissociation is the most likely explanation for the results. Spontaneous dissociative experiences are independent of all major socioeconomic conditions, other than age, including income, education, employment status, household size, importance of religion, and place of birth (Ross et al., 1990). It is likely then that endogenous and not psychosocial factors primarily account for dissociation, as should be the case for an innate psychological defense. Neural plasticity appears to favor dissociation, supported by how dissociative experiences decline as one gets older and level off around the fourth decade (Ross et al., 1990, 1991).

Like with positive cognitive distortions, dissociation provides a spectrum of psychological defense capacities from mild to extensive, diminishing the impact of negative emotional experiences. Returning briefly to classical psychological defense mechanisms, some have strong elements of dissociation, as mentioned. Examples include the following:

- Suppression: Provides a partial detachment from disturbing intrapsychic states.
- Repression and isolation: Separate ideation and affect, preserving in consciousness affect in the case of repression and ideation in the case of isolation.
- Intellectualization: Eliminates the emotional aspects from experience, leaving only ideation.
- Denial: Blocks awareness of adverse components of experience and can isolate affect.
- Schizoid fantasy: Detachment from reality into a world of fantasy.

While completely speculative, it is possible that dissociation might initially have evolved in carnivores who typically have more intelligence than the herbivores they eat, to detach from the suffering of the animal they are eating, who often is still alive as the meal starts.

Additional psychological defenses:

Consistent with Freud's comment that he touched upon one of the greatest secrets in nature with psychological defense mechanisms (Personal communication to his friend Wilhelm Fliess, cited in Masson (1985)) there are an even more extensive array than the ones looked at so far, that we will now consider.

Grieving process

I have proposed that the grieving process evolved as a defense to help manage losses (Bowins, 2004, 2010a). Given that loss of some form is involved in traumatic experiences, such as a loss of control, freedom, mental or physical well-being, relationships, trust, and valued objects, the grieving process also helps manage trauma (Bowins, 2004, 2010a). This process likely operates, at least in part, by fusing the cognitive and emotional components of the experience: it has been found that the repetition of thoughts and feelings during grieving produces a sense of control or mastery (Levy, 2000), in contrast to that associated with post-traumatic stress disorder (PTSD). When a traumatic experience is too painful to process consciously, the various components remain dissociated (Bowins, 2010a). While this dissociative response is protective in the moment safeguarding sensitive conscious system functioning, in the longer run it contributes to PTSD, because thoughts, feelings, memories, and the like repeat endlessly as dissociated elements (Bowins, 2010a). Activating the grieving process by focusing on losses associated with trauma assists with fusion of the dissociated elements (Bowins, 2010a).

Hypomania

Hypomania has been described as a defense against sadness and depression (Bowins, 2008; French et al., 1996). In the Activity chapter, we considered hypomania related to the behavioral approach/activation system (BAS) and behavioral inhibition system (BIS). While depression involves low BAS and high BIS inhibiting behavior, hypomania having the reverse profile of high BAS and low BIS counters depression (Akiskal and Pinto, 1999; Bowins, 2008; Meyer et al., 1999). Hypomania with 1–3 days of increased physical, social, and mental behavior can defensively override depressive inhibition in the moment to restore adaptive functioning (Bowins, 2008). It can also override inhibited states arising from anxiety, characterized by high BIS. Relative to depression, and even normal functioning in some instances, hypomania is mostly highly adaptive (Akiskal, 2005; Akiskal and Pinto, 1999; Bowins, 2008; Eckblad and Chapman, 1986; Jamison et al., 1980; Johnson et al., 2000; Koukopoulos et al., 2003). Furthermore, as a personality variant known as hyperthymia or hyperthymic personality it confers success across the lifespan and resilience to depression (Akiskal and Pinto, 1999). When hypomania progresses to mania, likely due to negative symptoms (see the Human-specific cognition chapter) and psychoactive substances impairing regulation over the hypomanic defense, it is typically dysfunctional (Bowins, 2008).

Personality-based defenses

I have proposed (Bowins, 2010b) that extreme and enduring expressions of certain defense mechanisms produce personality disorders: avoidant, narcissistic, obsessive-compulsive, and dependent. The underlying defensive processes and their transformation into personality disorders consist of the following.

Avoidance

Avoiding threatening agents is a survival defense. If a predator or dangerous person is detected it is natural to avoid these threats. Problems arise, though, when people avoid situations that are not objectively threatening and offer the potential for reward (Olsson and Dahl, 2012). Extreme and enduring avoidance involving situations that are not objectively threatening and offer the potential for reward produces Avoidant Personality Disorder (Bowins, 2010b). However, milder versions of avoidance constitute a crucial defense for survival and well-being. There are elements of dissociation, given that psychological and typically physical detachment from a situation occurs.

Narcissism

Applying strengths to compensate for insecurities and weaknesses is a natural defense. For example, if you hurt your left arm, you will use your right arm more. If insecure about your academic ability but great at sports, you will likely focus more on athletic pursuits at school. When the insecurities/weaknesses are severe the compensation tends to be excessive, a counterbalancing of sorts that generates problems in terms of excessive self-focus with a lack of empathy, resulting in behavior that annoys and distresses other people (Bowins, 2010b). For instance, a person, who comes from severe poverty producing a sense of inferiority, might become ruthless and uncaring in pursuing financial success to compensate, if a strength is business acumen. Extensive insecurities/weaknesses with enduring intense overcompensation produces Narcissistic Personality Disorder. Milder degrees of narcissism characterize mental health, given that it is adaptive to apply strengths to compensate for weaknesses. In addition, the occasional "narcissistic fantasy" to counter the struggles of life can be inspiring.

Obsessive-compulsive

Obsessions entail anxiety, while compulsive behavior contains it through repetition of the physical or mental activity. Compulsive ritualistic behavior has been found to maintain tension at a manageable level (Rachman and Hodgson, 1980). From an evolutionary perspective, obsessive-compulsive type behavior serves the defensive function of minimizing risk by maintaining order (Brune, 2006), or managing various other threats such as contamination or resource depletion (Polimeni et al., 2005). In a milder form, obsessive-compulsive behavior is a defense designed by nature to contain and manage anxiety (Bowins, 2010b). Defensive containment of anxiety takes the form of mild compulsive-type behavior. For example, clinicians usually feel at least a slight degree of anxiety arising from the threat of complaints to regulating bodies or lawsuits. A typical response is to keep fairly detailed and organized records that will enable an effective response if either eventuality arises, with the record keeping mild compulsive behavior containing the anxiety. If stressed many people find cleaning, tidying, and organizing their place calming as the mild compulsive behavior contains the anxiety.

Obsessions also play a defensive role when more diffuse threats are funneled into a specific obsession, and compulsive behavior manages the anxiety. For example, vague fears of death and illness might be funneled into a fear of contamination, and handwashing manages the anxiety. Obsessive-compulsive experiences and symptoms have been reported in 90% of healthy adults and children as might be expected if there is a defensive function (Boyer and Lienard, 2006). For example, almost everyone demonstrates a compulsive habit such as biting nails or twirling hair that soothes in the moment. When the anxiety is more intense and obsessive-compulsive behavior extreme and enduring, then dysfunction occurs as the person is consumed to the point of inflexibility blocking adaptive responses—Obsessive-Compulsive Personality

Disorder (Bowins, 2010b). However, in a mild form it provides defensive containment of anxiety.

Dependence

We are a social species (see the Social connectedness chapter) and relying on others is a defense against threats, helping to regulate fears and anxiety. Solitary animals such as tigers do not have such a need. Humans evolving in hunting-gathering groups naturally turn to other people when fearful or hurt. This is a very basic defensive response to stress, and we consider loners and hermits to be odd and less equipped to handle stress. When dependence in response to perceived threats takes the form of extreme and enduring reliance on others, such that the person cannot function individually, it becomes Dependent Personality Disorder (Bowins, 2010b). Milder degrees of reliance on others provide an ongoing defense against threats helping to manage anxiety.

Resilience

The concept of resilience is complex and there is no real uniformity derived from research or standard definition. Perspectives gravitate around coping with adversity, such that stressors are resisted or rebounded (Davydov et al., 2010; Rutten et al., 2013). Hence, there is the notion of adapting to challenging circumstances. Resilience is a multifaceted entity with various levels including societal, social, psychological, and biological (Rutten et al., 2013). At a societal level, organizations and even norms can help an individual resist or recover from stress. For example, if you are shot at one of the seemingly endless mass shootings, then support from organizations that promote gun control and are trying to establish this as a norm, might help with recovery. Likewise, friends and family provide valuable social support. Biological processes heal the wound and neurochemical changes might facilitate emotional healing. Psychological aspects align with defense mechanisms (Davydov et al., 2010).

A couple of concepts from material science relate to resilience as a psychological defense: tensile strength and elasticity. Tensile strength refers to resistance of a material to breaking under tension. Elasticity is the ability of a material to resume its normal shape after being stretched or compressed, and the ability to change and adapt underscoring the importance of adaptability (see the Adaptability chapter for information regarding this important topic). We commonly describe these capacities in people or animals as toughness under stress and flexibility/adaptability in returning to normal functioning. Individual people and animals vary in their resilience generally or in response to specific forms of stress. As a psychological defense mechanism there are different options, one being that it stands alone as inner strength and elasticity. Another is that it arises from optimal functioning of the other defense mechanisms. For instance, a person who naturally has a positivity bias (positive cognitive distortions) and primarily utilizes mature classical defense mechanisms, will be far more able to resist the impact of stressors, and rebound from any functional deviation fast. Still another possibility is that the defensive capacity of resilience derives from many inputs and processes. Rutten et al. (2013) in a review of the literature identify secure attachment, positive emotions, and purpose in life as three key influences contributing to enhanced resilience. Regulation might be another key ingredient as secure attachment advances self-regulation capacity, and emotional regulation counters severe emotional fluctuations (see the Regulation chapter). Perhaps it includes all the above, but regardless of what it entails, resilience does enhance psychological and biological defensive capacity.

Summary note

Psychological defense mechanisms constitute a crucial component of good mental health. Beyond the classical psychological defense mechanisms identified by Freud and elaborated on by Vaillant, there appears to be the major defense mechanism templates of positive cognitive distortions and dissociation. Classical psychological defense can be subsumed under positive cognitive distortions, with some having strong elements of dissociation. Occurring on a continuum the classical defenses vary in maturity levels, and this is inversely associated with the degree of cognitive distortion: as the maturity level increases the degree of cognitive distortion decreases. Generally speaking, milder positive distortions and dissociation are more adaptive, and extreme variants less so except when under intense stress. Additional psychological defenses include the grieving process, hypomania, and personality variants—avoidance, narcissism, obsessive-compulsive behavior, dependence, and resilience. The extensive array of psychological defense mechanisms enables humans to function despite emotional stress, largely by reducing the burden of negative emotions and favoring positive emotions, thereby enhancing mental health.

References

Allen, J., Lolafaye, C., 1995. Dissociation and vulnerability to psychotic experience: the dissociative experiences scale and the MMPI-2. J. Nerv. Ment. Dis. 183 (10), 615–622.

Akiskal, H.S., 2005. Searching for behavioral indicators of bipolar II in patients presenting with major depressive episodes: the "red sign," the "rule of three" and other biographic signs of temperamental extravagance, activation and hypomania. J. Affect. Disord. 84, 279–290.

Akiskal, H.S., Pinto, O., 1999. The evolving bipolar spectrum: prototypes I, II, III, and IV. Psychiatr. Clin. North Am. 22, 517–534.

Beck, A., 1991. Cognitive therapy: a 30-year retrospective. Am. Psychol. 46 (4), 368–375.

Beck, A., Clark, D., 1997. An information processing model of anxiety: automatic and strategic processes. Behav. Res. Ther. 35 (1), 49–58.

Bowins, B.E., 2004. Psychological defense mechanisms: a new perspective. Am. J. Psychoanal. 64, 1–26.

Bowins, B., 2008. Hypomania: a depressive inhibition override defense mechanism. J. Affect. Disord. 109, 221–232.

Bowins, B.E., 2010a. Repetitive maladaptive behavior: beyond repetition compulsion. Am. J. Psychoanal. 70, 282–298.

Bowins, B.E., 2010b. Personality disorders: a dimensional defense mechanism approach. Am. J. Psychother. 64 (2), 153–169.
Bowins, B.E., 2012. Therapeutic dissociation: compartmentalization & absorption. Couns. Psychol. Q. 25 (1), 307–317.
Bowins, B.E., 2016. Mental Illness Defined: Continuums, Regulation, and Defense. Routledge, New York & London.
Boyer, P., Lienard, P., 2006. Why ritualized behavior? Precaution systems and action parsing in developmental, pathological and cultural rituals. Behav. Brain Sci. 29, 595–613.
Brune, M., 2006. The evolutionary psychology of obsessive-compulsive disorder. Persp. Biol. Med. 49 (3), 317–329.
Castillo, R.J., 2003. Trance, functional psychosis, and culture. Psychiatry 66 (1), 9–21.
Cohen, L., 1989. Attributional asymmetries in relation to dysphoria and self-esteem. J. Pers. Indiv. Differ. 10 (10), 1055–1061.
Davydov, D.M., Stewart, R., Ritchie, K., Chaudieu, I., 2010. Resilience and mental health. Clin. Psychol. Rev. 30 (5), 479–495.
Eckblad, M., Chapman, L.J., 1986. Development and validation of a scale for hypomanic personality. J. Abnorm. Psychol. 95, 214–222.
French, C.C., Richards, A., Scholfield, E.J., 1996. Hypomania, anxiety, and the emotional Stroop. Psychol. Psychother. 35 (4), 617–626.
Freud, S., 1894/1964 . The neuro-psychosis of defense. In: Strachey, J. (Ed.), The Standard Edition of the Complete Psychological Works of Sigmund Freud, vol. 3. Hogarth Press, London.
Freud, S., 1895/1964. Studies on hysteria. In: Strachey, J. (Ed.), The Standard Edition of the Complete Psychological Works of Sigmund Freud, vol. 2. Hogarth Press, London.
Freud, S., 1915/1949. Repression. In: Collected Papers, vol. IV. The Hogarth Press, London.
Freud, S., 1964. The neuro-psychosis of defense. In: Strachey, J. (Ed.), The Standard Edition of the Complete Psychological Works of Sigmund Freud, vol. 3. Hogarth Press, London, pp. 45–61.
Jamison, K., Gerner, R., Hammen, C., Padesky, C., 1980. Clouds and silver linings: positive experiences associated with primary affective disorders. Am. J. Psychiatry 137, 198–202.
Johnson, S.L., Sandrow, D., Meyer, B., Winters, R., Miller, I., Solomon, D., Keitner, G., 2000. Increases in manic symptoms after life events involving goal attainment. J. Abnorm. Psychol. 109, 721–727.
Kaplan, H., Saddock, B., Grebb, J., 1994. Synopsis of Psychiatry: Behavioral Sciences Clinical Psychiatry, Seventh Edition. Williams & Wilkins, Baltimore.
Kihlstrom, J., Glisky, M., Angiulo, M., 1994. Dissociative tendencies and dissociative disorders. J. Abnorm. Psychol. 103 (1), 117–124.
Kingdon, D., Turkington, D., 1994. Cognitive-Behavioural Therapy of Schizophrenia. Lawrence A. Earlbaum Associates, Hillsdale.
Koukopoulos, A., Sani, G., Koukopoulos, A.E., Minnai, G.P., Girardi, P., Pani, L., et al., 2003. Duration and stability of the rapid-cycling course: a long-term personal follow-up of 109 patients. J. Affect. Disord. 73, 75–85.
Landa, Y., Silverstein, S., Schwartz, F., Savitz, A., 2006. Group cognitive behavioral therapy for delusions: helping patients improve reality testing. J. Contemp. Psychother. 36 (1), 9–17.
Levy, M., 2000. A conceptualization of the repetition complulsion. Psychiatry 63, 45–53.
Marmar, C.R., Weiss, D.S., Schlenger, W.E., Fairbank, J.A., Jordan, J.A., Kulka, R.A., Hough, R.L., 1994. Peritraumatic dissociation and posttraumatic stress in male Vietnam theater veterans. Am. J. Psychiatry 151, 902–907.
Masson, J.M., 1985. The Complete Letters of Sigmund Freud to Wilhelm Fliess, 1887-1904. Harvard University Press, Cambridge, MA, p. 45.

Merckelbach, H., Rassin, E., Muris, P., 2000. Dissociation, schizotypy, and fantasy proneness in undergraduate students. J. Nerv. Ment. Dis. 188 (7), 428–431.

Meyer, B., Johnson, S.L., Carver, C.S., 1999. Exploring behavioral activation and inhibition sensitivities among college students at risk for bipolar spectrum symptomatology. J. Psychopathol. Behav. Assess. 21, 275–292.

Morgan, C., 2001. Symptoms of dissociation in humans experiencing acute, uncontrollable stress: a prospective investigation. Am. J. Psychiatry 158 (8), 1239–1247.

Nelson, R., Craighead, W., 1977. Selective recall of positive and negative feedback, self-control behaviors, and depression. J. Abnorm. Psychol. 86, 379–388.

Nijenhuis, E., Spinhoven, P., Van Dyck, R., Van Der Hart, O., Vanderlinden, J., 1996. The development and psychometric characteristics of the somatoform dissociation questionnaire (SDQ-20). J. Nerv. Ment. Dis. 184 (11), 688–694.

Olsson, I., Dahl, A.A., 2012. Avoidant personality problems—their association with somatic and mental health, lifestyle, and social network. A community-based study. Compr. Psychiatry 53 (6), 813–821.

Polimeni, J., Reiss, J.P., Sareen, J., 2005. Could obsessive-compulsive disorder have originated as a group-selected adaptive trait in traditional societies. Med. Hypothesis 65, 655–664.

Putman, F.W., 1985. Dissociation as an extreme response to trauma. In: Kluft, R.P. (Ed.), Childhood Antecedents of Multiple Personality. American Psychiatric Press, Washington, DC, pp. 66–97.

Rachman, S., Hodgson, R., 1980. Obsessions and Compulsions. Prentice-Hall, Englewood Cliffs.

Ross, C., Joshi, S., Currie, R., 1990. Dissociative experiences in the general population. Am. J. Psychiatry 147 (11), 1547–1552.

Ross, C., Joshi, S., Currie, R., 1991. Dissociative experiences in the general population: a factor analysis. Hosp. Community Psychiatry 42 (3), 297–301.

Ross, C., Joshi, S., Currie, R., 1992. Paranormal experiences in the general population. J. Nerv. Ment. Dis. 180 (6), 357–361.

Rutten, B.P., Hammels, C., Geschwind, N., Menne-Lothmann, C., Pishva, E., Schruers, K., et al., 2013. Resilience in mental health: linking psychological and neurobiological perspectives. Acta Psychiatrica Scand. 128 (1), 3–20.

Simeon, D., 1997. Feeling unreal: 30 cases of DSM-III-R depersonalization disorder. Am. J. Psychiatry 154 (8), 1107–1113.

Steiner, H., Araujo, K., Koopman, C., 2001. The response evaluation measure (REM-71): a new instrument for the measurement of defenses in adults and adolescents. Am. J. Psychiatry 158 (3), 467–473.

Tiger, L., 1979. Optimism: The Biology of Hope. Simon & Schuster, New York.

Trijsburg, R., Van Spiijker, A., Van, H.L., Hesselink, A.J., Duivenvoorden, H.J., 2000. Measuring overall defensive functioning with the defense style questionnaire. J. Nerv. Ment. Dis. 188 (7), 432–439.

Vaillant, G., 1977. Adaptation to Life. Little, Brown and Company, Boston.

Vaillant, G., 1994. Ego mechanisms of defense and personality psychopathology. J. Abnorm. Psychol. 103 (1), 44–50.

Van Der Hart, O., Friedman, B., 1989. A reader's guide to Pierre Janet on dissociation: a neglected intellectual heritage. Dissociation 2, 3–16.

Waelde, L.C., 2004. Dissociation and meditation. J. Trauma Dissociation 5 (2), 147–162.

Wastell, C., 1999. Defensive focus and the defense style questionnaire. J. Nerv. Ment. Dis. 187 (4), 217–223.

Watkins, J.G., Watkins, H.H., 1997. Ego states: Theory and Therapy. W.W. Norton, New York, NY.

Weinberger, D., 1990. The construct validity of the repressive coping style. In: Repression and Dissociation. University of Chicago Press, Chicago, pp. 200-222.

Chapter 4

Social connectedness

Human evolution has been dynamic producing many changes but one constant is social contact that took the form of hunting–gathering groups for about 95% of the total, then agricultural settlements, then towns and cities. The reason is crystal clear: given our lack of body weaponry compared to many other animals, solitary behavior would not have worked out well. In hunting–gathering groups there was safety, the option of cooperative hunting and gathering, and finding mates was much easier. This 200,000 plus years of social contact has given us a social brain, such that we view the world in social terms and rely on others. Lack of social connectedness leaves a person feeling lonely and usually vulnerable. It then follows that social connectedness characterizes mental health, whereas social disconnection will be more consistent with mental illness, or at least lesser mental health. Of course, negative social contact as with bullying, discrimination, or being relegated to a very low social status, can result in worse mental health, but we will focus on positive social contact. Social connectedness implies social contact that is positive. I am referring to social connectedness here to capture the sense of belonging and being linked to others in a positive way. In the Activity chapter, social activity was left out and reserved for this chapter, but social activity is important for mental health. We will first look at the mental health impact of social disconnection and then that for social connectedness.

Social disconnection

When people feel disconnected from others loneliness is a common reaction, but reality and perception both appear to play a role: loneliness and isolation are often thought to be synonymous, but they do not always equate. It is possible to be fairly isolated and not feel lonely, or have people around and feel lonely due to a sense of not being connected to them. Demonstrating how loneliness and isolation are not synonymous, Coyle and Dugan (2012) studied 11, 825 participants from the Leave Behind Questionnaire of the Health and Retirement Study in 2006 and 2008. Loneliness was associated with greater odds of having a mental health problem, and isolation to self-reported poor health. They did find some overlap but loneliness and isolation were not highly correlated.

Research does demonstrate that loneliness is linked to worse mental health. For example, suicidal behavior is associated with loneliness based on a study

States and Processes for Mental Health. DOI: 10.1016/C2020-0-00574-8

by Stickley and Koyanagi (2016), who applied the Adult Psychiatric Morbidity Survey with information from 7403 households. Common mental disorders were evaluated using the Clinical Interview Schedule Revised, and the respondents were questioned about perceived loneliness and lifetime, as well as past year, suicide ideation and attempts. Loneliness was associated with suicidal behavior (ideation and attempts), and participants reporting the most severe degree of loneliness had a 3.45 greater odds ratio for lifetime suicide attempts, and 17.37 greater odds ratio for past year suicide attempts. The researchers adjusted for the influence of conditions such as depression that could account for suicidal behavior and the results still held.

Dementia is another mental illness that appears to be linked to loneliness but not isolation, based on a study by Holwerda et al. (2014) who examined 2173 nondemented community-living older persons as part of the Amsterdam Study of the Elderly, following them for 3 years. The criteria for social isolation included living alone, unmarried, or without social support, while feelings of loneliness were self-reported. The Mental State Automated Geriatric Examination for Computer-Assisted Taxonomy measured dementia. While isolation was not linked to dementia, those reporting feelings of loneliness were more likely to develop dementia after taking into consideration other risk factors.

Additional research reveals that mental health is diminished and formal mental illness worsened by loneliness. For example, Meltzer et al. (2013) evaluated 7461 randomly selected participants as part of the 2007 Adult Psychiatric Morbidity Survey in England, with common mental disorders assessed using the Clinical Interview Schedule and psychosis by the Schedules of the Clinical Assessment of Neuropsychiatry. The Social Functioning Questionnaire was applied to assess feelings of loneliness that turned out to be associated with all mental disorders, but mostly depression. An even larger sample survey investigating the impact of loneliness on mental health was conducted in Switzerland by Richard et al. (2017), with the Swiss Health Survey 2012/2013 involving 20,841 individuals ranging from 15 to 70+ years of age. Psychological distress was assessed by the Mental Health Inventory-5 (MHI-5), depression by the Patient Health Questionnaire-9, and loneliness by the question—How often do you feel lonely? Loneliness was correlated with moderate to high psychological distress and depression. Focusing on adolescents, Shevlin et al. (2014) utilized data from the Young Life and Times Survey of North Irish adolescents with loneliness assessed by the UCLA Loneliness Scale. Their results revealed loneliness to be associated with risk of psychiatric problems, and this relationship increased from low to high loneliness ratings. In assessing what accounted for this relationship, specific isolation experiences and disconnectedness stood out. Alienation and disconnection can characterize some adolescents as they shift from family to peer identities.

Research then reveals that loneliness, but not necessarily isolation, is linked to mental illness, but why not isolation when it seemingly generates a sense of loneliness? Different scenarios might account for this, with a major one being compensation. For example, some isolated people feel a sense of connection to television or movie fictional characters, or those in books. Perhaps more significant are pets. Demonstrating how pets can compensate for contact with people, Stanley et al. (2014) assessed 830 older adults (greater than 60 years old) in a primary care health setting, discovering that pet owners were 36% less likely to report loneliness, even after factors such as age, living status (alone versus not alone), happy mood, and seasonal residency, were taken into account. Pet ownership and living status (somewhat related to degree of isolation for these people) interacted in that living alone and not owning a pet was associated with the greatest odds of feeling lonely.

Ascribing human-like qualities to nonhuman objects, including pets and nonliving entities, is another way that people compensate for isolation that otherwise would likely produce feelings of loneliness. This process was demonstrated in a very interesting study by Bartz et al. (2016), who initially assessed 178 individuals with the UCLA Loneliness Scale. Experimental group participants were then primed to recall an important and meaningful relationship in their life, whereas control group participants were asked to recall an acquaintance, but not a close friend. All subjects next completed a gadget task consisting of rating them on a number of social and nonsocial traits, and the pet task, whereby they selected traits that best described a pet of theirs or one known to them. Participants from both groups who scored higher on loneliness anthropomorphized to a greater extent, showing that attributing human-like tendencies to pets and even inanimate objects helps to compensate for loneliness. For those participants who were reminded of a close relationship, a reduced tendency to anthropomorphize emerged, likely due to how the reminder of closeness to another person lowered any feelings of loneliness. The results from this study demonstrate that we ascribe human-like traits to animals and inanimate objects to compensate for feelings of loneliness, and that even being reminded of a close relationship can reduce such feelings and hence motivation to anthropomorphize.

Social connectedness

If social disconnection and the resulting feeling of loneliness worsens mental health, then it follows that social connectedness will advance mental health. Indeed, research backs up this assertion. A concept that has arisen with research on social activity and connectedness is social capital, broadly defined as a type of "capital" resulting from social relationships between people, including physical health, mental health, life skills, and perceptions of wellbeing. There is debate regarding whether it is valid as a single conceptual entity and what it actually entails, but it is applied in research.

The link between social capital and mental health has been investigated in the work setting, such as by Gao et al. (2014) who evaluated 2796 employees from 35 diverse workplaces in Shanghai. Social capital was measured by a validated and tested 8-item instrument, and mental health by the World Health Organization-Five Well-Being Index. Workers in the top quartile of social capital were compared to those in the remaining quartiles: those in the top quartile had significantly lower odds of poor mental health, even after controlling for variables such as sex, age, marital status, education level, occupational status, smoking, physical activity, and job stress. A similar result emerged when female poultry line workers in Brazil were studied by Pattussi et al. (2016). They found that higher workplace social capital was linked to lower stress, fewer common mental health problems like depression and anxiety, and better health-related behaviors.

Most research examining social connectedness involves group activities, such as that by Jones et al. (2013), who conducted a before and after evaluation of the South West Well-Being programme in England, consisting of 10 organizations providing leisure, exercise, cooking, befriending, arts and crafts social activities. A total of 687 adults with a wide range of ages were assessed prior to and at the conclusion of the given program. Results showed that social and mental wellbeing, and also self-reported mental health improved significantly from before the given social activity commenced to after completion. Although the nature of the activity did not impact on the outcome, structured practitioner support was strongly associated with higher mental health at the conclusion of the given activity. This result supports the perspective that good quality social contact benefits mental health. In the Activity chapter, social connectedness was one of the key themes for how art and hobby activity improves mental health.

Collective bonding can be more significant that one-to-one connections, as revealed by Pearce et al. (2016) who longitudinally evaluated both collective bonding and relational (one-to-one) bonding within singing and creative writing or crafts groups. Eighty-four individuals in four singing classes were compared to 51 participants in three creative writing or crafts classes, assessed at 1, 3, and 7 months. At baseline and each follow-up period mental health was assessed with the 7-item Generalised Anxiety Disorder Scale and the 9-item Patient Health Questionnaire, while wellbeing was evaluated using the Flourishing and Satisfaction with Life scales. The pictorial Inclusion of Other in Self scale was applied to measure collective bonding, and relational bonding was assessed by asking participants to list all the names of fellow group members they could remember and how connected they felt to each. At 7 months, collective bonding was associated with greater wellbeing and lower anxiety, but bonding to individuals within the groups (relational bonding) did not produce any significant results. A limitation of their study was that mental health of the participants was quite high making it challenging to assess positive changes in terms of both collective and individual bonding, but the positive results for the former do support the value of group bonding.

Social connectedness can also be considered in terms of social cohesion, as with a study by Van Dyck et al. (2015) who studied 3965 middle-aged and older adults as part of the Wellbeing, Eating and Exercise for a Long Life study in Victoria, Australia. Neighborhood social cohesion was linked to mental health quality of life. Related to social cohesion is social networks. Windsor et al. (2016) assessed 2001 mid-life and older age people regarding diversity of their social networks based on partner status, network size, contact frequency, and activity engagement. Greater social network diversity was associated with self-reported mental health, and restricted social networks to poor mental health, even after the influence of age, sex, education, and employment status was taken into account.

The research reviewed so far has focused on adults, but what about younger people? VanKim and Nelson (2013) assessed 14,706 college students from a national United States sample of 94 undergraduate schools, part of the Harvard School of Public Health Study of College Health Behavior. Social connectedness was evaluated by two questions pertaining to the number of close friends, dichotomized into five or more and less than five, and the amount of time spent socializing, dichotomized into 2 or more hours per day and less than 2 hours per day. Low socializing was associated with greater odds of poor mental health and perceived stress for both female and male students. Focusing on even younger individuals, Rothon et al. (2012) assessed 15,770 randomly selected households in 2004 when the primary participants were 13–14 years old, and 13,539 households at follow-up a year later, as part of the Longitudinal Study of Young People in England. Mental health was measured by the 12-item General Health Questionnaire, with a score of 4 or greater indicating depression and/or anxiety. Social involvement was based on social capital including family social capital evaluated in terms of quality of parent–child relationships/adult interest in the child, and monitoring of the adolescent's activities (parenteral surveillance) pertaining to how often the parents know where the adolescent is in the evening and setting curfew on school nights. Community social capital consisted of parental social networks, adolescent's sociability, and adolescent's involvement in activities outside the home. Family social capital, but not community social capital produced about a third less risk of mental illness for both male and female adolescents. These results suggest that at least for young to mid age adolescents, social connectedness to parents is very important for their mental health.

Young people, as well as older individuals, use social media, and although this is currently a hotly debated subject, it appears that good social media connections help with mental health. Bessiere et al. (2010) found that online communication with friends and family (mostly social media) is actually associated with lower depression. In a 2014 review, Pantic concluded that there is no clear evidence that social media impairs mental health and might help, although results are inconclusive (Pantic, 2014). Given that social connectedness of various forms has been shown to advance mental health, it is likely that social media has mental health benefits as well.

Highlighting how important social connectedness is, the quality of social bonding from the early years of life impacts on mental health. There are different attachment (bonding) styles, but the main division is secure and insecure, with the former arising from supportive, sensitive, and responsive parenting (Bee and Boyd, 2004). Secure attachment provides a person with a sense of being socially worthy and trusting that others will be reliable, while insecure attachment occurs when caregivers are nonresponsive, inconsistent, and fail to support the young child producing doubts about oneself and others (Atwool, 2006).

Although it can be tenuous to link later life mental health outcomes to early attachment style (Gittleman et al., 1998), there does appear to some influence. Analyzing data from the National Comorbidity Survey Replication involving 5692 people over 18 years of age, Palitsky et al. (2013) found that insecure attachment is associated with greater odds of suicide ideation, suicide attempts, and all mental disorders analyzed. Secure attachment is associated with a decreased likelihood of these mental illness manifestations. The results for insecure and secure attachment held after controlling for confounding variables. In a review of the relevant literature, Beatson and Taryan (2003) conclude that secure attachment reduces activation of the hypothalamic–pituitary–adrenal axis during a critical period of development, and from this reduces the risk of depression later on. Securely attachment individuals grow to become more resilient (Rutten et al., 2013), the psychological aspect we considered as a defense in the Psychological defense mechanism chapter.

Summary note

Due to our evolution in hunting–gathering groups and reliance on others, we benefit psychologically from social connectedness. Loneliness worsens mental health, and isolation likely does in the absence of compensation strategies, such as pets. Bonding of various forms, such as group, individual, social cohesion, social networks, and probably social media, seems to counter mental illness and advance mental health in the general population. Underscoring the significance of social connectedness, early life attachment styles influence later life mental health, such as by fostering resilience.

References

Atwool, N., 2006. Attachment and resilience: implications for children in care. Child Care Pract. 12, 315–330.

Bartz, J.A., Tchalova, K., Fenerci, C., 2016. Reminders of social connection can attenuate anthropormorphism: a replication and extension of Epley, Akalis, Waytz, and Cacioppo (2008). Psychol. Sci. 27 (12), 1644–1650.

Beatson, J., Taryan, S., 2003. Predisposition to depression: the role of attachment. Aust. N. Z. J. Psychiatry 37 (2), 219–225.

Bee, H.L., Boyd, D., 2004. The Developing Child, Tenth ed. Allyn & Bacon, Boston.

Bessiere, K., Pressman, S., Kiesler, S., 2010. Effects of internet use on health and depression: a longitudinal study. J. Med. Internet Res. 12 (1), e6. doi:10.2196/jmir.1149.

Coyle, C.E., Dugan, E., 2012. Social isolation, loneliness and health among older adults. J. Aging Health 24 (8), 1346–1363.

Gao, J., Weaver, S.R., Dai, J., Jia, Y., Liu, X., Jin, K., et al., 2014. Workplace social capital and mental health among Chinese employees: a multi-level, cross-sectional study. Plos One 9 (1), e85005.

Gittleman, M.G., Klein, M.H., Smider, N.A., Essex, M.J., 1998. Recollections of parental behaviour, adult attachment and mental health: mediating and moderating effects. Psychol. Med. 28 (6), 1443–1455.

Holwerda, T.J., Deeg, D.J., Beekman, A.T., Van Tilburg, T.G., Stek, M.L., Jonker, C., et al., 2014. Feelings of loneliness, but not social isolation, predict dementia onset: results from the Amsterdam Study of the Elderly (AMSTEL). J. Neurol. Neurosurg. Psychiatry 85 (2), 135–142.

Jones, M., Kimberlee, R., Deave, T., Evans, S., 2013. The role of community centre-based arts, leisure and social activities in promoting adult well-being and healthy lifestyles. Int. J. Environ. Res. Public Health 10 (5), 1948–1962.

Meltzer, H., Bebbington, P., Dennis, M.S., Jenkins, R., McManus, S., Brugha, T.S., 2013. Feelings of loneliness among adults with mental disorders. Soc. Psychiatry Psychiatr. Epidemiol. 48 (1), 5–13.

Palitsky, D., Mota, N., Afifi, T.O., Downs, A.C., Sareen, J., 2013. The association between adult attachment style, mental disorders, and suicidality: findings from a population-based study. J. Nervous Mental Disord. 201 (7), 579–586.

Pantic, I., 2014. Online social networking and mental health. Cyberpsychol. Behav. Soc. Netw. 17 (10), 652–657.

Pattussi, M.P., Olinto, M.T., Canuto, R., Da Silva, G.A., Paniz, V.M., Kawachi, I., 2016. Workplace social capital, mental health and health behaviors among Brazilian female workers. Soc. Psychiatry Psychiatr. Epidemiol. 51 (9), 1321–1330.

Pearce, E., Launay, J., Machin, A., Dunbar, R.I.M., 2016. Is group singing special? Health, well-being and social bonds in community-based education classes. J. Community Appl. Soc. Psychol. 26 (6), 518–533.

Richard, A., Rohrmann, S., Vandeleur, C.L., Schmid, M., Barth, J., Eichholzer, M., 2017. Loneliness is adversely associated with physical and mental health and lifestyle factors: results from a Swiss national survey. Plos One 12 (7), e0181442.

Rothon, C., Goodwin, L., Stansfeld, S., 2012. Family social support, community "social capital" and adolescents' mental health and educational outcomes: a longitudinal study in England. Soc. Psychiatry Psychiatr. Epidemiol. 47 (5), 697–709.

Rutten, B.P., Hammels, C., Geschwind, N., Menne-Lothmann, C., Pishva, E., Schruers, K., et al., 2013. Resilience in mental health: linking psychological and neurobiological perspectives. Acta Psychiatr. Scand. 128 (1), 3–20.

Shevlin, M., Murphy, S., Murphy, J., 2014. Adolescent loneliness and psychiatric morbidity in the general population: identifying "at risk" groups using latent class analysis. Nordic J. Psychiatry 68 (8), 633–639.

Stanley, I.H., Conwell, Y., Bowen, C., Van Orden, K.A., 2014. Pet ownership may attenuate loneliness among older adult primary care patients who live alone. Aging Mental Health 18 (3), 394–399.

Stickley, A., Koyanagi, A., 2016. Loneliness, common mental disorders and suicidal behavior: findings from a general population survey. J. Affect. Disord. 197, 81–87.

Van Dyck, D., Teychenne, M., McNaughton, S.A., De Bourdeaudhuij, I., Salmon, J., 2015. Relationship of the perceived social and physical environment with mental health-related quality of life in middle-aged and older adults; mediating effects of physical activity. Plos One 10 (3), e0120475.

VanKim, N.A., Nelson, T.F., 2013. Vigorous physical activity, mental health, perceived stress, and socializing among college students. Am. J. Health Promot. 28 (1), 7–15.

Windsor, T.D., Rioseco, P., Fiori, K.L., Curtis, R.G., Booth, H., 2016. Structural and functional social network attributes moderate the association of self-rated health with mental health in midlife and older adults. Int. Psychogeriatr. 28 (1), 49–61.

Chapter 5

Regulation

Biological entities could never survive and thrive without regulation over essential processes. For mammals and primates, physiological parameters such as electrolyte composition, blood sugar level, temperature, and blood pressure are tightly controlled. Whenever this regulation falters disease occurs, as with diabetes involving deficient control of blood sugar levels and hypertension-sustained high blood pressure. Even the growth of cells is controlled by various signals to keep the system in balance, and cancer arises when cells remove themselves from this regulation and divide without restraint. Physiological homeostasis transpires when regulatory processes are functioning effectively.

Natural biological regulation also occurs at the ecosystem level. For example, if deer populations increase due to abundant vegetation, wolves will eat well diminishing the deer population, thereby preserving the vegetation deer feed on. Competition between wolfs will, in turn, limit their number in a given area. Salmon mature in rivers and then enter the sea where they live for a few years, before returning to the same river system they grew up in. After spawning they die, their bodies providing a crucial source of nitrogen and carbon for their developing offspring and other animals such as bears that eat the salmon. Partially eaten salmon and the feces of animals that eat them return minerals to the soil enabling the growth of trees and plants, that, in turn, shade the river cooling the water so that salmon can survive. Healthy ecosystems achieve this self-regulation through extensive interconnectedness. If regulation is necessary for healthy biological functioning, both at individual organism and ecosystem levels, then it follows that it is highly relevant for psychological functioning and mental health, given that psychological processes ultimately have a biological basis. Indeed, research has demonstrated that neural structures are involved in psychological regulation based on top-down connectedness, with the prefrontal cortex (PFC) prominent (Arnsten, 2009; Arnsten, 2011; Beauregard et al., 2006; Brambilla et al., 2005; Goldin, 2009; Goldin et al., 2009; Hartley and Phelps, 2010; Philippot and Brutoux, 2008; Salzman and Fusi, 2010; Schardt et al., 2010). The pattern of connections within the brain has been referred to as the connectome (Sporns et al., 2005). We will now look at the different forms of psychological regulation consistent with good mental health.

States and Processes for Mental Health. DOI: 10.1016/C2020-0-00574-8

Emotion regulation

Emotions are brief responses to internal and external stimuli, and as discussed in the Activity chapter, there are several that are primary and universal: fear, sadness, anger, disgust, shame, happiness, interest, and surprise. In addition, there are secondary emotions as either combinations of primary ones or points on a continuum of each (Izard, 1992). For example, contempt arises from a combination of anger and disgust, and contentment a point on the happiness continuum (Izard, 1994). Mammals and primates likely have at least the primary emotions, but the evolution of human intelligence has amplified emotions by making the cognitive activating appraisals (unconscious and conscious triggering thoughts) more intensive, extensive, and adding a temporal dimension—the Amplification Effect (Bowins, 2004). Beyond the initial amplification, mutually reinforcing cycles of thoughts and emotions further amplify the emotional state. For instance, cognitive activating appraisals detecting threat or danger produce fear, creating an emotional climate for further fear-related thoughts, triggering more fear, and so on (Izard, 1992). The same process applies to other primary emotions, such as anger when excessive and enduring thoughts pertaining to violations amplify this emotion, creating an emotional climate conducive to more violation themes, generating more anger. At some point the amplification of anger can overwhelm emotion regulation leading to aggression. This amplification of emotions has made us the most emotional of animals, which is great on the positive side, but a burden on the negative side.

The impact of amplified negative emotions is actually much more significant than for positive emotions, due to a couple of processes. First, simply the number of negative emotions relative to positive emotions: of the eight possible primary emotions five are generally negative in feeling tone (fear, sadness, anger, disgust, shame), one (surprise) either positive or negative, and only two (happiness and interest) are clearly positive in feeling tone. Regarding secondary emotions, the five primary negative emotions can combine in configurations of two or three to produce a complex array of additional negative emotions. As points on a continuum of primary emotions, there will also be more manifestations for the five negative primary emotions, than the two positive primary emotions. The second related reason is how evolution has equipped us to perceive negative over positive stimuli, for the basic reality that negative circumstances typically have greater survival implications (Ledoux, 1994). For example, failure to detect a predator is going to impact on the survival of yourself and/or your children much more than is failure to detect one potential food source. Hence, emotionally we are weighted in a sense for negative emotions over positive emotions! This would be impactful enough without the amplification effect of human intelligence on primary and secondary emotions, but with it we are burdened by negative emotions.

In the Psychological defense mechanism chapter, we examined how the burden of negative emotions led to the evolution of these defenses safeguarding psychological functioning. Psychological defense mechanisms help us regulate emotions. For example, milder positive cognitive distortions such as self-enhancing spins on events reconfigure negative circumstances that trigger sadness, anger, fear, disgust, and shame, thereby attenuating these reactions. Defenses involving greater degrees of cognitive distortion, such as the immature classic defense mechanisms, can also regulate negative emotions, although typically in a much less functional way, as with projection transferring negative qualities of oneself, including anger/aggression to other people. Positive cognitive distortions facilitate emotion regulation by altering perceptions and perspectives favoring negative emotions, shifting them to those favoring more positive emotions. Dissociation also limits negative emotions by distancing a person psychologically from negativity and fostering positivity via absorption in positive pursuits.

Aside from defense mechanisms, emotion regulation involves several other psychological processes mitigating, adjusting, and maintaining a given emotion (Fiore et al., 2014; Racine and Wildes, 2016). Clarifying the nature of emotional dysregulation and facilitating its evaluation, Gratz and Roemer (2004) developed the Difficulties in Emotion Regulation Scale (DERS). Various aspects of emotional dysregulation are assessed via six subscales consisting of lack of awareness of emotional responses, lack of clarity of emotional responses, non-acceptance of emotional responses, limited access to emotion regulation strategies perceived as effective, difficulties controlling impulses when experiencing negative emotions, and difficulties engaging in goal-directed behaviors when experiencing negative emotions (Gratz and Roemer, 2004). The converse of emotional dysregulation provides for effective regulation of emotions: awareness of emotional responses, clarity of emotional responses, acceptance of emotional responses, access to emotion regulation strategies perceived as effective, controlling impulses when experiencing negative emotions, and engaging in goal-directed behaviors when experiencing negative emotions. High emotion regulation capacities provide for solid emotional intelligence.

Considering the six aspects of emotion regulation identified by Gratz and Roemer (2004), it is clear that they can and do help regulate excessive negative emotions. Awareness of emotional responses motivates and activates conscious processes that counter disturbing emotional states. Being clear as to what an emotion represents, such as distinguishing sadness from fear, assists with appropriate regulation responses, as for example, compensating for a loss when sadness arises and managing threats in the case of fear. Accepting emotions and working with them, as opposed to consciously rejecting them or unconsciously converting them into somatic states, fosters effective regulation. Controlling impulses is a crucial aspect of regulation, as impaired regulation of impulses results in negative outcomes worsening emotional states. For example, not containing an impulse to shout at your boss is going to result in detrimental outcomes. Engaging in goal-directed behaviors brings into play absorption in positive activities we covered in the Psychological defense mechanism chapter, highlighting how this mild form of dissociation is a powerful way to disconnect from negative emotions via immersion in positive pursuits. An additional crucial emotion regulation strategy consists of frustration tolerance, providing the capacity to delay gratification for when it is appropriate and feasible.

Demonstrating how deficiencies of these emotional regulation strategies detract from mental health, eating disorders entail various deficiencies. For example, binge eating and recurrent purging are linked to difficulties controlling impulses when experiencing negative emotions (Racine and Wildes, 2013). Racine and Wildes (2016) found that emotional dysregulation predicted change in anorexia symptom severity, but not the reverse. Alexithymia involving a lack of awareness of emotional responses, is present in anorexia to a greater extent than in controls (Gilboa-Schechtman et al., 2006). Anorexic individuals also have difficulty recognizing emotions in others, making it difficult to regulate their own emotional reactions (Harrison et al., 2009). Emotion regulation deficiencies also apply to bulimia. Lavender et al. (2014) administered the DERS to 80 adults (90% women) with bulimia, and found that the global DERS score correlated significantly with eating disorder behavior, and more specifically, the difficulties engaging in goal-directed behaviors when experiencing negative emotions subscale, was associated with the frequency of purging and driven exercise. Negative urgency, defined as the tendency to act impulsively in response to negative affect, is increased when there is binging and purging (Fischer et al., 2008), highlighting an undercontrolled component. Regarding childhood obesity, Aparicio et al. (2016) in a review ascertained that emotion regulation strategies mediate the relationship between stress and weight gain, in that ineffective strategies contribute to emotional eating and a sedentary lifestyle, while effective emotion regulation strategies produce behaviors countering weight gain when stress is present. Emotional dysregulation is also involved in adult obesity via impulsive food consumption (Micanti et al., 2017).

Impaired emotion regulation plays a role in other mental illnesses. For example, borderline personality disorder (BPD) involves deficient regulation of impulses and excessive negative emotions, and even at times positive emotions, producing extreme swings in emotional states. Comparing emotional regulation dysfunction, problematic relations, and nonintegrated self, Cheavans et al. (2012) discovered that the former had the strongest relationship to BPD symptoms. Herr et al. (2013) studying a BPD adult sample ascertained that emotional regulation mediates the relationship between BPD symptom severity and interpersonal dysfunction. In a review of the literature, Berking and Wupperman (2012) indicate that deficiencies in emotion regulation contribute to depression, borderline personality disorder, substance-abuse disorders, eating disorders, somatoform disorders, and other psychopathological symptoms. Regarding somatoform (somatic) disorders, failure to process emotions efficiently leads to their expression in bodily forms producing a range of difficult to manage physical symptoms.

Effective emotion regulation in terms of awareness of emotional responses, clarity of emotional responses, acceptance of emotional responses, access to emotion regulation strategies perceived as effective, controlling impulses when experiencing negative emotions, engaging in goal-directed behaviors when experiencing negative emotions, and frustration tolerance, fosters mental health while deficiencies favor mental illness. Healthy psychological defense mechanism functioning also provides for intact emotion regulation safeguarding mental health. Impaired emotion regulation transpires with depression, anxiety, eating disorders, borderline personality disorder, substance abuse, and somatic disorders. Emotion dysregulation results in negative emotions exceeding positive emotions (negative affectivity over positive affectivity). Robust emotion regulation greatly limits negative emotions, in effect cleaning up the signal so that they arise when circumstances really warrant them, such as clear threats producing fear. Positive emotions are then favored over negative emotions. Hence, emotion regulation in and of itself entails positive emotions exceeding negative emotions, or positive affectivity over negative affectivity, on an ongoing and sustainable basis.

Higher cortical centers appear to be involved in emotion regulation facilitated by defense mechanisms and other psychological processes, toning down the excessive limbic system activity occurring with intense emotions. A key higher cortical structure involved in this emotion regulation is the PFC, representing the brain's master controller accounting for a third of the human cortex (Arnsten, 2009; Arnsten, 2011). Depression and anxiety seem to arise when there is impaired top-down regulation of limbic system activity. For example, in the case of depression deficient PFC, and frontal cortices more generally, regulation of excessive limbic-based feelings of sadness and related emotions transpires (Arnsten, 2009; Arnsten, 2011; Beauregard et al., 2006; Brambilla et al., 2005; Hartley and Phelps, 2010; Philippot and Brutoux, 2008; Salzman and Fusi, 2010; Schardt et al., 2010). Neuroimaging studies reveal excessive activation of limbic and other emotion-related structures, and attenuated activity of frontal regions implicated in emotion regulation (Arnsten, 2009; Arnsten, 2011; Beauregard et al., 2006; Cusi et al., 2012; Dunlop and Mayberg, 2014; Hamilton et al., 2012; Kaiser, 2015). Beauregard et al. (2006) found that compared to nondepressed controls, depressed subjects demonstrated impaired down-regulation of sad feelings, ensuring that they had difficulty containing depression-related emotions. Suggestive of a "scar" on cognitive regulatory processes, deficits pertaining to cognitive control might even increase with each depressive episode and persist after remission (Vanderhasselt and DeRaedt, 2009). Additional evidence points to excessive connectivity within the limbic affective network including the amygdala and hippocampus during negative thoughts, as would be expected if the limbic system is overly active and negative thoughts and emotions are mutually reinforcing one another (Chalah and Ayache, 2018).

Regarding anxiety, there is amplified activity in limbic and paralimbic structures, and decreased activity in the PFC (Delgado et al., 2006; Freitas-Ferrari, et al., 2010; Goldin, 2009; Goldin et al., 2009; Hartley and Phelps, 2010; Larson, et al., 2006; Martin et al., 2009). This pattern is typically interpreted as the PFC failing to exert sufficient top-down regulation of limbic system fear/anxiety responses (Arnsten, 2009; Arnsten, 2011; Goldin, 2009; Goldin et al., 2009; Hartley and Phelps, 2010; Kim and Hamann, 2007; Larson, et al., 2006; Martin et al., 2009). With both anxiety and depression, a negative feedback loop appears to occur, whereby with sufficient stress the regulatory function of the PFC is impaired resulting in excessive emotional responses that generate additional stress, further impairing PFC regulation and so on and so forth (Arnsten, 2009; Arnsten, 2011). Research also suggests that the PFC plays a role in the extinction of established fear responses, restoring emotional homeostasis (Maroun, 2013).

Emotion regulation is then clearly based on patterns of neural connectivity, with effective top-down regulation promoting good mental health and deficient regulation of excessive negative emotions, namely sadness and fear, playing a role in these emotions amplifying to depression and anxiety, respectively. The balance between emotion intensity and higher cortical regulation capacity is relevant, as when the former exceeds the latter emotions escalate to levels consistent with depression and anxiety (Heatherton and Wagner, 2011). Bottom-up regulation is fostered from intact psychological emotion regulation processes including defense mechanisms, because they greatly limit negative emotions while favoring positive emotions, thereby attenuating limbic system activity and, in particular, that pertaining to negative emotions. These same processes also advance top-down regulation by facilitating cortical regulation of limbic system activity, such as short-circuiting feedback loops between negative emotions and thoughts.

Psychosis

Reality congruency or reality testing is a very important component of mental health. Try and imagine going to work and believing that coworkers are acting on behalf of the devil to destroy you, and hearing voices of the devil detailing how this will occur. Functioning is severely impaired by psychosis, and the capacity to discern reality is a key feature of optimal functioning. Psychosis involves extreme variants of thought content, thought form, and sensory-perceptual experiences (Bowins, 2011; Kingdon and Turkington, 1994; Landa et al., 2006). Each of these cognitive capacities occurs on a continuum, with thought content consisting of cognitive distortions, that as we noted in the Psychological defense mechanism chapter range from mild to extensive, the more extreme versions comprising delusions (Kingdon and Turkington, 1994; Landa et al., 2006). Thought form, likewise, ranges from tight logical thinking to circumstantial and tangential to very loose associations. Sensory-perceptual experiences extend from highly reality congruent to reading patterns in sensory perceptions, such as clouds representing images, to illusions or misinterpretation of stimuli, and, in an extreme form, hallucinations perceiving things that are not there.

A very interesting aspect of cognitive distortions, thought form, and sensory-perceptual experiences, is that the more extensive expressions are uncommon during the conscious and awake state. When they do occur during this state psychosis is present, with impaired reality congruency (testing) diminishing functioning. I have proposed that to facilitate reality congruency maintaining evolutionary fitness, psychotic level cognitions are regulated from the conscious and awake state (Bowins, 2011). During dreaming psychotic equivalents are commonly experienced, likely due to the relevant cognitive regulatory processes being relaxed: during sleep these expressions do not detract from evolutionary fitness, and the regulatory processes undoubtedly need a rest. Dreams involve extreme ideas and scenarios, thought form is very loose, and we hear and see things that are not at all real. The cognitive regulatory processes can also be relaxed to facilitate defensive functioning. For instance, an evaluation of 293 widowed people found that 14% had a visual hallucination of their deceased spouse, 13% experienced an auditory hallucination, and 47% had the more general hallucinatory event of feeling the presence of the deceased spouse (Olson et al., 1985). Given that the vast majority of these people were mentally healthy, it appears that the hallucinations defensively restored the lost sensory and emotional stimuli (Bowins, 2011, 2012). Brief reactive psychosis occurring with extreme stress, such as with kidnapping, can also represent a defensive response. For example, the belief, possibly along with sounds and images, that God is rescuing you.

Regulation over psychotic level cognitions relies on connectivity between brain regions, as with emotional regulation. The frontal cortices, and, in particular, the PFC, appear to be instrumental in this crucial regulation capacity. Different lines of neuroscience evidence support this proposition. Psychedelic drugs were believed to induce psychosis by increasing brain activity, but it appears that reduced cognitive control is involved. Carhart-Harris et al. (2012) discovered that psilocybin, the hallucinogenic in magic mushrooms, reduces activity in control centers of the brain such as the PFC, thalamus, and anterior and posterior cingulated cortices, and that the greater the reduction in activity within these control regions, the more intense the self-reported psychedelic experiences. During dreaming when psychotic equivalents are expressed there is less PFC activity (Solms and Turnbill, 2002), and the bizarreness of a dream is directly related to the degree of hypofunction of the PFC (Hobson et al., 2000). Creativity has often been linked to psychotic thought capacity, and this linkage appears related to regulation, or reductions thereof, over cognitive distortions: during creative idea generation, the PFC is less active, but more active when the products of creative thought are implemented (Chrysikou and Thompson-Schill, 2011).

When psychosis occurs, aside from dreaming during sleep and for defensive functioning, there must be impairment in the neural connectivity necessary for adequate regulation over cognitive distortions, thought form, and sensory-perceptual experiences. Evidence supports neural dysconnectivity impairing the connectivity required for adequate regulation (Bowins, 2016), a topic we will explore further in the Human specific cognition chapter. The perspective that regulatory impairments play a pivotal role is more apparent when we consider how with psychosis there is often deficient regulation over inappropriate and maladaptive behaviors and emotional states. For instance, aggressive and sexual impulses are often expressed without inhibitory control, and the PFC is involved in this regulation (Dietrich, 2003; Lhermitte et al., 1986). Hence, with intact mental health regulatory control processes appear to scrub psychotic level cognitive distortions, thought form, and sensory perceptual experiences from the conscious and awake state to facilitate reality congruency necessary for adaptive functioning.

Hypomania–mania

A continuum occurs consisting of subthreshold hypomania (equivalent to normal heightened physical, social, and mental activity) to hypomania to subthreshold mania to mania. As a rule of thumb, when dysfunction > functionality, or certainly, dysfunction >> functionality, a shift to mania is occurring. In the Activity chapter, we looked at how hypomania involves high behavioral approach/activation (BAS) and low behavioral inhibition (BIS) consistent with the requirements of our evolution, and also how in its modal duration of 1–3 days it rarely progresses to mania being approximately equivalent in frequency of occurrence to depression. Coverage of hypomania continued in the Psychological defense mechanism chapter with the perspective that it represents a defense against depression, and also anxiety, temporarily overriding depressive and anxiety-based inhibition to restore adaptive functioning in the moment (Bowins, 2008). Hypomania achieves this outcome largely by shifting the depressive profile of low BAS and high BIS to high BAS and low BIS, and in the process, restores adaptive levels of activity. Hyperthymia or hyperthymic personality, as a personality variant of hypomania, confers success across the lifespan and resilience to depression (Akiskal and Pinto, 1999). This personality variant highlights how hypomania–mania is a separate continuum, enabling expressions in the absence of depression.

Hypomania provides a solid defensive response to depression, generating a level of behavioral activation and reinforcement that is typically very adaptive relative to that found with depression, and also relative to the normal state of many people. Given the demands on people in modern industrial society it might even be the case that genes for hyperthymia are spreading, conferring the level of activity required for ongoing success (Bowins, 2008). This sounds all good for the most part, but the downside is with mania where activity increases to unsustainable levels, sleep diminishes, and adaptive functioning declines. Why might hypomania progress to mania? As with psychosis it appears that impaired regulation is pivotal, in this case removing the brakes so to speak on hypomania. In many instances, alcohol, illicit drugs, antidepressants, and combinations of these are involved, impairing healthy regulatory capacity. Furthermore, neural dysconnectivity appears to play a key role, compromising the connectivity required for healthy regulation of hypomania (Bowins, 2016), a topic we will explore in the Human specific cognition chapter. With intact regulation over the hypomanic defensive response to depression (and anxiety), physical, social, and mental activity is increased in a limited way, countering the behavioral inhibition of depression and anxiety, consistent with the high BAS and low BIS profile providing for evolutionary success.

Summary note

Biological regulation is well-defined at both the individual organism and ecosystem level, supporting the case for psychological regulation. Emotion regulation occurs with higher cortical, and most prominently the PFC, exerting control over the emotion generating limbic system to dampen excessive emotional states. This process regulates sadness and fear helping prevent the amplification to depression and anxiety, respectively. The balance between limbic system activity and regulation of this activity is crucial, because when the former exceeds the latter negative emotions amplify to levels consistent with mental illness. Emotion regulation entails both the bottom-up and top-down aspects, the former limiting negative emotions and the latter diminishing excessive negative emotions.

Key ingredients to effective emotion regulation include: awareness of emotional responses, clarity of emotional responses, acceptance of emotional responses, access to emotion regulation strategies perceived as effective, controlling impulses when experiencing negative emotions, engaging in goal-directed behaviors when experiencing negative emotions, and frustration tolerance. Various forms of mental illness entail deficiencies in these regulation strategies. Psychological defense mechanisms play a major role in regulating emotions, particularly milder positive cognitive distortions including mature classic defense mechanisms, and dissociative absorption. Impaired emotion regulation results in negative emotions exceeding positive emotions (negative affectivity over positive affectivity), whereas robust emotion regulation ensures that positive emotions exceed negative emotions in an ongoing and sustainable fashion. This benefit transpires via reduced negative emotions and cleaning up the signal for their occurrence. Regulation extends to psychosis and bipolar disorder (hypomania–mania), with psychotic level cognitions regulated out of the conscious and awake state, and hypomania blocked from progressing to mania. When these forms of regulation are impaired psychosis and mania transpire. Regulation over psychotic level cognitions facilitates reality congruency (reality testing) necessary for adaptive functioning, and regulation over hypomania yields an effective defensive response to depression.

References

Akiskal, H., Pinto, O., 1999. The evolving bipolar spectrum: prototypes I, II, III, and IV. Psychiatr. Clin. North Am. 22, 517–534.

Aparicio, E., Canals, J., Arija, V., De Henaux, S., Michels, N., 2016. The role of emotion regulation in childhood obesity: implications for prevention and treatment. Nutr. Res. Rev. 29 (1), 17–29.

Arnsten, A., 2009. Stress signaling pathways that impair prefrontal cortex structure and function. Nat. Rev. Neurosci. 10, 410–422.

Arnsten, A., 2011. Prefrontal cortical network connections: key sites of vulnerability in stress and schizophrenia. Int. J. Dev. Neurosci. 29 (3), 215–223.

Beauregard, M., Paquette, V., Levesque, J., 2006. Dysfunction in the neural circuitry of emotional self-regulation in major depressive disorder. Neuroreport 17 (8), 843–846.

Berking, M., Wupperman, P., 2012. Emotion regulation and mental health: recent findings, current challenges, and future directions. Curr. Opin. Psychiatry 25 (2), 128–134.

Bowins, B.E., 2004. Psychological defense mechanisms: a new perspective. Am. J. Psychoanal. 64, 1–26.

Bowins, B., 2008. Hypomania: a depressive inhibition override defense mechanism. J. Affect. Disord. 109, 221–232.

Bowins, B.E, 2011. A cognitive regulatory control model of schizophrenia. Brain Res. Bull. 85, 36–41.

Bowins, B.E., 2012. Psychosis: a synthesis of motivational and defect perspectives. Am. J. Psychoanal. 72, 152–165.

Bowins, B.E., 2016. Mental Illness Defined: Continuums, Regulation, and Defense. Routledge, New York & London.

Brambilla, P., Glahn, D., Balestrieri, M., Soares, J., 2005. Magnetic resonance findings in bipolar disorder. Psychiatr. Clin. North Am. 28 (2), 443–467.

Carhart-Harris, R., Erritzoe, D., Williams, T., Stone, J., Reed, L., Colasanti, A., et al., 2012. Neural correlates of the psychedelic state as determined by fMRI studies with psilocybin. Proc. Natl. Acad. Sci. USA 109 (6), 2138–2143.

Chalah, M.A., Ayache, S.S., 2018. Disentangling the neural basis of cognitive behavioral therapy in psychiatric disorders: a focus on depression. Brain Sci. 8 (8). doi:10.3390/brainsci8080150.

Cheavens, J.S., Strunk, D.R., Chriki, L., 2012. A comparison of three theoretically important constructs: what accounts for symptoms of borderline personality disorder? J. Clin. Psychol. 68 (4), 477–486.

Chrysikou, E., Thompson-Schill, S., 2011. Dissociable brain states linked to common and creative object use. Hum. Brain Mapp. 32 (4), 665–675.

Cusi, A., Nazarov, A., Holshausen, K., MacQueen, G., McKinnon, M., 2012. Systematic review of the neural basis of social cognition in patients with mood disorders. J. Psychiatry Neurosci. 37 (3), 154–169.

Delgado, M.R., Olsson, A., Phelps, E.A., 2006. Extending animal models of fear conditioning to humans. Biol. Psychol. 73 (1), 39–48.

Dietrich, A., 2003. Functional neuroanatomy of altered states of consciousness: the transient hypofrontality hypothesis. Conscious Cogn. 12, 231–256.

Dunlop, B.W., Mayberg, H.S., 2014. Neuroimaging-based biomarkers for treatment selection in major depressive disorder. Dialogues Clin. Neurosci. 16 (4), 479–490.

Fiore, F., Ruggiero, G.M., Sassaroli, S., 2014. Emotional dysregulation and anxiety control in the psychopathological mechanism underlying drive for thinness. Front. Psychiatry 5, 43–49.

Fischer, S., Smith, G.T., Cyders, M.A., 2008. Another look at impulsivity: A meta-analytic review comparing specific dispositions to rash action in their relationship to bulimic symptoms. Clin. Psychol. Rev. 28, 1413–1425.

Freitas-Ferrari, M.C., Hallak, J.E., Trzesniak, C., Filho, A.S., Machado-De-Sousa, J.P., Chagas, M.H., Nardi, A.E., Crippa, J.A., 2010. Neuroimaging in social anxiety disorder: a systematic review of the literature. Prog. Neuropsychopharmacol. Biol. Psychiatry 34 (4), 565–580.

Gilboa-Schechtman, E., Avnon, L., Zubery, E., Jeczmien, P., 2006. Emotional processing in eating disorders: specific impairment or general distress related deficiency? Depress. Anxiety 23, 331–339.

Goldin, P., 2009. Effects of cognitive–behavioral therapy on neural bases of emotion regulation in social anxiety disorder. Biol. Psychiatry 65 (Suppl. 1), 1215–1221.

Goldin, P.R., Manber, T., Halimi, S., Canli, T., Gross, J., 2009. Neural bases of social anxiety disorder: emotional reactivity and cognitive regulation during social and physical threat. Arch. Gen. Psychiatry 66 (2), 170–180.

Gratz, K.L., Roemer, L., 2004. Multidimensional assessment of emotion regulation and dysregulation: development, factor structure, and initial validation of the difficulties in emotion regulation scale. J. Psychopathol. Behav. Assess. 26, 41–54.

Hamilton, J., Etkin, A., Furman, D., Lemus, M., Johnson, R., Gotlib, I., 2012. Functional neuroimaging of major depressive disorder: a meta-analysis and new integration of baseline activation and neural response data. Am. J. Psychiatry 169 (7), 693–703.

Harrison, A., Sullivan, S., Tchanturia, K., Treasure, J., 2009. Emotion recognition and regulation in anorexia nervosa. Clin. Psychol. Psychother. 16, 348–356.

Hartley, C., Phelps, E., 2010. Changing fear; the neurocircuitry of emotion regulation. Neuropsychopharmacology 35, 136–146.

Heatherton, T.F., Wagner, D.D., 2011. Cognitive neuroscience of self-regulation failure. Trends Cogn. Sci. 15 (3), 132–139.

Herr, N.R., Rosenthal, M.Z., Geiger, P.J., Erikson, K., 2013. Difficulties with emotional regulation mediate the relationship between borderline personality disorder symptom severity and interpersonal problems. Personal. Ment. Health 7 (3), 191–202.

Hobson, J., Pace-Schott, E., Stickhold, R., 2000. Dreaming and the brain: towards a cognitive neuroscience of conscious states. Behav. Brain Sci. 23, 793–866.

Izard, C., 1992. Basic emotions, relations among emotions, and emotion-cognition relations. Psychol. Bull. 99 (3), 561–565.

Izard, C., 1994. Innate and universal facial expressions: evidence from developmental and cross-cultural research. Psychol. Bull. 115 (2), 288–299.

Kaiser, R.H., 2015. Large-scale network dysfunction in major depressive disorder: a meta-analysis of resting-state functional connectivity. JAMA Psychiatry 72 (6), 603–611.

Kim, S., Hamann, S., 2007. Neural correlates of positive and negative emotion regulation. J. Cogn. Neurosci. 19 (5), 776–798.

Kingdon, D., Turkington, D., 1994. Cognitive-Behavioural Therapy of Schizophrenia. Lawrence A. Earlbaum Associates, Hillsdale.

Landa, Y., Silverstein, S., Schwartz, F., Savitz, A., 2006. Group cognitive behavioral therapy for delusions: helping patients improve reality testing. J. Contemp. Psychother. 36 (1), 9–17.

Larson, C., Schaefer, H., Siegle, G., Jackson, C., Anderle, M., Davidson, R., 2006. Fear is fast in phobic individuals; amygdala activation in response to fear-relevant stimuli. Biol. Psychiatry 60 (4), 410–417.

Lavender, J.M., Wonderlich, S.A., Peterson, C.B., Crosby, R.D., Engel, S.G., Mitchell, J.E., et al., 2014. Dimensions of emotion dysregulation in bulimia nervosa. Eur. Eat. Disord. Rev. 22 (3), 212–216.

Ledoux, J., 1994. "Cognitive-Emotional Interactions in the Brain." Nature of Emotions. Oxford University Press, Oxford.

Lhermitte, F., Pillon, B., Serdaru, M., 1986. Human autonomy and the frontal lobes. Part I: imitation and utilization behavior: a neuropsychological study of 75 patients. Ann. Neurol. 19, 326–334.

Maroun, M., 2013. Medial prefrontal cortex: multiple roles in fear and extinction. Neuroscientist 19 (4), 370–383.

Martin, E.I., Ressler, K.J., Binder, E., Nemeroff, C.B., 2009. The neurobiology of anxiety disorders: brain imaging, genetics, and psychoneuroendocrinology. Psychiatry Clin. North Am. 32 (3), 549–575.

Micanti, F., Iasevoli, F., Cucciniello, C., Costabile, R., Loiarro, G., Pecoraro, G., et al., 2017. The relationship between emotional regulation and eating behavior: a multidimensional analysis of obesity psychopathology. Eat. Weight Disord. 22 (1), 105–115.

Olson, P.R., Suddeth, J.A., Peterson, P.J., 1985. Hallucinations of widowhood. J. Am. Geriatr. Soc. 33, 543–547.

Philippot, P., Brutoux, F., 2008. Induced rumination dampens executive processes in dysphoric young adults. J. Behav. Ther. Exp. Psychiatry 39 (3), 219–227.

Racine, S.E., Wildes, J.E., 2013. Emotion dysregulation and symptoms of anorexia nervosa: the unique roles of lack of emotional awareness and impulse control difficulties when upset. Int. J. Eat. Disord. 46 (7), 713–720.

Racine, S.E., Wildes, J.E., 2016. Dynamic longitudinal relations between emotion regulation difficulties and anorexia nervosa symptoms over the year following intensive treatment. J. Consult. Clin. Psychol. 83 (4), 785–795.

Salzman, D., Fusi, S., 2010. Emotion, cognition, and mental state representation in amygdala and prefrontal cortex. Annu. Rev. Neurosci. 33, 173–202.

Schardt, D., Erk, S., Nusser, C., Nothen, M., Cichon, S., Rietschel, M., et al., 2010. Volition diminishes genetically mediated amygdala hyperreactivity. Neuroimage 53 (3), 943–951.

Solms, M., Turnbill, O., 2002. The Brain and the Inner World. Other Press, New York.

Sporns, O., Tononi, G., Kotter, R., 2005. The human connectome: a structural description of the human brain. PLOS Comput. Biol. https://journals.plos.org/ploscompbiol/article?id=10.1371/journal.pcbi.0010042.

Vanderhasselt, M., DeRaedt, R., 2009. Impairments in cognitive control persist during remission from depression and are related to the number of past episodes: an event related potentials study. Biol. Psychiatry 81 (3), 169–176.

Chapter 6

Human-specific cognition

Humans are distinct from other species both in regard to appearance and behavior, but what characteristics distinguish us? In terms of appearance this is relatively easy to describe, but behavior is more challenging. Cognition is crucial to understanding this distinction with several features representing human-specific cognition (Bowins, 2011, 2016; Burns, 2009; Fiszdon et al., 2007). Evolution builds on pre-existing traits due to how natural selection conserves resources by utilizing what has come before (Darwin, 1858/1958), but the degree of capacity provides for unique features distinguishing humans from other species. Of relevance for mental health, intact human-specific cognition contributes to a healthy state, while deficits play a major role in mental illness, a topic that has been quite neglected. Human-specific cognition involves basic cognition, social cognition, and motivational states.

Basic cognition involves executive functions at its core, and additional capacities including problem solving, the ability to generalize beyond past experience, and overall or fluid intelligence (Ashby et al., 1999; Bilder et al., 2000; Elvevag and Goldberg, 2000; Fiszdon et al., 2007; Gross and Grossman, 2010; Ivleva et al., 2012; Keefe and Fenton, 2007; Morice and Delahunty, 1996; Reichenberg et al., 2010). Executive functions consist of:

- Working memory—the ability to hold information in short term memory allowing time to process it as required for the given mental activity
- Initiation—the capacity to begin a task or activity, or independently generate ideas
- Inhibition—the ability to stop behavior including thoughts, actions, and impulses
- Cognitive flexibility (set shifting)—being able to flexibly shift from one thought or behavior to another, in line with the demands of the situation
- Task completion—the ability to carry through with a task to its endpoint without distraction
- Attention—being able to focus on a mental or physical task sufficiently long enough to complete it
- Planning—the capacity to anticipate future events and prepare accordingly
- Organization—the ability to arrange thoughts, items, and behavior in an orderly and logical fashion or sequence
- Monitoring—assessing performance during and after a task to ensure completion
- Multitasking—the capacity to perform different functions during the same short time frame

States and Processes for Mental Health. DOI: 10.1016/C2020-0-00574-8

(Ashby et al., 1999; Bilder et al., 2000; Bowins, 2016; Elvevag and Goldberg, 2000; Fiszdon et al., 2007; Gross and Grossman, 2010; Keefe and Fenton, 2007; Morice and Delahunty, 1996; Reichenberg et al., 2010).

Executive functions do not exist in isolation from one another with several relying on others, for example, cognitive flexibility or set shifting relying on the ability to inhibit prior actions and responses (Gross and Grossman, 2010). Working memory is crucial for a diverse range of cognitive abilities (Johnson et al., 2013). Several capacities including inhibition, set shifting, attention, monitoring, organizing, and task completion contribute to multitasking (Gross and Grossman, 2010). Broader capacities like problem solving, the ability to generalize, and overall intelligence rely extensively on executive functions (Bilder et al., 2000; Elvevag and Goldberg, 2000; Fiszdon et al., 2007; Gross and Grossman, 2010; Ivleva et al., 2012; Keefe and Fenton, 2007; Morice and Delahunty, 1996; Reichenberg et al., 2010).

Social cognition comprises a variety of capacities including how people think about themselves, others, social situations and interactions (so-called Theory of Mind abilities), emotional information processing, understanding complex social–emotional scenarios such as irony and sarcasm, and social drive limitations (Bediou et al., 2007; Combs et al., 2013; De Jong et al., 2013; Fett et al., 2011; Fiszdon et al., 2007; Kirkpatrick and Buchanan, 1990; Rapp et al., 2014). With good mental health understanding complex social scenarios seems automatic, such as deciphering or intuiting the intentions of others, appreciating one's own social resources or capital, and how interactions might play out. Intact social cognition relies on emotion information processing with facial expression recognition a key component (Bediou et al., 2007). Being able to recognize at least primary emotions—anger, sadness, fear, shame, disgust, surprise, happiness and interest—greatly influences the success of social encounters. Requiring more advanced social information processing, the ability to understand complex social–emotional scenarios as with irony and sarcasm, assists in processing and navigating more involved social interactions. For example, if you cannot distinguish between humor and sarcasm, it is difficult to know what reaction is appropriate. With social interactions moderation and knowing reasonable limitations is healthy. For example, I recently heard a story where a man and his male friend were conversing with two attractive women in a high-end bar. Noting "hookers" outside the bar on the street, the man asked the women, "Are you one of those?" Almost needless to say opportunity and potential success rapidly descended into embarrassment and failure. The various social cognitive capacities seem almost natural to most people, although we all struggle at times given the complexity of many social interactions, a testimony to the role of these capacities in good mental health.

Motivation is another category of human-specific cognition that is so automatic for the most part that it is easy to miss (Bowins, 2016). However, without motivation to act both generally and in regard to specific tasks failure is almost guaranteed. Human-specific cognition includes motivation to strive for knowledge, self-improvement, self-actualization, career accomplishments, friends, romantic partners, and more basic needs such as food, water, and shelter. Motivation is crucial for success, and seems to arise naturally, because it has evolved as part of human-specific cognition. Clearly, all animal species have motivation, but building on more fundamental motivations humans strive for self-actualization, career and financial success, and other rarified goals.

The composite of basic cognition, social cognition, and motivation, is what really distinguishes humans from other animal species behaviorally. These diverse and crucial capacities unfold so naturally and unconsciously with intact mental health that it is easy to omit them when considering mental illness. This is particularly the case given how the focus of mental illness research is on psychopathology only, and typically ignores what constitutes good mental health. We will now take a look at what transpires when human-specific cognition is impaired.

Human-specific cognition deficits

Considering the importance of basic cognition, social cognition, and motivation to mental health, it is not surprising that impairments are fundamental to understanding various mental illnesses. Those covered here are not necessarily exhaustive, and future research might address the full role of negative symptoms in all forms of mental illness. When there is a deficit or impairment in the positive functional capacities provided by human-specific cognition, the term negative symptom is appropriate.

Autism spectrum disorder

This condition involves global deficits in social cognition (Owen, 2012; Waltereit et al., 2014). People with autism, even milder versions such as so-called Asperger syndrome, are impaired in their ability to process and navigate social interactions, struggling with capacities such as facial expression recognition and emotion information processing, understanding the intentions of others and their own social resources or capital, and are lost in regard to complex social–emotional scenarios like irony and sarcasm. Given the pronounced impairments to social cognition and the importance of social interactions, most people with autism do not succeed relative to conventional standards. For example, barely 55% have any employment, including volunteer and part-time work, 6 years after leaving high school, with the rate of employment higher for those with intellectual disability (Volkmar and Wolf, 2013). Improvements always entail some enhanced social cognition capacity, such as making enough eye contact to process facial expressions.

Intellectual disability

Formerly known as developmental delay and mental retardation, intellectual disability involves global deficits in basic cognition (Owen, 2012; Waltereit et al., 2014). These individuals have deficits in regard to executive functions, problem solving, the ability to generalize beyond past experience, and overall or fluid intelligence. Meanwhile, their social cognition is relatively intact despite their information processing deficits. They routinely try to interact with others, make eye contact, can usually distinguish fundamental facial expressions such as anger, sadness, and happiness, and can often appreciate humor. Given our social nature as a species it is then understandable that they usually fare better than autistic people, matched for the degree of impairment to basic cognition and social cognition respectively, obtaining and retaining marginal employment for the simple reason that they engage and connect with people, such that employers and coworkers feel more comfortable with them (Volkmar and Wolf, 2013). On a milder scale, specific forms of learning impairments, such as for math or language, result from focal deficits in basic cognition, such as verbal information processing deficits with language impairments (Owen, 2012; Waltereit et al., 2014).

Attention deficit hyperactivity disorder

Select deficits in executive functioning, such as attention, task completion, monitoring, inhibition, set shifting, organization, planning, and multitasking characterize attention deficit hyperactivity disorder (ADHD) (Oades, 1998; Owen, 2012; Purper-Ouakil and Franc, 2011). At the core of the condition, there are significant problems in terms of attending to a task long enough to complete it without being distracted. Worsening outcomes, the ability to assess performance during and after a task to ensure completion is too much of a challenge. Difficulty is also encountered in terms of inhibiting behavior including thoughts, actions, and impulses, and then flexibly shifting from one thought or behavior to another, in line with the demands of the situation. Without these more fundamental executive functioning capacities, more complex cognitive abilities, such as organizing, planning, and multitasking are virtually impossible to be successful at. ADHD might also involve select social cognition limitations related to emotional information processing (Owen, 2012; Waltereit et al., 2014).

Schizophrenia

Symptoms characterizing schizophrenia consist of positive and negative, the former psychosis, and the latter deficits in basic cognition, social cognition, and motivational states. With substantial impairment to all three forms of human-specific cognition, schizophrenia is understandably a very severe form of mental illness. Frequently, the focus is on psychosis and schizophrenia is considered to be much improved when antipsychotic medications eliminate or remove these manifestations. However, the more detrimental long-term impact is with the negative symptoms involving pronounced impairments to basic cognition, social cognition, and motivation. Regarding motivational, or what have been referred to as absence states, apathy, avolition, anhedonia, alogia, motor retardation, affective flattening, and absence of play and curiosity, transpires (Ballmaier et al., 2008; Bemporad, 1991; Mahurin et al., 1998). These motivation deficits contribute to the deficit syndrome consisting of restricted affect, poverty of speech, reduced interests, and diminished sense of purpose (Amador et al., 1999; Kirkpatrick et al., 1989; Kulhara and Chandiramani, 1990).

The distinction between positive and negative symptoms has been questioned but is valid based on differences in course of illness, symptoms, response to treatment, neurochemistry relevant to pharmacological intervention, neurobiology, neuropsychological functioning, family history, premorbid adjustment, and risk factors (Arango et al., 2004; Carpenter et al., 1999; Fanous et al., 2001; Fenton and McGlashan, 1994; Horan and Blanchard, 2003; Kirkpatrick et al., 2001; Kirkpatrick et al., 2000; Klemm et al., 2006; Lahti et al., 2001; Malaspina and Coleman, 2003; Pogue-Gelle and Harrow, 1984; Vaiva et al., 2002). In addition, positive symptoms involve distortions and typically added mental activity beyond what is normal, whereas negative symptoms entail something removed from what is normal, and usually reduced mental activity (Arango et al., 2004; Bowins, 2011; Langdon et al., 2014).

As pertains to course and treatment, psychosis (positive symptoms) is usually episodic and responds very well to antipsychotic medications acting via dopamine blockage, while negative symptoms develop gradually in a long prodromal phase and are quite resilient to treatment, with extensive efforts such as cognitive remediation often producing limited gains that frequently do not generalize beyond the task (Addington and Addington, 2009; Amador et al., 1999; Arango et al., 2004; Dickinson et al., 2010; Galletly, 2009). Dopamine blockage does little for negative symptoms, and alternative neurochemical receptors and transmitters, such as serotonin receptors (including 5HT-1A and 5HT-2A), glycine, and glutamate are more involved in negative symptoms (Galletly, 2009; Goff and Coyle, 2001; Gupta and Kulhara, 2010; Javitt, 2008; Lane et al., 2005; Uchida et al., 2011).

One of the major reasons why most people, mental health professionals included, focus more on psychosis than negative symptoms and overweigh their contribution to schizophrenia, is that hallucinations, delusions, and disordered thought form is far more dramatic being difficult to miss. Additionally, psychosis greatly impairs functioning in the moment. Negative deficit symptoms are far less dramatic and colorful, and erode functioning in a more insidious fashion. So far, the discussion suggests that these two forms of symptoms are unrelated, but they are actually very closely linked. Schizophrenia typically begins with a lengthy prodromal phase of negative symptoms and declining functioning, often lasting for several years, followed by positive symptoms (Donohoe et al., 2006; Fenton and McGlashan, 1994; Hemmingsen et al., 1999). I have proposed that the disease process underlying negative symptoms impairs regulation over psychotic level cognitions, resulting in psychosis manifesting in the conscious and awake state (Bowins, 2011, 2016). This process likely involves neural connectivity and dysconnectivity. In the Regulation chapter, we looked at how connectivity between brain regions is integral to mental health, and is impaired in mental illness, such as with depression and clinical level anxiety. Evidence was also presented for how psychosis results from impaired regulation. Neural dysconnectivity is pronounced with negative symptoms, and this dysconnectivity appears to impair the connectivity required for healthy regulation of psychotic level cognitions (Bowins, 2016). Hence, negative symptoms lead to positive symptoms (psychosis) likely via advancing dysconnectivity, impairing the connectivity necessary for adequate regulation of psychotic level cognitions.

Bipolar disorder

In the Regulation chapter, it was suggested that regulation deficits are involved in largely adaptive hypomania progressing to mostly dysfunctional mania. As with depression, anxiety, and psychotic level cognitions, neural connectivity must be involved in this regulation. By interfering with the connectivity required for adequate regulation, the dysconnectivity associated with negative symptoms is a likely candidate for what might impair regulation over the hypomania defense to depression (and anxiety). Although negative symptoms are more commonly associated with schizophrenia, they also appear to be prominent in BPI disorder (depression and mania), but not BPII (depression and hypomania) beyond what might be present with depression, consistent with the adaptive value of hypomania (Ancin et al., 2013; Blanchard et al., 1994; Brandt et al., 2014; Kuswanto et al., 2013; Nieto and Castellanos, 2011; Simonsen et al., 2008).

When negative symptoms are combined with alcohol, illicit drugs, and/or antidepressants, it is understandable that regulation over hypomania could become impaired. In my extensive clinical experience managing bipolar disorder, I have encountered numerous people who have multiple hypomanic episodes that never progress to mania unless regulation impairing substances are involved. A common occurrence with bipolar disorder is that those having prominent and recurrent mania struggle to maintain functioning at prior levels, even when free of depression and mania. This might transpire because negative symptoms diminish their capacity to function effectively. For example, a lawyer with bipolar disorder had frequent manic episodes, and reported difficulty functioning even prior to these mental illness issues, having to get others to check his work. Related to an insurance claim, I proposed that psychological testing addressing executive functions be conducted. Not to my surprise, the results indicated significant impairments on several executive functioning parameters, highly consistent with the struggles he encountered in his career. It appears that negative symptoms associated with bipolar disorder can manifest over time, and impair functioning and regulation. The regulation impairments likely arise from the dysconnectivity inherent in negative symptoms, compromising the connectivity necessary for adequate regulation over hypomania, allowing its progression to full-blown mania.

Mental illness and negative symptoms

Based on the evidence for autism spectrum disorder, intellectual disability, ADHD, schizophrenia, and bipolar disorder, negative symptoms are definitely involved and in a prominent way, being largely responsible for many of the manifestations. In severe depression, at least with psychotic manifestations, negative symptoms likewise seem to play a significant role (Harvey, 2011). Confounding the picture somewhat, depression often entails secondary negative symptoms arising from the depressed state, such as amotivation and impairments in basic cognition. While negative symptoms are not as dramatic and obvious as psychosis and mania, they act in a very insidious fashion to produce mental illness. In the case of autism spectrum disorder, intellectual disability, and ADHD, negative symptoms manifest during early development, whereas with schizophrenia, bipolar disorder, and possibly depression and even anxiety, they typically manifest somewhat later. Neural dysconnectivity is a key feature of negative symptoms.

Dysconnectivity and mental illness

Given how the emphasis has been on neural dysconnectivity, and the role it plays in negative symptoms, it is important to take a brief look at what the evidence shows. Regarding executive functions, both structures and intact connections (connectivity) between different brain regions are necessary for healthy functioning (Eisenberg and Berman, 2010; Gross and Grossman, 2010). In terms of structures the frontal lobes, and particularly the prefrontal cortex, are very important. Connectivity between various cortical structures (cortical–cortical), and cortical and subcortical (cortical–subcortical) play a prominent role. (Gross and Grossman, 2010). Based on functional neuroimaging studies, frontoparietal connections are critical to several executive functions, including working memory, set shifting (cognitive flexibility), and inhibition (Collette et al., 2005; Gross and Grossman, 2010; Smith and Jonides, 1997). Connections between cortical regions and the basal ganglia (subcortical) are required for planning (Gross and Grossman, 2010; Monchi et al., 2006). Gray and white matter integrity is also crucial for executive functions, with white matter being the basis for connectivity (Eisenberg and Berman, 2010). Gray matter and white matter connectivity can be viewed as neural networks or neural circuits, with particular patterns of structures and connections associated with each executive function (Eisenberg and Berman, 2010; Gross and Grossman, 2010). Impairment to the neural networks associated with executive functions, impacts negatively on these functions, and in turn adaptive behavior (Eisenberg and Berman, 2010; Gross and Grossman, 2010; Mateer, 1999). Social cognition also relies on neural connectivity, as demonstrated by connections between the amygdala and both the PFC and temporal cortex necessary for facial expression recognition (Bediou et al., 2007).

As pertains to specific forms of mental illness, there is evidence for dysconnectivity between brain regions with deficient, or in some instances excessive, connectedness a common finding in mental illnesses involving negative symptoms (Adler et al., 2004; Bartfeld et al., 2014; Hong et al., 2015; Knochel et al., 2014; Kumar et al., 2014; Mamah et al., 2013; Meda et al., 2012; Skudlarski et al., 2013). For example, in the case of ADHD, reduced dorsal caudate functional connectivity with the superior and middle PFC, and reduced putamen connectivity with the parahippocampal cortex have been identified (Hong et al., 2015). Intrinsic dysconnectivity is linked to hyperactivity, impulsivity, and depression (Bartfeld et al., 2014).

The best evidence of dysconnectivity comes from schizophrenia and bipolar disorder research with both overlap and distinct patterns evident. In terms of overlap, white matter tracts essential for linking brain regions demonstrate substantial dysconnectivity in both conditions (Kumar et al., 2014; Skudlarski et al., 2013), and there is a loss of white matter coherence in the PFC (Adler et al., 2004). Reduced connectivity occurs in frontoparietal control networks (Baker et al., 2014), and fronto/occipital connectivity to anterior default mode/PFC seems to be impaired in both conditions (Meda et al., 2012). Mamah et al. (2013) found decreased connectivity in both illnesses for cingulo-opercular to cerebellar neural networks, with a somewhat greater reduction in the schizophrenic group. In terms of different outcomes for schizophrenia and bipolar disorder, Meda et al. (2012) discovered meso/paralimbic to sensory-motor connectivity only altered in schizophrenia, and mesoparalimbic to frontotemporal/paralimbic altered just in bipolar disorder (Meda et al., 2012). Decreased cerebellar to salience network connectivity distinguishes bipolar disorder patients, whereas decreased cingulo-opercular to salience network, cingulo-opercular to frontoparietal, and frontoparietal to cerebellar characterizes schizophrenic subjects (Mamah et al., 2013).

Dysconnectivity frequently appears to be more intense in schizophrenia than bipolar disorder. For example, Argyelan et al. (2014) comparing global connectivity in schizophrenics, bipolar disorder patients, and normal individuals, found least impairment in the latter group, and greatest global dysconnectivity in the schizophrenic group. Likewise, reductions in functional connectivity within the hippocampal network seem to be present in both schizophrenia and bipolar disorder, but more in the former (Knochel et al., 2014). The Mamah et al. (2013) study mentioned above uncovered greater reductions in cingulo-opercular to cerebellar neural network connectivity in their schizophrenic subjects. Considering the widespread impairments in basic cognition, social cognition, and motivational states in schizophrenia, it is understandable that more extensive dysconnectivity is likely with this illness. Overlap will occur in part because mania often entails psychosis, and hence the pattern of dysconnectivity associated with psychosis.

The coverage of neural dysconnectivity might seem intimidating for psychotherapists, and is difficult to decipher for even neuroscientists, but is important to consider given the notion that human-specific cognition in terms of basic cognitive capacities, social cognition, and motivational states relies on healthy neural connectivity. It is also important due to how dysconnectivity plays out in various forms of mental illness. At a basic level this is almost common sense, because functionality relies on connections, such as the shoulder-arm-elbow-forearm-hand connection necessary for manual tasks. Likewise, brain regions must connect for mental functions, with this healthy connectivity disrupted when mental illness issues arise, much as hand tasks are compromised if the elbow is damaged. The reasons for why dysconnectivity occurs impairing human-specific cognition are complex but likely involve general processes: the relatively recent evolutionary origin of human-specific cognition making these capacities less stable than say olfaction, how entropy (order to disorder) naturally erodes complex structures such as human-specific cognition particularly when they are not well established genetically, and complexities associated with biological algorithms required to develop these capacities in each person (Bowins, 2016). In addition, a multitude of specific contributing influences, such as infections and genetic mutations, undoubtedly play a role (Bowins, 2016).

Summary note

Various basic cognitive capacities with executive functions prominent, social cognitive abilities, and motivational process, provide for human-specific cognition forming the basis of what distinguishes humans behaviorally from other species. Reductions in these capacities constitute negative symptoms, that are actually integral to many forms of mental illness, and certainly, autistic spectrum disorder, intellectual disability (and specific forms of learning disorders), ADHD, schizophrenia, and bipolar disorder, with the very real possibility of substantial involvement in depression, anxiety, and still other forms of mental illness. Regarding schizophrenia, bipolar disorder, depression, and anxiety, impaired regulation plays a key role. Neural dysconnectivity underlying negative symptoms appears to impair the connectivity required for healthy regulation resulting in mental illness. Solid connectivity, on the other hand, yields robust human-specific cognition and from these capacities, mental health.

References

Addington, J., Addington, D., 2009. Three-year outcome of treatment in an early psychosis program. Can. J. Psychiatry 54, 626–630.

Adler, C.M., Holland, S.K., Schmithorst, V., Wilke, M., Weiss, K.L., Pan, H., Strakowski, S.M., 2004. Abnormal frontal white matter tracts in bipolar disorder: a diffusion tensor imaging study. Bipolar Disord. 6 (3), 197–203.

Amador, X.F., Kirkpatrick, B., Buchanon, R.W., Carpenter, W.T., Marcinko, L., Yale, S.A., 1999. Stability of the diagnosis of deficit syndrome in schizophrenia. Am. J. Psychiatry 156 (4), 637–639.

Ancin, I., Cabranes, J.A., Santos, J.L., Sanchez-Moria, E., Barabash, A., 2013. Executive deficits: a continuum schizophrenia-bipolar disorder or specific to schizophrenia? Psychiatry Res. 47 (11), 1564–1571.

Arango, C., Buchanan, R., Kirkpatrick, B., Carpenter, W., 2004. The deficit syndrome in schizophrenia: implications for the treatment of negative symptoms. Eur. Psychiatry 19, 21–26.

Argyelan, M., Ikuta, T., DeRosse, P., Braga, R.J., Burdick, K.E., John, M., et al., 2014. Resting-state fMRI connectivity impairment in schizophrenia and bipolar disorder. Schizophr. Bull. 40 (1), 100–110.

Ashby, F.G., Isen, A.M., Turken, U., 1999. A neuropsychological theory of positive affect and its influence on cognition. Psychol. Rev. 106 (3), 529–550.

Baker, J.T., Holmes, A.J., Masters, G.A., Yeo, B.T., Krienen, F., Buckner, R.L., Ongur, D., 2014. Disruption of cortical association networks in schizophrenia and psychotic bipolar disorder. JAMA Psychiatry 71 (2), 109–118.

Ballmaier, M., Schlagenhauf, F., Toga, A.W., Gallinat, J., Koslowski, M., Zoli, M., et al., 2008. Regional patterns and clinical correlates of basal ganglia morphology in non-medicated schizophrenia. Schizophr. Res. 106 (2-3), 140–147.

Bartfeld, P., Petroni, A., Baez, S., Urquina, H., Sigman, M., Cetkovich, M., et al., 2014. Fiunctional connectivity and temporal variability of brain connections in adults with attention deficit/hyperactivity disorder and bipolar disorder. Neuropsychobiology 69 (2), 65–75.

Bediou, B., Asri, F., Brunelin, J., Krolak-Salmon, P., D'Amato, T., Saoud, M., Tazi, I., 2007. Emotion recognition and genetic vulnerability to schizophrenia. Br. J. Psychiatry 191, 126–130.

Bemporad, J.R., 1991. Dementia praecox as a failure of neoteny. Theor. Med. 12, 45–51.

Bilder, R.M., Goldman, R.S., Robinson, D., Reiter, G., Bell, L., Bates, J.A., et al., 2000. Neuropsychology of first-episode schizophrenia: initial characterization and clinical correlates. Am. J. Psychiatry 157, 549–559.

Blanchard, J.J., Bellack, A.S., Mueser, K.T., 1994. Affective and social-behavioral correlates of physical and social anhedonia in schizophrenia. J. Abnorm. Psychol. 103 (4), 719–728.

Bowins, B.E, 2011. A cognitive regulatory control model of schizophrenia. Brain Res. Bull. 85, 36–41.

Bowins, B.E., 2016. Mental Illness Defined: Continuums, Regulation and Defense. Routledge, New York & London.

Brandt, C.L., Eichele, T., Melle, I., Sundet, K., Server, A., Agartz, I., et al., 2014. Working memory networks and activation patterns in schizophrenia and bipolar disorder: comparison with healthy controls. Br. J. Psychiatry 204, 290–298.

Burns, J.K., 2009. Reconciling 'the new epidemiology' with an evolutionary genetic basis for schizophrenia. Med. Hypothesis 72, 353–358.

Carpenter, W., Arango, C., Buchanan, R., Kirkpatrick, B., 1999. Deficit psychopathology and a paradigm shift in schizophrenic research. Biol. Psychiatry 46, 352–360.

Collette, F., Van der Linden, M., Laureys, S., 2005. Exploring the unity and diversity of the neural substrates of executive functioning. Hum. Brain Mapp. 25 (4), 409–423.

Combs, D.R., Finn, J.A., Wohlfahrt, W., Penn, D.L., Basso, M.R., 2013. Social cognition and social functioning in nonclinical paranoia. Cogn. Neuropsychiatry 18 (6), 531–548.

Darwin, C., 1858/1859. On the Origin of Species. Signet Classic, New York.

De Jong, J.J., De Gelder, B., Hodiamont, P.P., 2013. Sensory processing, neurocognition, and social cognition in schizophrenia: towards a cohesive cognitive model. Schizophr. Res. 146 (1-3), 209–216.

Dickinson, D., Tenhula, W., Morris, S., Brown, C., Peer, J., Spencer, K., et al., 2010. A randomized controlled trial of computer-assisted cognitive remediation for schizophrenia. Am. J. Psychiatry 167, 170–180.

Donohoe, G., Corvin, A., Robertson, I.H., 2006. Evidence that specific executive functions predict symptom variance among schizophrenic patients with a predominantly negative symptom profile. Cogn. Neuropsychiatry 11, 13–32.
Eisenberg, D.P., Berman, K.F., 2010. Executive function, neural circuitry, and genetic mechanisms in schizophrenia. Neuropsychopharmacology 35 (1), 258–277.
Elvevag, B., Goldberg, T.E., 2000. Cognitive impairment in schizophrenia is the core of the disorder. Crit. Rev. Neurobiol. 14, 1–21.
Fanous, A., Gardner, C., Walsh, D., Kendler, K., 2001. Relationship between positive and negative symptoms of schizophrenia and schizoptypal symptoms in nonpsychotic relatives. Arch. Gen. Psychiatry 58 (7), 669–673.
Fenton, W.S., McGlashan, T.H., 1994. Antecedents, symptom progression, and long-term outcome in the deficit syndrome in schizophrenia. Am. J. Psychiatry 151, 351–356.
Fett, A.K., Viechtbauer, W., Dominguez, M.D., Penn, D.L., Van Os, J., Krabbendam, L., 2011. The relationship between neurocognition and social cognition with functional outcomes in schizophrenia: a meta-analysis. Neurosci. Biobehav. Rev. 35 (3), 573–588.
Fiszdon, J.M., Richardson, R., Greig, T., Bell, M.D., 2007. A comparison of basic and social cognition between schizophrenia and schizoaffective disorder. Schizophr. Res. 91, 117–121.
Galletly, C., 2009. Recent advances in treating cognitive impairment in schizophrenia. Psychopharmacology 202, 1302–1309.
Goff, D.C., Coyle, J.T., 2001. The emerging role of glutamate in the pathophysiology and treatment of schizophrenia. Am. J. Psychiatry 158 (9), 1367–1377.
Gross, R.G., Grossman, M., 2010. Executive resources. Continuum 16 (4), 140–152.
Gupta, S., Kulhara, P., 2010. What is schizophrenia: a neurodevelopmental or neurodegenerative disorder or combination of both. A critical analysis. Indian J. Psychiatry 52 (1), 21–27.
Harvey, P.D., 2011. Mood symptoms, cognition, and everyday functioning: in major depression, bipolar disorder, and schizophrenia. Innov. Clin. Neurosci. 8 (10), 14–18.
Hemmingsen, R., Madsen, A., Glenthoj, B., Rubin, P., 1999. Cortical brain dysfunction in early schizophrenia: secondary pathogenetic hieracrchy of neuroplasticity, psychopathology and social impairment. Acta Psychiatry Scand. 99 (Suppl.395), 80–88.
Hong, S.B., Harrison, B.J., Fornito, A., Sohn, C.H., Song, I.C., Kim, J.W., 2015. Functional dysconnectivity of corticostriatal circuitry and differential response to methylphenidate in youth with attention-deficit/hyperactivity disorder. J. Psychiatry Neurosci. 40 (1), 46–57.
Horan, W.P., Blanchard, J.J., 2003. Neurocognitive, social, and emotional dysfunction in deficit syndrome schizophrenia. Schizophr. Res. 65, 125–137.
Ivleva, E.I., Shohamy, D., Mihalakos, P., Morris, D.W., Carmody, T., Tamminga, C.A., 2012. Memory generalization is selectively altered in the psychosis dimension. Schizophr. Res. 138 (1), 74–80.
Javitt, D.C., 2008. Glycine transport inhibitors and the treatment of schizophrenia. Biol. Psychiatry 63, 6–8.
Johnson, M.K., McMahon, R.P., Robinson, B.M., Harvey, A.N., Hahn, B., Leonard, C.J., et al., 2013. The relationship between working memory capacity and broad measures of cognitive ability in healthy adults and people with schizophrenia. Neuropsychology 27 (2), 220–229.
Keefe, R.S., Fenton, W.S., 2007. How should DSM-V criteria for schizophrenia include cognitive impairment? Schizophr. Bull. 33, 912–920.
Kirkpatrick, B., Buchanan, R.W., 1990. The neural basis of the deficit syndrome of schizophrenia. J. Nerv. Ment. Dis. 178, 545–555.

Kirkpatrick, B., Buchanan, R.W., McKenney, P.D., Alpha, L.D., Carpenter, W.T., 1989. The schedule for the deficit syndrome: an instrument for research in schizophrenia. Psychiatry Res. 30 (2), 119–123.

Kirkpatrick, B., Buchanan, R.W., Ross, D.E., Carpenter, W.T., 2001. A separate disease within the syndrome of schizophrenia. Arch. Gen. Psychiatry 58, 165–171.

Kirkpatrick, B., Ross, D.E., Walsh, D., Karkowski, L., Kendler, K.S., 2000. Family characteristics of deficit and nondeficit in schizophrenia in Roscommon Family Study. Schizophr. Res. 45, 57–64.

Klemm, S., Schmidt, B., Knappe, S., Blanz, B., 2006. Impaired working speed and executive functions as frontal lobe dysfunctions in young first-degree relatives of schizophrenic patients. Eur. Child Adolesc. Psychiatry 15, 400–408.

Knochel, C., Stablein, M., Storchak, H., Reinke, B., Jurcoane, A., Prvulovic, D., et al., 2014. Multimodal assessments of the hippocampal formation in schizophrenia and bipolar disorder: evidence from neurobehavioral measures and functional and structural MRI. Neuroimaging Clin. 23 (6), 134–144.

Kulhara, K., Chandiramani, T., 1990. Positive and negative subtypes of schizophrenia. Schizophr. Res. 3 (2), 107–116.

Kumar, J., Iwabucchi, S., Oowise, S., Balain, V., Palaniyappan, L., Liddle, P.F., 2014. Shared white-matter dysconnectivity in schizophrenia and bipolar disorder with psychosis. Psychol. Med. 4, 1–12.

Kuswanto, C.N., Sum, M.Y., Sim, K., 2013. Neurocognitive functioning in schizophrenia and bipolar disorder: clarifying concepts of diagnostic dichotomy vs. continuum. Front. Psychiatry 5 (4), 162–169.

Lahti, A.C., Holocomb, H.H., Medoff, D.R., Weiler, M.A., Tamminga, C.A., Carpenter, W.T., 2001. Abnormal patterns of regional cerebral blood flow in schizophrenia with primary negative symptoms during an auditory recognition task. Am. J. Psychiatry 158, 1797–1808.

Lane, H., Chang, Y., Liu, Y., Chiu, C., Guochan, T., 2005. Sarcosine or d-serine add-on treatment for acute exacerbation of schizophrenia. Arch. Gen. Psychiatry 62 (11), 1196–1204.

Langdon, R., Still, M., Connors, M., Ward, P., Catts, S., 2014. Jumping to delusions in early psychosis. Cogn. Neuropsychiatry 19 (3), 241–256.

Mahurin, R.K., Velligan, D.I., Miller, A.L., 1998. Executive-frontal lobe cognitive dysfunction in schizophrenia: a symptom subtype analysis. Psychiatry Res. 79, 139–149.

Malaspina, D., Coleman, D., 2003. Olfaction and social drive in schizophrenia. Arch. Gen. Psychiatry 60, 578–584.

Mamah, D., Barch, D.M., Repovs, G., 2013. Resting state functional connectivity of five neural networks in bipolar disorder and schizophrenia. J. Affect Disord. 150 (2), 601–609.

Mateer, C.A., 1999. Executive function disorders: rehabilitation challenges and strategies. Semin. Clin. Neuropsychiatry 4 (1), 50–59.

Meda, S.A., Gill, A., Stevens, M.C., Lorenzoni, R.P., Glahn, D.C., Calhoun, V.D., Sweeney, J.A., et al., 2012. Differences in resting-state functional magnetic resonance imaging functional network connectivity between schizophrenia and psychotic bipolar probands and their unaffected first-degree relatives. Biol. Psychiatry 71 (1), 881–889.

Monchi, O., Petrides, M., Strafella, A.P., 2006. Functional role of the basal ganglia in the planning and execution of actions. Annu. Neurol. 59 (2), 257–264.

Morice, R., Delahunty, A., 1996. Frontal/executive impairments in schizophrenia. Schizophr. Bull. 22, 125–137.

Nieto, R.G., Castellanos, F.X., 2011. A meta-analysis of neuropsychological functioning in patients with early onset schizophrenia and bipolar disorder. J. Clin. Child Adolesc. Psychol. 40 (2), 266–280.

Oades, R.D., 1998. Frontal, temporal and lateralized brain function in children with attention-deficit hyperactivity disorder: a psychophysiological and neuropsychological viewpoint on development. Behav. Brain Res. 94 (1), 83–95.

Owen, M.J., 2012. Intellectual disability and major psychiatric disorders: a continuum of neurodevelopmental causality. Br. J. Psychiatry 200 (4), 268–269.

Pogue-Gelle, M., Harrow, M., 1984. Negative and positive symptoms in schizophrenia and depression: a follow-up. Schizophr. Bull. 10 (3), 371–387.

Purper-Ouakil, D., Franc, N., 2011. Emotional dysfunction in attention deficit hyperactivity disorder. Arch. Pediatr. 18 (6), 679–685.

Rapp, A.M., Langohr, K., Mutschler, D.E., Wild, B., 2014. Irony and proverb comprehension in schizophrenia: do female patients "dislike" ironic remarks? Schizophr. Res. Treatment 84, 10–18.

Reichenberg, A., Caspi, A., Harrington, H., Houts, R., Keefe, R., Murray, R., et al., 2010. Static and dynamic cognitive deficits in childhood preceding adult schizophrenia: a 30-year study. Am. J. Psychiatry 167, 160–169.

Simonsen, C., Sundet, K., Vaskinn, A., 2008. Neurocognitive profiles in bipolar I and bipolar II disorder: differences in pattern and magnitude of dysfunction. Bipolar Disord. 10, 245–255.

Skudlarski, P., Schretlen, D.J., Thaker, G.K., Stevens, M.C., Keshavan, M.S., Sweeney, J.A., et al., 2013. Diffusion tensor imaging white matter endophenotypes in patients with schizophrenia or psychotic bipolar disorder and their relatives. Am. J. Psychiatry 170 (8), 886–898.

Smith, E.E., Jonides, J., 1997. Working memory: a view from neuroimaging. Cogn. Psychol. 33 (1), 5–42.

Uchida, H., Takeuchi, H., Graff-Guerrero, Suzuki, T., Watanabe, K., Mamo, D.C., 2011. Dopamine D2 receptor occupancy and clinical effects: a systematic review and pooled analysis. J. Clin. Psychopharmacol. 31 (4), 497–502.

Vaiva, G., Cottencin, O., Llorca, P.M., 2002. Regional cerebral blood flow in deficit/nondeficit types of schizophrenia according to SDS criteria. Prog. Neuro-psychophathol. 26, 481–485.

Volkmar, F.R., Wolf, J.M., 2013. When children with autism become adults. World Psychiatry 12 (1), 78–80.

Waltereit, R., Banaschewski, T., Meyer-Lindenberg, A., Poustka, L., 2014. Interaction of neurodevelopmental pathways and synaptic plasticity in mental retardation, autistic spectrum disorder and schizophrenia: implication for psychiatry. World J. Biol. Psychiatry 15 (7), 507–516.

Chapter 7

Self-acceptance

Accepting oneself is a very important component of mental health, and conversely not liking who you are favors mental illness. People who like themselves seem to be more resilient to stress, and negative outcomes. Of course, the other direction could apply such that those who are mentally healthy might view themselves better, and with good outcomes it is easier to like oneself. However, even intuitively it does follow that accepting yourself will contribute to better mental health. Conceivably, both directions might transpire in a mutually reinforcing fashion with self-acceptance favoring better outcomes and those outcomes fostering greater self-acceptance.

The notion of self-acceptance is very psychological and yokes to several other psychological constructs including self-esteem, self-worth, self-concept, self-efficacy, self-actualization, empowerment, self-respect, and self-affirmation. There is quite a bit of overlap between these constructs, but for the most part they do seem to capture different aspects of the self. Some appear to occur on the same continuum, as with self-efficacy very specific and self-concept global. Some are more action oriented as with self-actualization and empowerment. They can also be divided based on evaluation and perspective, with self-esteem and self-worth evaluative, whereas self-concept and self-efficacy represent perspectives on the self. Regardless of what they actually represent, the overall composite weighs in on whether or not, and to what extent, a person accepts themselves. We will now look at what research shows for these various components of self-acceptance, focusing on their role in mental health and mental illness.

Self-esteem

Of all the psychological constructs contributing to self-acceptance the most evidence exists for self-esteem. Evaluation of a global and longer standing nature is the hallmark of self-esteem (Engel, 1959; Mann et al., 2004). In a classic study of adolescent self-esteem, Engel (1959) found that it only shifts gradually over a 2-year period, and since adolescence is an age of rapid change, it follows that self-esteem will only shift very gradually in adulthood. Self-esteem refers to a person's global appraisal of his/her positive or negative value, based on evaluations in more specific areas, and is equivalent to self-regard, self-estimation, and self-worth (Lakey et al., 2014; Mann et al., 2004). Research covers

States and Processes for Mental Health. DOI: 10.1016/C2020-0-00574-8

many facets of self-esteem relevant to mental health, and it is helpful to divide it into that pertaining to mental illness and that focused on mental health. Much of the research is correlational in nature, preventing any conclusion regarding direction and causation. Some is longitudinal and although still correlational it increases confidence in the assertion that self-esteem impacts mental health and mental illness.

Mental illness

In line with the notion of cognitive distortions (see the Psychological defense mechanism chapter), self-esteem influences positive and negative evaluations. Looking at cognitive and emotional reactions to daily events and the role of self-esteem, Campbell et al. (1991) found that low self-esteem participants viewed daily events more negatively, and negative life events as more important, than did high self-esteem subjects. Low self-esteem participants were also more likely to attribute negative events to stable and global internal characteristics relevant to self-esteem, than to external and transient events less relevant to self-esteem. Meanwhile, high self-esteem participants attributed positive events to stable and global internal features (Campbell et al., 1991). These attributions in turn reinforce self-esteem: negative evaluations intensify low self-esteem, whereas positive ones strengthen self-esteem. Although the research is correlational it does appear that there is a link between attribution style, self-esteem, and the so-called internalizing forms of mental illness (Abramson et al., 1989; Hammen and Goodman-Brown, 1990; Mann et al., 2004).

Research investigating the relationship between self-esteem and mental illness tends to separate into internalizing and externalizing forms. Internalizing includes depression, suicide, anxiety, eating disorders, and psychosis, whereas externalizing consists of conduct problems, aggression, school issues, and antisocial behavior.

Internalizing forms of mental illness

Low self-esteem does show a consistent relationship with internalizing forms of mental illness, from both cross-sectional and longitudinal research. Longitudinal studies have found that low self-esteem in the age range from childhood to early adulthood, is a predictor of later depression (Iancu et al., 2015; Isomaa et al., 2013; Reinherz et al., 1993; Teri, 1982; Wilhelm et al., 1999). Isomaa et al. (2013) assessed 2070 female and male adolescents in 2002–2003 when they were 15 years old and then conducted a 2-year follow-up. Based on Rosenberg Self-Esteem Scale scores, low self-esteem was related to depression and social anxiety. Trzesniewski et al. (2006) followed adolescents for 11 years into adulthood, finding that low self-esteem predicted depression and clinical anxiety, after controlling for several variables that might account for the findings. Additional research has also uncovered a link between low self-esteem and anxiety problems (Beck et al., 2001; Fickova, 1999; Ginsburg et al., 1998). For instance, Ginsburg et al. (1998) found that low self-esteem is associated with social anxiety in children, and good self-esteem seems to defensively buffer it.

Although most research does show a strong link between low self-esteem and mental illness in the forms of depression and anxiety, some outcomes are more limited regarding the role of self-esteem. For example, Miller et al. (1989) found that self-esteem alone does not have an impact, but does via buffering stress responses. Countering this finding, Orth et al. (2009) using data from a couple of longitudinal studies of adolescents and young adults, discovered that self-esteem did not buffer stress, but both low self-esteem and stress act as independent risk factors for depression. An interesting meta-analysis of longitudinal studies by Sowislo and Orth (2013) addressed the direction issue of low self-esteem and both depression and anxiety. They evaluated 77 longitudinal studies on depression and 18 on anxiety, finding that the effect of self-esteem on depression is significantly stronger than the effect of depression on self-esteem. Results for anxiety were more balanced with self-esteem influencing anxiety and anxiety impacting on self-esteem approximately equally (Sowislo and Orth, 2013).

Eating disorders are another internalizing form of mental illness linked to low self-esteem, at least for females (Fisher et al., 1994; Hartmann et al., 2014; Smolak et al., 1998; Vohs et al., 2001). Hartmann et al. (2014) compared 47 participants with either anorexia or body dysmorphic disorder to 22 healthy controls, finding that clinical participants had significantly lower self-esteem. Low self-esteem appears to be a risk factor for eating disorders (Fisher et al., 1994; Smolak et al., 1998; Vohs et al., 2001). While depression, anxiety, and eating disorders can be severe, suicide and psychosis are typically more extreme forms of mental illness, and often with dire outcomes. There is some evidence that suicidal ideation and actions are linked to low self-esteem (Bhar et al., 2008; Overholser et al., 1995). For instance, Bhar et al. (2008) assessed 338 psychiatric outpatients for self-esteem, hopelessness, suicidal ideation, and depression, finding that low self-esteem correlated with suicidal ideation even after controlling for the influence of depression and hopelessness. Lakey et al. (2014) also found that among college students, low self-esteem is linked to suicidal behavior, and also depression.

Regarding psychosis and self-esteem, an empirical study I conducted with a colleague earlier in my career is highly relevant. The study focused on the relationship between the content of delusions and hallucinations and self-esteem (Bowins and Shugar, 1998). Forty actively psychotic individuals (mostly schizophrenic) on inpatient wards were assessed for delusions and hallucinations with the Present State Examination, and the Coopersmith Self-Esteem Inventory was applied. Independent raters assessed the content of all reported delusions and hallucinations for probable self-enhancing and self-diminishing content. The results revealed a very robust positive correlation between global self-esteem and self-enhancing content, but only for delusions: the better a participant's self-esteem, the more self-enhancing the content of the delusion, and likewise lower self-esteem meant more self-diminishing content. We surmised that these results did not extend to the content of hallucinations as they are sensory-perceptual in nature, while delusions are more cognitive. Although the results are correlational and so cannot indicate direction, self-esteem was focused on in part because it only changes gradually (Engel, 1959), whereas the content of delusions and hallucinations can shift rapidly; hence, it is most logical that self-esteem would influence the content of delusions. Backing up these results, Kesting and Lincoln (2013) conducted a systematic review of studies examining persecutory delusions and self-esteem, finding that low global self-esteem correlated with negative self-schemas in persecutory delusions. Like with our study, they concluded that delusions reflect self-esteem.

Externalizing forms of mental illness

Low self-esteem is linked to conduct problems, aggression, antisocial behavior, and school problems, at least for younger people. For example, applying a longitudinal design Jessor et al. (1998) found that among high-school adolescents, low self-esteem predicted problem behavior of various forms. Low self-esteem correlates with violence and gang membership (Schoen, 1999). The same study found that both bullies and those bullied have low self-esteem (Schoen, 1999). Additionally, dropping out of school is linked to low self-esteem (Muha, 1991).

Donnellan et al. (2005) examined the link between self-esteem and externalizing issues over a few studies of adolescents and college students, conducted in the United States and New Zealand. Based on self-report, teacher ratings, and parent ratings, a robust relationship was uncovered between low self-esteem and externalizing problems such as aggression (Donnellan et al., 2005). Both from cross-sectional and longitudinal studies, the relationship held after controlling for potential confounding variables including supportive parenting, parent-child relationships, peer relationships, achievement test scores, IQ scores, narcissism, and socioeconomic status! The Trzesniewski et al. (2006) longitudinal study mentioned for depression, also found that low self-esteem predicted tobacco dependence, criminal convictions, school dropout, and money/work problems for adolescents over the 11 years of follow-up into adulthood.

Mental health

In the Psychological defense mechanism chapter, we looked at how positive cognitive distortions represent a major psychological defense mechanism template (Bowins, 2004). These positive cognitive distortions include self-evaluations influencing self-esteem, even to the point of overestimating oneself (Mann et al., 2004). For example, mastery is facilitated by an exaggerated sense of self-worth resulting in better mental health (Seligman, 1995). Mental health involves distorting reality in a direction that protects and enhances self-esteem

(Mann et al., 2004). Depression and anxiety entail an absence of these self-enhancing distortions (Beck, 1991; Bowins, 2004; Mann et al., 2004). Of course, extreme cognitive distortions approaching the psychotic range tend to impair functioning, and are less adequate as defenses except under extreme circumstances (Bowins, 2004). The defensive function of self-esteem plays out in terms of resilience (Mann et al., 2004). Self-esteem functions as an internal moderator of stressors while social support represents an external moderator (Mann et al., 2004).

Consistent with the defensive function of self-esteem, various aspects of good mental health are associated with better self-esteem. For example, Rouse (1998) found that adolescents with higher self-esteem are more resilient to stress than their lower self-esteem peers. Adolescents with high self-esteem are also less likely to engage in self-destructive behavior, such as drug and alcohol abuse (Crump et al., 1997; Jones and Heaven, 1998). There is evidence that high-risk sexual behaviors are less likely if a person has high self-esteem (Somali et al., 2001). Academic success has quite consistently been linked to high self-esteem applying both cross-sectional and longitudinal research designs (Adams, 1996; Hay et al., 1998). Job satisfaction later in middle age also relates to higher self-esteem in the younger years of life (Judge et al., 2000). Hence, higher self-esteem fosters actions and choices that favor better mental health.

Summary note for self-esteem

The major self-evaluative construct relevant to mental health is self-esteem, with self-regard, self-estimation, and self-worth equivalent to it. Low self-esteem is associated with and even predictive of various mental health problems, both internalizing and externalizing. Higher self-esteem correlates with success and more optimal functioning consistent with good mental health. Although the results are correlational, given that it would be unethical to deliberately induce low self-esteem in subjects, the overall consistency of the results including longitudinal studies controlling for confounding variables, does yield solid evidence that higher self-esteem provides for good mental health. Self-esteem can be viewed as a defensive entity involving positive cognitive distortions, in that it represents a positive self-enhancing psychological construct not always completely grounded in reality. It constitutes a major internal defensive buffer against stress and challenges to the self.

Self-concept and self-efficacy

Whereas self-esteem is evaluative, self-concept and self-efficacy represent perspectives pertaining to oneself (Mann et al., 2004). Self-concept can be viewed as the sum of an individual's beliefs and knowledge regarding personal attributes and qualities, and is equivalent to self-image and self-perception (Mann et al., 2004). Self-efficacy is much more focused referring to beliefs regarding specific behaviors such as math ability (Mann et al., 2004). Compared to the extensive research evidence for self-esteem and mental health, evidence for self-concept and self-efficacy is limited. To a certain extent this makes sense, in that the evaluative component (self-esteem) seems closer to emotional states highly relevant to mental health. Self-concept and self-efficacy are more detached from emotional states representing self-perspectives. However, a negative self-concept does tend to link with mental illnesses such as depression and suicidal tendencies, whereas positive self-concept is more associated with good mental health (Andersson et al., 2014; Mann et al., 2004; Orbach, 2007). For instance, Andersson et al. (2014) conducted a cross-sectional study of 3981 adults finding that those with low global self-efficacy (self-concept) were more likely to suffer from mental illness than those with high global self-efficacy.

A key issue that emerges with linking psychological constructs including self-concept, self-efficacy, and self-esteem to mental health in a causal fashion, is what Swann et al. (2007) refer to as the specificity-matching principle, indicating that predictions are best when the predictor variable and outcome match with regard to specificity, and that more specific predictor variables and outcomes produce the strongest results. The first part of the specificity-matching principle suggests that trying to link global predictor variables such as self-concept and self-esteem to a specific outcome like math performance, is not going to yield a strong result. Linking a general predictor variable to a general outcome, on the other hand, will result in a stronger correlation, assuming that the linkage is valid (Swann et al., 2007). Hence, self-esteem and self-concept link to mental health, and even conditions like depression and anxiety which are quite general. The second component—that more specific predictor variables and outcomes produce the strongest results—is quite intuitive, in that a specific aspect of functioning is likely to result in a tighter correlation with outcomes of that type. For example, high self-efficacy regarding math ability will likely correlate well to math performance, unless the self-perspective pertaining to math ability is completely uninformed.

In line with the specificity-matching principle, self-efficacy does link well to specific outcomes, such as academic achievement. A meta-analysis that illustrates this is by Robbins et al. (2004) who examined 109 prospective studies of psychosocial and study skills linked to academic success, revealing that academic self-efficacy predicted grade point average and academic persistence, the correlations emerging as robust. Research has demonstrated that as the specificity of the predictor and outcome variables increase, so does the strength of the relationship. For example, in a meta-analysis of prospective studies, Hansford and Hattie (1982) found that specific academic self-concepts predicted academic success better than did global self-esteem. Marsh et al. (2006) discovered that math self-concept, equivalent to self-efficacy for math, strongly predicted several math outcomes but global self-esteem was not closely linked.

Select research studies suggest that self-efficacy plays a mediating role in mental illness. For example, Cardenas et al. (2013) found that for schizophrenic patients, relatively high self-efficacy mediated between skills capacity and functional outcomes, but low self-efficacy is common in this condition. Coping self-efficacy might buffer the impact of trauma, at least in terms of fewer negative memory intrusions (Brown et al., 2012). Experience with specific outcomes such as martial arts can enhance self-efficacy, and that, in turn, improves performance in the specific area. Interestingly, it has been suggested that too high self-efficacy might impair performance is some instances by overmotivating and adding stress (Schonfeld et al., 2017), although this proposition is in need of experimental confirmation. Believing that you are efficacious in various tasks contributes to a good self-concept, and not feeling efficacious contributes to poor self-concept.

Self-acceptance

Self-esteem represents a global evaluation of oneself while self-concept is a global perspective regarding oneself, with self-efficacy beliefs pertaining to capacity in specific tasks contributing to self-concept. Self-acceptance is a global affirmation of self with good self-esteem and self-concept feeding into it: when a person generates a positive evaluation of the self and has positive beliefs about the self, self-affirmation follows. In turn, self-acceptance likely influences self-evaluation and self-perspectives fostering even higher self-esteem and self-concept, respectively. Additional variables, such as empowerment and self-actualization might also play a role in these mutually reinforcing cycles, in that with better self-esteem, self-concept, and self-acceptance, a person is more likely to engage in actions that empower and promote self-actualization, leading to improved self-evaluation and self-perspectives, and from these further self-affirmation and hence self-acceptance. Self-respect might represent a higher level of self-acceptance occurring when self-affirmation involves actual pride and confidence in oneself. They appear to be on the same continuum with self-respect higher, given that it is possible to have self-acceptance without actual self-respect, but inconceivable to have self-respect without self-acceptance, and both involve self-affirmation. Acceptance of the self, even if the self-affirmation does not reach the level of actual self-respect, produces a comfort and peace with oneself that aligns with good mental health.

References

Abramson, L.Y., Metalsky, G.I., Alloy, L.B., 1989. Hopelessness depression: a theory based subtype of depression. Psychol. Rev. 96, 358–372.

Adams, M.J., 1996. Youth in crisis: an examination of adverse risk factors effecting children's cognitive and behavioral-emotional development, children's ages 10-16. Diss. Abstr. In. A: Hum. Social Sci. 56 (A-8), 3313–3389.

Andersson, L.M., Moore, C.D., Hensing, G., Krantz, G., Staland-Nyman, C., 2014. General self-efficacy and its relationship to self-reported mental illness and barriers to care: a general population study. Commun. Mental Health 50 (6), 721–728.

Beck, A., 1991. Cognitive therapy: a 30-year retrospective. Am. Psychol. 46 (4), 368–375.

Beck, A.T., Brown, G.K., Steer, R.A., Kuyken, W., Grisham, J., 2001. Psychometric properties of the Beck Self-Esteem Scales. Behav. Res. Ther. 39, 115–124.
Bhar, S., Ghahramanlou-Holloway, M., Brown, G., Beck, A.T., 2008. Self-esteem and suicide ideation in psychiatric outpatients. Suicide Life Threat. Behav. 38 (5), 511–516.
Bowins, B.E., 2004. Psychological defense mechanisms: a new perspective. Am. J. Psychoanal. 64, 1–26.
Bowins, B., Shugar, G., 1998. Delusions and self-esteem. Can. J. Psychiatry 43, 154–158.
Brown, A.D., Joscelyne, A., Dorfman, M.L., Marmar, C.R., Bryant, R.A., 2012. The impact of perceived self-efficacy on memory for aversive experiences. Memory 20 (4), 374–383.
Campbell, J.D., Chew, B., Scrathley, L., 1991. Cognitive and emotional reactions to daily events: the effects of self-esteem and self-complexity. J. Personality Social Psychol. 59, 473–505.
Cardenas, V., Abel, S., Bowie, C.R., Tiznado, D., Depp, C.A., Patterson, T.L., et al., 2013. When functional capacity and real-world functioning converge: the role of self-efficacy. Schizophr. Bull. 39 (4), 908–916.
Crump, R., Lillie-Blanton, M., Anthony, J., 1997. The influence of self-esteem on smoking among African American school children. J. Drug Educ. 27, 277–291.
Donnellan, M.B., Trzesniewski, K.H., Robins, R.W., Moffitt, T.E., Caspi, A., 2005. Low self-esteem is related to aggression, antisocial behavior, and delinquency. Psychol. Sci. 16 (4), 328–335.
Engel, M., 1959. The stability of the self-concept in adolescence. J. Abnorm. Social Psychol. 58, 211–215.
Fickova, E., 1999. Personality dimensions and self-esteem indicators relationship. Stud. Psychol. 41, 323–329.
Fisher, M., Pastore, P., Schneider, M., Pegler, C., Napolitano, B., 1994. Eating attitudes in urban and suburban adolescents. Int. J. Eat. Disord. 16, 67–74.
Ginsburg, G.S., La Greca, A.M., Silverman, W.K., 1998. Social anxiety in children with anxiety disorders: relation with social and emotional functioning. J. Abnorm. Child Psychol. 26, 175–185.
Hammen, C., Goodman-Brown, T., 1990. Self-schemas and vulnerability in specific life stress in children at risk for depression. Cogn. Theory Res. 14, 215–227.
Hansford, B.C., Hattie, J.A., 1982. The relationship between self and achievement/performance measures. Rev. Educ. Res. 52, 123–142.
Hartmann, A.S., Thomas, J.J., Greenberg, J.L., Matheny, N.L., Wilhelm, S., 2014. A comparison of self-esteem and perfectionism in anorexia nervosa and body dysmorphic disorder. J. Nervous Mental Disord. 202 (12), 883–888.
Hay, I., Ashman, A.F., Van Kraayenoord, C.E., 1998. Educational characteristics of students with high or low self-concept. Psychol. Schools 35, 391–400.
Iancu, I., Bodner, E., Ben-Zion, I.Z., 2015. Self-esteem, dependency, self-efficacy and self-criticism in social anxiety disorder. Comprehen. Psychiatry 58, 165–171.
Isomaa, R., Vaananen, J.M., Frojd, S., Kaltiala-Heino, R., Marttunen, M., 2013. How low is low? Low self-esteem as an indicator of internalizing psychopathology in adolescence. Heath Educ. Behav. 40 (4), 392–399.
Jessor, R., Turbin, M.S., Costa, F.M., 1998. Risk and protection in successful outcomes among disadvantaged adolescents. Appl. Dev. Sci. 2, 194–208.
Jones, S., Heaven, P., 1998. Psychosocial correlates of adolescent drug-taking behavior. J. Adolescence 21, 127–134.
Judge, T.A., Bono, J.E., Locke, E.A., 2000. Personality and job satisfaction: the mediating role of job characteristics. J. Appl. Psychol. 85, 237–249.
Kesting, M.L., Lincoln, T.M., 2013. The relevance of self-esteem and self-schemas to persecutory delusions: a systematic review. Comprehen. Psychiatry 54 (7), 766–789.

Lakey, C.E., Hirsch, J.K., Nelson, L.A., Nsamenang, S.A., 2014. Effects of contingent self-esteem on depressive symptoms and suicidal behavior. Death Stud. 38 (6–10), 563–570.
Mann, M., Hosman, C.M., Schaalma, H.P., De Vries, N.K., 2004. Self-esteem in a broad-spectrum approach for mental health promotion. Health Educ. Res. 19 (4), 357–372.
Marsh, H.W., Trautwein, U., Ludtke, O., Koller, O., Baumert, J., 2006. Integration of multidimensional self-concept and core personality constructs: construct validation and relations to well-being and achievement. J. Personality 74, 403–456.
Miller, P.M., Kreitman, N.B., Ingham, J.G., Sashidharan, S.P., 1989. Self-esteem, life stress and psychiatric disorder. J. Affective Disord. 17, 65–75.
Muha, D.G., 1991. Dropout prevention and group counselling. High School J. 74, 76–80.
Orbach, I., 2007. Self-destructive processes and suicide. Isr. J. Psychiatry Related Sci. 44 (4), 266–279.
Orth, U., Robins, R.W., Meier, L.L., 2009. Disentangling the effects of low self-esteem and stressful events on depression: findings from three longitudinal studies. J. Personality Social Psychol. 97 (2), 307–321.
Overholser, J.C., Adams, D.M., Lehnert, K.L., Brinkman, D.C., 1995. Self-esteem deficits and suicidal tendencies among adolescents. J. Am. Acad. Child Adolescent Psychiatry 34, 919–928.
Reinherz, H.Z., Giaconia, R.M, Pakiz, B., Silverman, A.B., Farst, A.K., Lefkowitz, E.S., 1993. Psychological risk of major depression in later adolescence. J. Am. Acad. Child Adolescent Psychiatry 32, 1155–1163.
Robbins, S.B., Lauver, K., Le, H., Langley, R., Carlstrom, A., 2004. Do psychosocial and study skill factors predict college outcomes? A meta-analysis. Psychol. Bull. 130, 261–288.
Rouse, K.A., 1998. Longitudinal health endangering behavior among resilient and nonresilient early adolescents. J. Adolescent Health 23, 297–302.
Schoen, P., 1999. The etiology of violence and the voice of the perpetrator. Diss. Abstr. Int. B: Sci. Eng. 60 (2-B), 0875.
Schonfeld, P., Preusser, F., Margraf, J., 2017. Costs and benefits of self-efficacy: differences of the stress response and clinical implications. Neurosci. Biobehav. Rev. 75, 40–52.
Seligman, M.P., 1995. What You Can Change and What You Can't. Knopf, New York.
Smolak, L., Levine, M.P., Schermer, F., 1998. A controlled evaluation of an elementary school primary prevention program for eating problems. J. Psychosom. Res. 44, 339–353.
Somali, A., Kelley, J., Heckman, T., Hackl, K., Runge, L, Wright, C., 2001. Life optimism, substance abuse and AIDS-specific attitudes associated with HIV-risk behavior among disadvantaged inner city women. J. Women's Health Gender-Based Med. 9, 1101–1110.
Sowislo, J.F., Orth, U., 2013. Does low self-esteem predict depression and anxiety? A meta-analysis of longitudinal studies. Psychol. Bull. 139 (1), 213–240.
Swann, W.B., Chang-Schneider, C., McClarty, K.L., 2007. Do people's self-views matter? Self-concept and self-esteem in everyday life. Am. Psychol. 62 (2), 84–94.
Teri, L., 1982. Depression in adolescence: its relationship to assertion and various aspects of self-image. J. Clin. Child Psychol. 11, 101–106.
Trzesniewski, K., Donnellan, B., Moffat, T., Robbins, R., Poulton, R., Caspi, A., 2006. Low self-esteem during adolescence predicts poor health, criminal behavior, and limited economic prospects during adulthood. Dev. Psychol. 42, 381–390.
Vohs, K.D., Voelz, Z.R., Petiit, J.W., Bardone, A.M., Katz, J., Abramson, L.Y., 2001. Perfectionism, body dissatisfaction and self-esteem: an interactive model of bulimic symptom development. J. Social Clin. Psychol. 20, 476–497.
Wilhelm, K., Parker, G., Dewhurst-Savellis, J., Asghari, A., 1999. Psychological predictors of single and recurrent major depressive episodes. J. Affective Disord. 54, 139–147.

Chapter 8

Adaptability

The capacity to alter behavior in line with circumstances allows for optimal outcomes. Failure to inhibit maladaptive behavior and flexibly shift to alternative actions in keeping with current circumstances contributes to poor outcomes. Another way of looking at the action and outcome linkage is that adaptive/maladaptive outcomes are relative to circumstances necessitating flexible shifts in behavior. Better outcomes involve gains fostering good mental health, while poorer outcomes entail limitations and setbacks contributing to mental illness, at least when such outcomes repeat.

The mention of inhibiting maladaptive behavior and flexibly shifting to alternative actions might have brought to mind our earlier discussion of executive functions in the Human-specific cognition chapter. Executive functions, and indeed the other states and processes characterizing mental health, contribute greatly to adaptability, which is why I left this chapter for the last, although certainly not least. It might seem that for adaptability all that is required is shifting actions, but the prerequisite is to act in the first place, and it is at this level that many of the states and processes characterizing mental health play out. Hence, we will consider the capacity to act followed by altering behavior to fit circumstances, with the latter addressing the crucial topic of overcoming repetitive maladaptive behavior. Adaptability has a biological basis, known as neural plasticity, that will be covered to demonstrate how adapting to circumstances is facilitated and why dysfunction can be entrenched.

The capacity to engage in actions

Readers who are naturally active might have difficulty appreciating this first component of adaptability, but a person who does not engage in actions cannot possibly adapt to current circumstances, unless of course the circumstances favor inaction. This is a key reason why the prototypical chronic schizophrenic person, who mostly just sits watching television and smoking cigarettes, is considered to be inadequate—the person does not act sufficiently to adapt to changing circumstances. In line with Buddhist philosophy, the only thing that is constant is change. No matter how we wish for constant circumstances, they are always changing and a person has to engage in actions to have any hope of adapting to the changes.

The image of a person with chronic schizophrenia not acting drives home the point regarding the importance of engaging in actions, and also how deficiencies

States and Processes for Mental Health. DOI: 10.1016/C2020-0-00574-8

in regards to the states and processes characterizing mental health contribute to maladaptive and inflexible behavior. We looked at the importance of activity for mental health in the Activity chapter considering physical, nature, art/hobby, and music forms, and then social activity in the Social connectedness chapter. Activity of these various forms aligns with the higher behavioral activation and lower behavioral inhibition requirements of our evolution. In addition, given our evolution in hunting–gathering groups we rely on others for emotional and physical support, underscoring the importance of social activity. In the Psychological defense mechanism chapter, we looked at the crucial role of these defenses in reducing negative emotions and fostering positive emotional states, with the templates of positive cognitive distortions and dissociation focused on. Intact psychological defenses enable people to maintain positive emotional states in the face of stress, and hence enhance the capacity to act and adapt. Resilience as a psychological defense greatly contributes to adaptability.

The capacity to regulate emotions and behavior, covered in the Regulation chapter, is crucial when it comes to engaging in actions, given that excessive amplified fear producing anxiety favors inaction. One of the most detrimental things I have encountered over years of providing psychotherapy is avoidance, typically as a response to anxiety. People who avoid the challenges of life essentially fail by default. If you avoid an exam or class presentation out of fear, you fail to get a passing grade. People who fear the challenge of romantic relationships lose out on the benefits. If work is so anxiety provoking that a person avoids it, then the self-esteem and self-concept benefits of making a contribution are lost, not to mention the loss in terms of living in poverty. Research backs up the assertion that failure results from avoidance. For example, Olsson and Dahl (2012) compared 280 people with avoidant personality problems (not full-fledged avoidant personality disorder) to 1400 controls, finding that the avoidant participants were more likely to live alone, had lower levels of education, and lower income. They also experienced poorer self-rated health, more somatic symptoms, pain, mental distress, insomnia, and lower general self-efficacy. Avoidant responses limit self-control contributing to poor physical and mental health outcomes, highlighting how regulation is important for preventing avoidance and fostering adaptive behavior (Boals et al., 2011). Not being able to regulate fear and anxiety responses, and consequently not acting when it is required, clearly favors negative outcomes.

Human-specific cognition in terms of basic cognition, social cognition, and motivation is also crucial when it comes to engaging in actions. Returning to our example of the person with chronic schizophrenia, the lack of motivation in itself precludes acting at a level necessary for adaptability. Lacking the social cognition required for adequate interactions, people with autism usually do not engage with other people. Those with intellectual disability cannot perform the mental functions required for the many complex cognitive tasks required by modern-day society. The psychological constructs of self-esteem and self-concept providing for self-acceptance play a role in the capacity to engage in actions, given that when these are higher a person feels confident and capable encouraging activity, whereas with low levels confidence and a sense of being capable is absent favoring inaction.

The states and processes characterizing mental health that we have covered contribute to the capacity to engage in actions, as a prerequisite for adaptability. When these are impaired the requisite capacity to engage in actions is compromised. The world is in constant motion and change, and a person has to act to have any hope of flexibly adapting. Of course, actions in terms of quantity alone are not enough, given that these actions have to fit with circumstances for there to be adaptability.

Fitting actions to circumstances

Higher functioning people automatically adjust behavior to fit with changing circumstances, and given that the only constant is change, this is an ongoing process. The two major contributors to this capacity are human-specific cognition and not being trapped into repetitive maladaptive behavior, but the range of states and processes characterizing mental health contribute. Regarding activity of various forms, higher behavioral activation and lower behavioral inhibition typically mean a more extensive range of behaviors covering a greater number of scenarios. For example, if a person engages in sports activity, the capacity for more complex physical actions is present if required by current circumstances. Greater social connectedness produces more social confidence and experience to adjust social actions as required. For instance, conflictual situations can be managed when there is social confidence and prior experience with this scenario.

Healthy psychological defenses and additional emotion regulation capacities keep anxiety and other negative emotions at low enough levels to facilitate adequate adjustment to circumstances. If emotion regulation capacities are lacking, fear can escalate to levels that block flexible coping. Frequently, a person has to face circumstances that induce negative valence emotions like fear, sadness, anger, disgust, shame, and the ability to regulate them to moderate levels favors adjusting actions to adapt. For example, if a morally disgusting scenario is encountered such as the slaughter of endangered animals, regulating emotions such that a person engages in actions to reduce, contain, or eliminate the offending agent facilitates coping, as opposed to just avoiding it or not responding.

Believing in oneself is often necessary to act adaptively. In the Self-acceptance chapter, we noted how high self-esteem fosters mastery, resilience, and more positive responses to challenging circumstances. Furthermore, low self-esteem is associated with internalizing and externalizing forms of mental illness that impair coping capacity. For example, depression limits adaptability by impairing cognition, motivation, and hope. Aggression, an externalizing problem, while representing a very adaptive response to certain circumstances, favors costly consequences if applied without discretion. A self-concept consisting of positive perspectives regarding one's capabilities affords for a greater range of responses to circumstances and confidence in applying them. For instance, when a person believes in their capacity to lead, circumstances requiring leadership will be adapted to.

Human-specific cognition

Basic cognition, social cognition, and motivation not only fosters the capacity to engage in actions, but also fitting actions to circumstances. Observing a person with even mild autism attempt to romantically bond to another person, immediately confirms the value of intact social cognition for flexibly fitting behavior to circumstances. At one point in my career I worked part-time at a university health service encountering several individuals, each male and in math-related disciplines, who had "Asperger's Syndrome," and listening to how these people approached possible romance was painful. There was very little capacity to read the potential partner's facial expression and adjust behavior accordingly, nor understanding of appropriate topics, and when to advance and when to pull back. Social actions that most of us take for granted were sadly lacking.

Executive functions provide for several capacities relevant to flexibly adjusting behavior to fit circumstances. Of crucial significance, being able to inhibit one stream of actions, and flexibly shift to another plays a prominent role in adaptively adjusting to change. Attending to circumstances long enough to process them provides information that is required for modifying behavior. Those with attention deficit hyperactivity disorder are impaired in this regard, due to how attention is often not sustained long enough to process optimal actions. With more complex scenarios those with attention deficit hyperactivity disorder and intellectual disability falter due to impairments in organization, planning, monitoring, task completion, and multitasking, with the severity of the deficits largely determining the degree of behavioral impairment.

Social and basic cognition then foster adaptive and flexible adjustments of behavior to fit with circumstances. Since the environment involves people the social cognition component should not be underestimated: it is common to only focus on executive functions when considering adaptive shifts in behavior, and as crucial as this capacity is, understanding and processing social scenarios are equally important. Motivation is also critical as it provides the impetus to adaptively and flexibly adjust actions to fit with circumstances. A limitation of the capacities provided by human-specific cognition is that maladaptive behavior can be entrenched blocking flexible and adaptive alterations.

Repetitive maladaptive behavior

One of the most common occurrences in psychotherapy is maladaptive behavior that repeats. If behavior is adaptive then it is not a concern, and since psychotherapy is mostly focused on psychopathology it usually does not enter into discussions unless strengths are addressed. Maladaptive behavior that does not repeat is typically not a major concern, and even if the consequences are severe there is not much that psychotherapeutic interventions can do for it, given that it is a one-off occurrence. On the other hand, repetitive maladaptive behavior results in ongoing unfavorable outcomes detracting from mental health and worsening mental illness, and so is a common issue in those seeking psychotherapy.

I have proposed that repetitive maladaptive behavior can be divided into traumatic and nontraumatic forms (Bowins, 2010). The traumatic form represents a dissociative defense related to how the cognitive and emotional aspects of experience are automatically fused, based on a biologically based learning process (Bowlby, 1988; Kutz, 1989; Van Der Kolk, 1989). This process largely unfolds unconsciously, but traumatic occurrences must achieve conscious awareness to help ensure that the event is not repeated. If fusion of the cognitive and emotional aspects of the experience is too painful at a conscious level, then a defensive response is activated resulting in dissociation and endless repetition as flashbacks, images, partial memories, thoughts, dreams, emotions, somatic sensations, behavioral re-enactments, and the like. Although defensively relieving conscious pain in the moment when the various aspects of the traumatic experience are being fused, the endless fragmented expressions impair adaptive functioning by intruding into consciousness and distracting a person from a focus on current circumstances. In addition, responses to these fragmented occurrences can represent maladaptive behavior, such as if fear and avoidance arise when current circumstances favor approach behavior.

The nontraumatic form is hypothesized to arise from an evolutionary-based learning process, providing the capacity to internalize patterns of behavior from caregivers during the early years of life (Bowins, 2010). The patterns of behavior that are adaptive for a given environment will vary, but be displayed by caregivers. By internalizing these adaptive patterns a child is more likely to adjust to their physical and social environmental circumstances. Although the process is designed to facilitate the internalization of adaptive patterns of behavior, maladaptive ones can be acquired. During at least 95% of our evolution, we were in hunting–gathering groups where a child was exposed to several people who typically would display adaptive patterns of behavior, or if maladaptive then the group would likely have not survived. Aberrant child-rearing patterns would probably have been opposed as well. In our modern-day context of two and even one person raising a child, overexposure to maladaptive patterns of behavior is probably more likely to occur, and aberrant child-rearing patterns, such as abuse, can transpire without detection. In such a circumstance, these maladaptive patterns are not diluted by exposure to more adaptive ones, and hence are more likely to be internalized.

Internalized repetitive maladaptive patterns of behavior can take multiple forms including suspicion and anger, remaining aloof from people, not reciprocating, taking advantage of others, abusive behavior, being critical, and withdrawing instead of approaching. I believe that the fit with a person's early personality or temperament is relevant as to which patterns of behavior are internalized. For instance, if a person is open to experience, an approach pattern is much more likely to be internalized than a withdrawal pattern. Likewise, if a person is more agreeable, a pattern of getting close to other people will be acquired over one of suspicion and anger. Regardless of the maladaptive pattern of behavior acquired, it represents an implicit habit form of memory, and as such is engaged in as a default option. Hence, if a person has a pattern of withdrawal, whenever a novel scenario arises the person will automatically be predisposed to withdraw, regardless of the adaptive value in approaching. If a new person comes on the scene, then the individual who has internalized the suspicious and angry pattern is more likely to reject than embrace the newcomer. These repetitive maladaptive patterns of behavior can produce endless setbacks in a person's life by blocking flexible and adaptive behavioral responses to circumstances. Since they represent implicit habit memory the repetition is so automatic that it is very difficult to overcome (Bowins, 2010).

Aside from traumatic and nontraumatic repetitive maladaptive behavior, any instance of inflexible and rigid behavior can detract from flexibly and adaptively adjusting behavior to fit with circumstances. Excessive compulsive behavior for instance compromises adaptive responses. In the Psychological defense mechanism chapter, we looked at how milder compulsive behavior can help contain anxiety, but becomes dysfunctional at more intense levels because the person is consumed by the behavior, applying it when there is no adaptive benefit. The focus on compulsive behavior also compromises adaptive functioning by blocking awareness of what might constitute adaptive responses, and preventing such responses from being engaged in, at least when they conflict with the compulsive response.

Even consciously adopting rigid approaches to life can block flexible and adaptive coping. For instance, many people focus on the pursuit of happiness that can actually limit adaptive behavior: happiness represents a brief emotional response to gain (see the Activity chapter), and in a world and universe ruled by entropy (the natural progression of order to disorder) it is impossible to always be gaining, hence the pursuit of happiness is largely futile and misguided. Furthermore, the expectation of ongoing "happiness" can ironically make people feel worse, because if this is set out as a scenario to be expected and reality falls short people perceive a loss and sadness ensues. The same applies to the other positive universal emotion—interest—in response to potential reward, since this scenario cannot always be present. Instead of the pursuit of happiness, it is the happiness of pursuit, as by absorbing oneself in positive activities gains ensue producing feelings of happiness and interest! Additionally, in the longer range it is often necessary to persevere through challenges that definitely do not produce feelings of happiness or interest, to eventually achieve success. Consider how many successful academics and professionals have struggled through countless hours of study to achieve their goal, and although for some of these people study can be a form of positive absorption, I have not yet met anyone who loved it all the time, to say the least. Imagine for a moment the application of a new pharmaceutical agent that currently pharmaceutical company executives can only fantasize about, that makes a person so happy they do nothing, just sit around and feel happy. Would this constitute good mental health? If you answered yes, you probably work for such a company, but consider what would then happen if say the drug turned out to have severe long-term consequences and had to be stopped. The person would now be in a horrible state unable to cope with any stress or challenge, an emotional vegetable, lacking the resources to adapt and succeed.

A major component of flexible and adaptive coping ensuring that behavior fits with current circumstances, then includes not consciously adhering to rigid and often misguided approaches to life. Overcoming any repetitive maladaptive patterns of behavior, from both traumatic and nontraumatic sources, is another key component of adaptability. Given the automatic and largely unconscious nature of these repetitive maladaptive patterns of behavior, they are not likely to spontaneously change and require a great deal of conscious effort and usually psychotherapeutic support. Even misguided approaches to life can become automatic and hence resilient to change, requiring conscious effort and even psychotherapy. The reason why repetitions become resilient to change has to do with the neural basis of repetitive behavior, in that they become embedded in synaptic connections that strengthen with repetition. Fortunately, the brain does demonstrate plasticity that we will now briefly look at.

Neural plasticity

The capacity to encode behavior in synaptic connections between neurons provides for neural plasticity. This capacity represents a double-edged sword in that while enabling new forms of behavior to be laid down, the process can imbed maladaptive forms of behavior, thereby increasing the probability of repetition. This is why a key strategy in unlearning repetitive maladaptive behavior is to consciously overlearn the alternative, to gradually lay down a new more adaptive pattern (Bowins, 2010). To reveal how there is indeed a neural equivalent and basis for both flexible and rigid behaviors, we will briefly look at how neural plasticity works.

The central principle in the neural representation of behavior is known as Hebbian plasticity, and the well quoted saying that "neurons that fire together wire together" (Power and Schlaggar, 2016, p. 4). When behavior results in certain neurons firing together that behavior is represented at a neural level, and the more repetition the more robust the wiring (Power and Schlaggar, 2016). A striking example of this process occurs with musicians that play string instruments: neuroimaging has shown that sensory representations of the left playing fingers are larger than for those on the right hand (Elbert et al., 1995). This neural representation enables string musicians to play with greater ease, and the more playing the more robust the neural representation.

Neural representation of behaviors facilitates future adaptive responses for the particular circumstances, as it provides a template for responding that can be modified for novel scenarios. Reduced neural plasticity on the other hand compromises adaptability, and evidence reveals that this occurrence is linked to mental illness (Goto et al., 2010; Malykhin and Coupland, 2015; Meyer-Lindenberg and Tost, 2014; Pittenger and Duman, 2008; Schoenfeld and Cameron, 2015; Van Den Heuval et al., 2016; Waltereit et al., 2014). Waltereit et al. (2014) present evidence for impaired synaptic plasticity in autism spectrum disorder, mental retardation (intellectual disability), and schizophrenia, with the first two transpiring in early development; autism spectrum disorder involving reduced synaptic plasticity for social cognition, and intellectual disability plasticity issues with basic global cognition. Schizophrenia in contrast is characterized by the onset of synaptic plasticity problems in adolescence with both social and basic global cognition involved (Waltereit et al., 2014). Note that impaired synaptic connections are equivalent to dysconnectivity discussed in the Human-specific cognition chapter, associated with negative symptoms. Goto et al. (2010) present evidence for impaired prefrontal cortex plasticity so crucial to regulation, as discussed in the Regulation chapter, involved in various psychiatric disorders including schizophrenia, drug addiction, mood disorders, and Alzheimer's disease. Meyer-Lindenberg and Tost (2014) show how there is reduced neural plasticity longitudinally in both the prefrontal cortex and hippocampus with schizophrenia, arising from developmental abnormalities in neural circuits.

Reduced neural plasticity in the hippocampus, and even subfields within it, has been uncovered in depression (Malykhin and Coupland, 2015). Stress alone can reduce synaptic plasticity, theoretically increasing the likelihood of depression (Pittenger and Duman, 2008). In the case of depression, at least, the direction between reduced neural plasticity and illness is not entirely clear given the largely correlational and cross-sectional nature of the studies, and it is feasible that depression reduces neural plasticity (Schoenfeld and Cameron, 2015). Consistent with extensive compulsivity being dysfunctional and how psychopathology can influence neural plasticity, repetitive compulsive behavior appears to contribute to changes in the involved neural circuits ensuring chronicity of the compulsive actions (Van Den Heuval et al., 2016).

Evidence then supports the role of impaired neural plasticity in various forms of psychopathology, and also how psychopathology can entrench dysfunctional neuroplastic changes. The capacity for representing behavior in the form of synaptic connections, though, does contribute to adaptive learning. When the process goes well neural plasticity facilitates adjusting behavior to fit with circumstances, and also repeating these adaptive responses with similar circumstances. Hence, neural plasticity is a key component of adaptability.

Summary note

A crucial component of mental health is adaptability, involving both the capacity to engage in actions and fitting actions to circumstances. These two aspects rely on the other states and processes characterizing mental health discussed in previous chapters, consisting of activity, psychological defense mechanisms, social connectedness, regulation, human-specific cognition, and self-acceptance. Regarding fitting behavior to circumstances, human-specific cognition—basic cognition (largely executive functions), social cognition, and motivation—is all-important. An impediment to adaptability is entrenched maladaptive behavior in the form of both traumatic and nontraumatic repetitive maladaptive behavior, and more conscious rigid and inflexible approaches to life. The capacity for adaptability is based on neural plasticity, which enables adaptive behaviors to be encoded in synaptic connections and repeated with similar circumstances. Psychopathology of various forms is associated with impaired neural plasticity. Conversely, mental illness can entrench dysfunction in neural circuits. Behaviors consistent with mental health transpire when neural plasticity is not compromised and actions are adjusted in a flexible and adaptable way to fit with circumstances.

References

Boals, A., Vandellen, M.R., Banks, J.B., 2011. The relationship between self-control and health: the mediating role of avoidant coping. Psychol. Health 26 (8), 1049–1062.

Bowins, B.E., 2010. Repetitive maladaptive behavior: beyond repetition compulsion. Am. J. Psychoanal. 70, 282–298.

Bowlby, J., 1988. Developmental psychiatry comes of age. Am. J. Psychiatry 145, 1–10.

Elbert, T., Pantev, C., Wienbruch, C., Rockstroh, B, Taub, E., 1995. Increased cortical representation of the fingers of the left hand in string players. Science 270, 305–307.

Goto, Y., Yang, C.R., Otani, S., 2010. Functional and dysfunctional synaptic plasticity in prefrontal cortex: roles in psychiatric disorders. Biol. Psychiatry 67 (3), 199–207.

Kutz, I., 1989. Samson's complex: the compulsion to re-enact betrayal and rage. Br. J. Med. Psychol. 62, 123–134.

Malykhin, N.Y., Coupland, N.J., 2015. Hippocampal neuroplasticity in major depressive disorder. Neuroscience 309, 200–213.

Meyer-Lindenberg, A., Tost, H., 2014. Neuroimaging and plasticity in schizophrenia. Restorative Neurol. Neurosci. 32 (1), 119–127.

Olsson, I, Dahl, A.A., 2012. Avoidant personality problems—their association with somatic and mental health, lifestyle, and social network. A community-based study. Comprehen. Psychiatry 53 (6), 813–821.

Pittenger, C., Duman, R.S., 2008. Stress, depression, and neuroplasticity: a convergence of mechanisms. Neuropsychopharmacology 33 (1), 88–109.

Power, J.D., Schlaggar, B.L., 2016. Neural plasticity across the lifespan. Wiley Interdiscip. Rev. Dev. Biol. 6 (1). doi:10.1002/wdev.216.

Schoenfeld, T.J., Cameron, H.A., 2015. Adult neurogenesis and mental illness. Neuropsychopharmacology 40 (1), 113–128.

Van Den Heuval, O.A., Van Wingen, G., Soriano-Mas, C., Alonso, P., Chamberlain, S.R., Nakamae, T., et al., 2016. Brain circuitry of compulsivity. Eur. Neuropsychopharmacol. 26 (5), 810–827.

Van Der Kolk, B.A., 1989. The compulsion to repeat the trauma. Psychiatric Clin. North Am. 12, 389–411.

Waltereit, R., Banaschewski, T., Meyer-Lindenberg, A., Poustka, L., 2014. Interaction of neurodevelopmental pathways and synaptic plasticity in mental retardation, autistic spectrum disorder and schizophrenia: implication for psychiatry. World J. Biol. Psychiatry 15 (7), 507–516.

Chapter 9

Conclusion

Activity, psychological defense mechanisms, social connectedness, regulation, human-specific cognition, self-acceptance, and adaptability comprehensively characterize mental health, largely because each has a strong evolutionary rationale grounding them in a powerful framework. Without activity (behavioral activation > behavioral inhibition) humans would simply not have survived to become the dominant hominoid species. The evolution of human intelligence has amplified emotions such that negative valence ones detract from healthy functioning, necessitating the evolution of psychological defense mechanisms to reduce the burden of these emotions. Given our limited body weaponry we relied on hunting–gathering groups for survival and reproductive success, ensuring that our brains are wired for social connectedness. Regulation is a prominent feature of all biological systems, both at the individual and ecosystem level, and this extends to regulation over emotions and other psychological events such as psychotic level cognitions. Human-specific cognition in terms of basic cognition, social cognition, and motivation really defines what being "human" is, and it has been this combination of cognitive capacities that enabled us to outcompete other hominoid species. Self-acceptance, derived from positive self-esteem and self-concept, optimizes the psychological side of functioning consistent with the evolution of human intelligence and other cognitive capacities. Without adaptability a given organism or species loses by default, as there is just too much competition in natural settings, and successful outcomes are much more likely with cognitive and behavioral flexibility. Based on this evolutionary grounding, these states and processes advance mental health.

Intact functioning on the core states and processes for mental health translates into an absence of mental illness (robust mental health), whereas deficits produce mental illness, encompassing both formal and informal variants. Under activity, psychological defense mechanisms, social connectedness, regulation, human-specific cognition, self-acceptance, and adaptability, these expressions were presented, but will be summarized and in some instances elaborated on here, with further examples presented in Section 2:

Depression: Reduced activity with low behavioral activation and high behavioral inhibition. Impaired psychological defense mechanism functioning resulting in sadness-related emotions amplifying to depression. Social isolation and loneliness contribute to depression, and depression in turn usually further impairs social connectedness. Regulation over emotions is compromised resulting in an

States and Processes for Mental Health. DOI: 10.1016/C2020-0-00574-8

imbalance between limbic system activity and top-down regulation favoring the former. Negative symptoms likely contribute to depression (and most formal variants of mental illness). Impaired self-concept and self-esteem, and hence self-acceptance deficits, foster depression. Compromised adaptability, and in particular with repetitive maladaptive behavior, leads to dysfunctional outcomes producing losses, thereby contributing to depression.

Anxiety: High behavioral inhibition favoring avoidance over approach behavior, and hence further reductions in activity. Threat-related emotions escalate to anxiety due to impaired psychological defense mechanism functioning. Given our social nature as a species social isolation is perceived as a threat, fostering threat cognitions, furthering isolation, and fear/anxiety. Regulation over threat-related emotions is impaired allowing the escalation to anxiety. Negative symptoms might play a role in ongoing anxiety issues. Deficient self-concept and self-esteem (impaired self-acceptance) favor negative emotions generally including fear and anxiety. Recurrent failure due to impaired adaptability produces real and perceived threats, and hence fear and its amplification to anxiety is inevitable.

Psychosis: Extreme cognitive distortions, usually negative, transpire in part due to compromised mature psychological defense mechanism functioning. Social isolation favors suspicious thoughts given how during our evolution this occurrence was threatening. Regulation over psychotic level cognitions, including sensory-perceptual processes, is impaired allowing them to be routinely expressed in the conscious and awake state. Negative symptoms play a major role in impairing regulation over psychotic level cognitions, likely due to the dysconnectivity of negative symptoms impairing the connectivity required for healthy regulation. Low self-acceptance while not causing psychosis appears to influence the content of delusions making them more negative and self-depreciating. Psychosis in the conscious and awake state (as opposed to psychotic equivalents during sleep with dreaming) reduces adaptability, and the negative outcomes that follow worsen the other states and processes characterizing mental health, such as with social isolation.

Schizophrenia: Negative symptoms (impaired human-specific cognition), including basic cognition, social cognition, and motivation, are key to this severe mental illness, and appear to impair regulation over psychotic level cognition. Furthermore, issues with the other states and processes for mental illness that transpire with psychosis also play a role, given the co-occurrence of negative symptoms and psychosis in schizophrenia.

Mania: Negative symptoms play a major role in largely adaptive hypomania progressing to mostly dysfunctional mania. Psychosis also occurs in many instances bringing into play the impairments that transpire with it.

Autism spectrum disorders: Impaired social cognition is instrumental.

Intellectual disability: General deficits in basic cognition are prominent.

Attention deficit hyperactivity disorder: Select executive functioning impairments, such as with attention, response inhibition, and set shifting are central.

Post-traumatic stress disorder: Impaired psychological defense mechanism functioning in terms of dissociative fragmenting of the cognitive and emotional aspects of the traumatic experience, leading to endless repetition, despite the defensive value in the moment of trauma. Healthy grieving as a psychological defense mechanism is also impaired.

Dissociative disorders: Dissociation is one of the key defense mechanism templates, but extreme expressions often related to trauma are dysfunctional.

Personality disorders: Extreme and enduring expressions of psychological defenses, such as avoidance, dependence, and narcissism, occur resulting in ongoing dysfunction.

Eating disorders: Regulation impairments are prominent with mostly undercontrol but in some instances overcontrol, as with perfectionism in anorexia. Activity issues also play a role, such as anorexic individuals often engaging in excessive activity, and deficient activity in the case of obesity.

Addictions (reinforcement-based disorders): Defensive positive cognitive distortions maintain the dysfunctional behavior. Social connectedness is restricted to people likewise addicted, with this social scenario reinforcing the given behavior. Regulation over reinforcement parameters is compromised ensuring that the behavior persists. Impairments to human-specific cognition contribute in some instances, such as the behavior compensating for reduced executive functioning. Self-concept and self-esteem issues usually play a role in initiating and maintaining the dysfunctional behavior. Adaptability is compromised with the excessive focus on acquiring and using the given substance or engaging in the behavior, as with ongoing money problems resulting from gambling.

Informal mental illness: Aside from formal mental illness, the issues that people seek psychotherapy for involve reduced functioning in regards to one or more of the states and processes for mental health. The list is virtually endless, many examples indicated in this section and more in Section 2. Select instances, include: failure to progress in life resulting from deficient physical, social, or mental activity; immature psychological defense use in adulthood such as acting out, impairing relationships, and performance in other areas; deficient regulation of various urges; poor self-concept and self-esteem (self-acceptance) issues; repetitive maladaptive behavior compromising adaptability, resulting in repeated failure. Psychotherapy, by advancing the given state and process characterizing mental health, transforms formal and informal mental illness into mental health.

In the Introduction to this section it was noted that the omission of a happiness theme might surprise some readers, and in the Adaptability chapter we looked at why the pursuit of happiness is misguided and futile. In contrast, a scenario whereby positive emotions exceed negative emotions (positive affectivity over negative affectivity) is reasonable, and even at an intuitive level aligns with mental health. However, for this scenario to be sustainable it must follow from the states and processes for mental health, mainly because they consistently diminish negative emotions while enhancing positive emotions. Activity plays a prominent role, with behavioral activation and behavioral inhibition linked to positive affectivity and negative affectivity, respectively. Robust activity with high behavioral activation and low behavioral inhibition then translates into positive emotions > negative emotions. By managing excessive negative emotions, psychological defense mechanisms powerfully shift the balance in favor of positive emotions: positive cognitive distortions transform the negative framing characterizing depression, anxiety, and stress, fostering negative emotions, into positive perspectives eliciting positive emotions, while dissociation emotionally distances a person from negativity. Positive social contact (social connectedness) triggers and maintains positive emotional states, and reduces or eliminates negative emotions associated with loneliness. Emotion regulation plays a key role in positive affectivity over negative affectivity by greatly restricting negative emotions, thereby favoring positive emotions. Indeed, intact emotion regulation largely ensures that positive affectivity exceeds negative affectivity, and in an ongoing fashion. While less direct, human-specific cognition fosters positive emotions by contributing to success, which transpires in the social sphere via social cognition, and more generally from enhanced motivation. Self-acceptance arising from positive self-esteem and self-concept ensures that self-referential thoughts and ensuing emotions will be positive. Adaptability enables an individual to adjust to ever changing circumstances optimizing successful outcomes, producing more positive emotional reactions and diminishing negative emotions linked to dysfunctional behavior. These states and processes for mental health translate into positive affectivity exceeding negative affectivity in a sustainable fashion, as opposed to a brief elevation of positive emotions over negative emotions from a psychoactive substance or the time limited effect of a motivation enhancing psychological intervention.

With an understanding of how activity, psychological defense mechanisms, social connectedness, regulation, human-specific cognition, self-acceptance, and adaptability characterize mental health, it is time to explore the role of various psychotherapies, and also nonspecific factors. Are they actually able to advance the states and processes for mental health? If so then how might this transpire? Approaching a familiar topic from a different perspective is always challenging, so I encourage readers to recall how psychological flexibility and adaptability is so important for mental health.

Section II

Forms of psychotherapy and non-specific factors proof of concept

Chapter 10

Introduction

The purpose of this section is to determine if and how psychotherapy advances the states and processes for mental health—activity, psychological defense mechanisms, social connectedness, regulation, human-specific cognition, self-acceptance, and adaptability. This focus differs from the standard approach, whereby the distinguishing feature of a particular type of psychotherapy is thought to directly resolve psychopathology, thereby indirectly improving mental health. Instead, by directly advancing the states and processes characterizing mental health, the various forms of psychotherapy improve mental health and in the process, remedy mental illness. This unique focus has the capacity to explain why so many diverse forms of psychotherapy, each purportedly with unique actions, improve several types of mental illness. With ever-expanding forms of psychotherapy this concern is more paramount. Then there is the matter of nonspecific psychotherapy factors, including the placebo effect, that all psychotherapists, or hopefully all, are aware of but yet do not really grasp how they work, particularly if it is the special sauce of a given form of psychotherapy that counts. Could it be that these nonspecific factors, much like the various forms of psychotherapy, work by advancing the states and processes for mental health? We will examine this possibility.

Now that we have established the purpose of the second section, I will lay out how it has been approached to maximize objectivity. To start, I will indicate what will not be attempted:

- Although a comprehensive overview of each form of psychotherapy will be provided, an exhaustive description will not be. Entire books are devoted to the workings of a given form of psychotherapy, and any attempt to provide extensive coverage here would fall short of these descriptions. In addition, I can only justify having expertise in a few forms.
- Efficacy data for the given psychotherapy type will not be covered for a few reasons. First, efficacy is an extensive and complex topic requiring a lot of detailed attention. Second, how there is so much bias in the area: it is common for psychotherapy efficacy studies to be conducted by researchers with a vested interest in the particular form of psychotherapy, and the methodology is often questionable such as comparing the psychotherapy type to a waitlist control or treatment as usual, with only small number of participants. The ideal research study for psychotherapy consists of a large number of participants who are representative of the respective population,

States and Processes for Mental Health. DOI: 10.1016/C2020-0-00574-8

investigators not vested in the outcome (independent and objective), and random assignment to four conditions—psychotherapy type being investigated, another well-validated form of psychotherapy such as cognitive, active placebo condition consisting of some activity that at least at face value seems psychologically relevant, and waitlist. If the tested psychotherapy modality compares equally or better to the established form of psychotherapy, and both are superior to the active placebo and waitlist groups, then the outcome can be considered valid, although replication of this result is best. Rarely are these standards even attempted let alone realized. As a relevant side note, I find it quite amazing how evidence-based medicine is espoused almost as a reflexive response, without due consideration of the true quality of the evidence. The research literature for psychotherapy efficacy studies is saturated with highly limited studies at a high risk of bias; perhaps fewer very well-designed studies need to be conducted.

The third reason why I will not cover efficacy studies is due to how so many forms of psychotherapy seem to benefit some people. An occurrence that I suspect every experienced psychotherapist has encountered is clients indicating that they have previously benefited from a form of psychotherapy you have barely heard of, let alone know much about. When I ask the person how they benefited, the explanation seems in line with standard accounts regarding outcomes, such as "my depression resolved," "I became much less anxious," "it helped me understand myself," "I cope better." One thing that I have learned from conducting psychotherapy and pharmacotherapy for years, and general medicine prior to that, is never discount the experience of a client. Hence, when hearing a client report how some form of psychotherapy benefited them it would not be helpful to say, "No you could not have benefited from that type of therapy, as So and So et al, 2017 found that it is ineffective." This would be a sure way to alienate a new client from the start, and even if the benefit was via nonspecific factors it can be incredibly difficult to disentangle the various influences.

- Clustering of types of psychotherapy will not be attempted, such as for example relational, humanistic, cognitive (thought-based), and experiential categories. Each form of psychotherapy actually has quite diverse aspects that often overlap, and to try and slot these forms into distinct categories will not help with our understanding, despite our psychological preference for discrete entities to simplify information processing. Such an approach would also bias to certain clusters such as cognitive.
- General and very specific approaches to psychotherapy will not be covered. General approaches lack a circumscribed and well-defined set of principles and strategies, such as "supportive" psychotherapy involving a wide range of techniques depending on the therapist, with no clear focus. To a large extent, general approaches such as supportive psychotherapy rely on nonspecific factors (see the Non-specific factors chapter), although specific techniques are often applied including psychoeducation, medication counseling, reassurance,

feedback, and numerous others. Very specific approaches constitute psychotherapy techniques and not distinct forms of psychotherapy, such as exposure and response prevention.
- Group psychotherapy will not be covered, because most forms of psychotherapy can and are delivered both individually and in group formats, with the principles of the particular approach remaining the same. Individual, group, and Internet represent delivery modes of the particular form of psychotherapy.

Now for how I will cover the various forms of psychotherapy:

- Each form of psychotherapy will be presented in an alphabetical order so as not to bias by order of presentation; the alphabet does not bias. In researching this book, I was surprised and maybe even shocked, by how many forms of psychotherapy are out there. It is indeed a staggering number that seems to be increasing every decade for major forms, and yearly for subtypes. Hence, if I do not cover a form of psychotherapy that a reader practices or receives treatment in, an almost certain occurrence, hopefully this will be taken as evidence of how many forms there are. I have endeavored to cover the major types of psychotherapy. In addition to "forms of psychotherapy" nonspecific influences including placebo effects will be covered.
- Standard search terms have been applied to academic databases for each form of psychotherapy, to both reveal information and be objective. For example, mechanism of action, activity, psychological defense mechanisms, social connectedness, emotion regulation, executive functions, social cognition, motivation, self-esteem, self-concept, adaptability, cognitive flexibility. This extensive search has helped determine what evidence there is for the given form of psychotherapy advancing activity, psychological defense mechanisms, social connectedness, regulation, human-specific cognition, self-acceptance, and adaptability.
- Despite the lengthy searches for each form of psychotherapy often very little relevant information surfaced, perhaps not surprisingly given the routine focus on psychopathology and efficacy, necessitating creative exploration of how the given type of psychotherapy might advance the states and processes for mental health. This input aligns with my experience conducting theoretical research (Centre for Theoretical Research in Psychiatry and Clinical Psychology, Toronto, Canada), and also how there is a creative aspect to psychotherapy that I believe should never be sacrificed to manualized approaches. I typically practice eclectic psychotherapy adaptively fitting various approaches and strategies to the needs of a client at a particular point in time, although I am most familiar with behavioral therapy, cognitive therapy, and psychodynamic approaches listed alphabetically. My eclectic experience aligns with and facilitates a creative approach to psychotherapy. How a type of psychotherapy (and non-specific factors) furthers the states and processes for mental health is presented under the heading, "Enhancement of states and processes for mental health," in each chapter.

- For each way that a form of psychotherapy advances a state or process for mental health, it has a high probability of being true in my opinion, or if not this will be stated as a lesser probability for whatever reason. If the benefit is indirect this will also be mentioned. In some cases, the outcome depends on circumstances, such as for example if behavioral therapy includes social activity, then the probability of social connectedness is much higher than if solitary activity is recommended. I will mention when this scenario applies. Any research data relevant to the given point will be presented.
- When a "form" of psychotherapy has very distinct components I will cover each of these separately to the extent that it is possible, so for example cognitive therapy and behavioral therapy, instead of cognitive behavioral therapy (CBT), or instead of mindfulness CBT, cover mindfulness on its own.
- Resolution of mental illness follows from advancing the core states and processes for mental health, including positive affectivity over negative affectivity that ensues naturally from the others. The way that a given form of psychotherapy, and also nonspecific factors, achieves this will be discussed. For example, behavioral therapy resolving depression by advancing activity, and hence increasing behavioral activation while reducing behavioral inhibition.
- An occurrence I have noted is that people have a tendency to generate different versions of virtually everything. For example, major religions have split into numerous forms over time. Psychotherapy is not immune from this occurrence, and one of the only things that can be counted on is that with time subdivisions of a given form of psychotherapy will emerge. If a supposed type of psychotherapy is actually a clear variant of a major form then it is covered under that form, such as for example Behavioral Activation (BA) and Behavioral Activation Treatment for Depression, under behavioral therapy. In some instances, the name might suggest that it is distinct, whereas it is actually just a variant, and so will be subsumed under the parent form.

In conducting this research, a benefit has been learning a great deal about types of psychotherapy that in some instances I knew little about. The staggering diversity of approaches and the compelling ways that they seem to directly enhance the states and processes for mental health reinforce my notion that this is actually how psychotherapy ultimately works, but I will now have you the reader see how this perspective fits. The material presented might best be viewed as a proof of concept utilizing theory and relevant empirical evidence. An interesting outcome is what this approach contributes to synchronizing specific and nonspecific factors. The major forms of psychotherapy (along with nonspecific factors) that will now be examined to determine if and how they advance the states and processes for mental health consist of:

- Acceptance and Commitment Therapy
- Behavioral Therapy
- Cognitive Therapy

- Compassion-Focused Therapy
- Emotion-Focused Therapy
- Existential Psychotherapy
- Gestalt Therapy
- Interpersonal Psychotherapy
- Mindfulness-Based Therapy
- Narrative Therapy
- Person-Centered Therapy
- Positive Psychotherapy
- Problem-Solving Therapy
- Psychoanalytic Therapy
- Rational-Emotive Therapy
- Nonspecific Psychotherapy Factors

Chapter 11

Acceptance and commitment therapy

Overview

Avoiding psychological, and for that matter physical, pain is impossible: it is part of life. It has been said that the only things certain in life are death and taxes, but with offshore tax havens and the shadow economy more broadly, it is definitely possible to avoid taxes, although not for most of us. Hence, the only things certain in life are pain and death, quite negative but unfortunately true. The positive perspective on this reality is that how we relate to pain plays a key role in outcomes. This perspective is central to Acceptance and Commitment Therapy (ACT), and instead of trying to avoid or overcome psychological and physical pain, a person learns how to accept it and progress toward important goals in a committed way (Bramwell and Richardson, 2018; Dindo et al., 2017; Hayes and Follette, 2004; Yovel, 2009).

Two concepts that stand out are experiential avoidance and psychological flexibility. Experiential avoidance refers to an unwillingness to remain in contact with aversive experiences, such as anxiety; we try and avoid this contact (Bramwell and Richardson, 2018; Dindo et al., 2017; Hayes and Follette, 2004; Yovel, 2009). However, as with avoidance generally, outcomes can be undesirable despite short-term pain reduction. For instance, if a person is fearful of romance and intimacy, the anxiety is avoided by remaining single, a scenario that entails diminished rewards in exchange for short-term relief of the anxiety. If the person accepts the anxiety and moves toward romance and intimacy, then rewards will likely follow. Psychological flexibility is used somewhat differently than it is as an executive function, instead indicating the ability to flexibly adapt behavior in the service of valued goals (Bramwell and Richardson, 2018; Dindo et al., 2017; Hayes and Follette, 2004; Yovel, 2009). The term behavioral flexibility seems more to the point.

"Psychological flexibility" is achieved through six steps: flexibly and purposefully being mindful of psychological and physical states in the present moment, obviously drawing on mindfulness; ensuring balanced and broad perspectives so that adverse thoughts and feelings do not trigger maladaptive avoidance responses; clarifying values and goals; committing to these objectives; willingly accepting the adverse experiences that invariably arise in progressing to these goals; cognitive defusion, meaning stepping back from thoughts that

States and Processes for Mental Health. DOI: 10.1016/C2020-0-00574-8

lead to experiential avoidance, and seeing that they are not realities and truths (Dindo et al., 2017). Cognitive fusion, whereby many stimuli are linked often arbitrarily to negative feelings, is seen as fostering behavioral and psychological inflexibility (Yovel, 2009). The concept of committed action is also crucial and targeted behaviors are required for reaching valued goals (Yovel, 2009).

By accepting adverse emotional and physical feelings in the present moment, and not attempting to avoid these feelings, positive outcomes can follow. I often tell clients that one of the unique aspects of anxiety is that despite its unpleasantness no one dies from it, at least directly, and that if a person faces the anxiety-provoking stimulus in a constructive fashion the anxiety almost invariably diminishes. On the other hand, anxiety typically grows with avoidance. Indeed, short of medication the only solid way to reduce anxiety is to face the source. This reality seems to align well with ACT that also fosters committed actions to achieve valued goals with a reliance on psychological flexibility.

Enhancement of states and processes for mental health

ACT should by its very orientation increase **Activity,** based on committed action to achieve valued goals and overcoming experiential avoidance. For example, if a person values learning music then actions are taken to learn music, or to draw or socialize and the like. Research backs up this assertion for at least physical activity, the only form of activity really investigated. Moffit and Mohr (2015) randomly assigned 59 minimally active community participants to a 12-week pedometer-based walking program, or the same walking program plus an ACT DVD covering setting goals and other ACT principles. Postintervention the ACT group achieved significantly greater increases in physical activity based on pedometer values, and was more likely to achieve goals set. Focusing on a high-intensity constant work rate cycle exercise program, Ivanova et al. (2015) randomly assigned 39 low activity women to either an ACT plus music listening group, or just a music listening control group. Exercise tolerance time, perceived effort, and postexercise enjoyment were significantly better in the ACT plus music listening group. Another study investigating the impact of ACT on physical activity for women was conducted by Butryn et al. (2011). Random assignment was made to either an education or ACT group, both involving a couple of sessions. The ACT participants increased their physical activity level significantly more than did those in the education group.

Demonstrating that control conditions can also improve physical activity is a study by Kangasniemi et al. (2015) who randomly assigned 138 physically inactive adults 30–50 years of age to either a feedback or ACT plus feedback group. Participants in both groups significantly increased their objective and self-reported physical activity levels. Although it cannot be said that the ACT aspect worked given that the feedback alone did, cognitions fostering greater physical activity stability improved more with the ACT intervention. Setting goals that are valued and committing to actions that achieve these goals, while accepting negative experiences triggered in the process, intuitively will increase activity and certainly for forms of activity that advance mental health.

Psychological Defense Mechanisms are advanced with ACT in regards to adaptive dissociation. The fusion of stimuli to negative feelings (cognitive fusion) impairs psychological flexibility. Cognitive defusion entails stepping back from these thoughts fostering experiential avoidance to gain a more objective perspective, and seeing that they are not real or truthful. This stepping back or gaining psychological distance from cognitions fused to negative feelings is a form of adaptive psychological dissociation. For example, a person believes that intimacy can only lead to hurt, and from this particular cognitive fusion avoids intimate relationships. Based on the fusion the linkage between intimacy and hurt seems real and how things must unfold. By psychologically distancing oneself from this linkage, a more balanced perspective can be achieved, such that other options are possible as with intimacy and pleasure. Cognitive defusion achieves this psychological dissociation. As pertains to positive cognitive distortions, ACT is unlikely to directly advance this form of psychological defense, given that cognitions associated with negative feelings are not altered but accepted. However, by overcoming experiential avoidance and achieving outcomes previously not believed to be possible, cognitive perspectives relevant to the given focus are indirectly improved. Interestingly, sublimation a mature classical defense mechanism, whereby negative emotions are channeled into constructive pursuits, is very much facilitated by accepting negative feelings and redirecting the energy into committed action to achieve goals.

Social Connectivity is only likely to improve from ACT if a valued goal is improving social intimacy, and the person has avoided it due to fear. Accepting the fear and committed action can lead to real social connectedness. An occurrence I have noted many times over is that people who are fearful of social intimacy avoid it, and are often not really aware of the fear until they try and get close to another person. At this point the fear is activated and avoidance follows. From client reports it appears that online dating sites are loaded with people who engage in a futile cycle of wishing for a relationship and trying to approach one, only to pull back and avoid once a real possibility arises, due to fear of intimacy. Then as loneliness sets in the desire for closeness is triggered repeating the cycle. Accepting the anxiety and refraining from experiential avoidance on the path to real intimacy will help the person achieve social connectedness.

Enhanced **Regulation** appears to directly follow from the acceptance of disturbing feelings and thoughts component of ACT. Adverse internal experiences have a power to motivate based on negative reinforcement, whereby behavior that reduces or eliminates the adversity is reinforced. By accepting the adverse experience and not engaging in experiential avoidance, the negative reinforcement based motivation loses its influence. An area where this has been quite well studied is disordered eating. Forman et al. (2016) examined acceptance-based behavioral treatment for obesity, randomly assigning 190 participants to 25 sessions of ACT behavioral treatment or standard behavioral therapy extended over a year.

Weight, moderator, and mediating variable assessments were taken at baseline, 6 months, and 12 months posttreatment. Participants in the ACT behavioral treatment group attained a significantly greater reduction in weight at 12 months with a stable 10% reduction, whereas those in the standard behavioral therapy group initially lost weight but tended to regain it. Psychological acceptance of food-related urges was identified as a mediating influence for the ACT behavioral group, indicating improved self-regulation of urges to eat derived from tolerating discomfort (Forman et al., 2016). Forman and Butryn (2015) reviewing ACT for weight loss indicate that acceptance-based interventions are effective, and particularly for those who are most susceptible to eating in response to internal and external cues. They propose that this benefit is due to improved self-regulation of eating behavior. Investigating ACT for binge eating, Juarascio et al. (2017) conducted a small open trial involving 19 participants treated with Acceptance-Based Behavioral Therapy. They found that improvements in acceptance were strongly correlated to decreases in binge eating.

In addition to eating behavior, acceptance appears to enhance emotion regulation for children-adolescents (Burckhardt et al., 2016), aggression (Zarling et al., 2015), panic (Wang et al., 2016), and emotional responses to psychosis (Spidel et al., 2018). Burckhardt et al. (2016) randomly assigned 267 grade 10–11 students to an ACT and positive psychology group, or a control group, finding that those in the intervention group with depression, stress, and combined anxiety/depression experienced a reduction in these symptoms. They identified emotion regulation from ACT as being crucial for this benefit. Focusing on adult partner aggression, Zarling et al. (2015) randomly assigned 100 participants (68 females) to either an ACT or support and discussion intervention, both consisting of 12 weekly 2-hour sessions. Assessments of psychological and physical aggression were made pretreatment, during treatment, at the completion of treatment, and 3 months and 6 months later. Psychological and physical aggression levels diminished more in the ACT group, and a predictor was the level of emotion dysregulation: if it remained high indicating limited regulation gains aggression persisted. The researchers did not identify acceptance per se, but found that those who still demonstrated experiential avoidance indicating limited acceptance, did not benefit as much (Zarling et al., 2015).

Investigating the role of acceptance and emotion regulation for panic, Wang et al. (2016) randomly assigned 48 participants experiencing frequent panic attacks to either an emotion regulation intervention group, receiving only 5 min of acceptance training, or a no regulation group. ECG recordings were taken at baseline, while viewing aversive pictures, and during a resting state. These ECG recordings indicated that arousal from baseline to aversive pictures was significantly lower in the acceptance-based emotion regulation group. Studying psychosis combined with a history of childhood trauma, Spidel et al. (2018) randomly assigned 50 of these participants to an ACT or treatment as usual group. Participants in the ACT group improved in their ability to regulate their emotional reactions, and experienced less severe psychotic symptoms, overall symptoms, and anxiety.

Comparing cognitive and acceptance-based interventions from a theoretical perspective, Hoffman and Asmundson (2008) suggest that both improve emotion regulation, with CBT more antecedent focused by altering cognitions that trigger adverse emotional reactions, and ACT or more precisely the acceptance part, counteracting maladaptive responses to the adverse emotions. While this likely holds quite well, the picture is somewhat less clear based on the finding that cognitive defusion from ACT and cognitive reappraisal from CBT both can reduce smoking behavior, suggesting an antecedent action for ACT (Beadman et al., 2015). Presently the evidence for cognitive defusion is limited, but for acceptance appears quite robust, strongly supporting the capacity of ACT to enhance regulation. Regarding neuroscience evidence for ACT and regulation, research is in its infancy compared to cognitive and mindfulness-based therapies, but preliminary evidence supports top-down regulation involving enhanced prefrontal cortex-amygdala (limbic system) connectivity when anxiety is the focus (Young et al., 2019).

The role of ACT for **Human-Specific Cognition** is not clear at this point, but any benefit seems to be of lower probability. The only potential option appears to be inhibiting behavior, based on reducing experiential avoidance through acceptance. For instance, if a person repeatedly responds to hunger sensations with eating, then impaired inhibition is evident. By accepting the urges to eat and not acting on them, inhibition is improved. Psychological flexibility is a major component of ACT but given that it really fosters behavioral flexibility, the direct role in improving psychological flexibility might be limited. However, the steps consisting of flexibly and purposefully being mindful of psychological and physical states in the present moment, ensuring balanced and broad perspectives so that adverse thoughts and feelings do not trigger maladaptive avoidance responses, and clarifying values and goals, do seem to advance psychological flexibility.

Self-Acceptance might well be enhanced by ACT, from two sources. First, by accepting negativity and not engaging in experiential avoidance leading to detrimental outcomes, more positive options are feasible, that will in turn improve self-concept and self-esteem. Second, committed action to achieve valued goals will almost certainly yield better outcomes consistent with a person's values, enhancing self-concept and self-esteem. An example covering both components consists of a person who fears higher education based on self-doubts. With experiential avoidance, the person rationalizes not pursuing higher education and remains in lesser work roles, hindering self-concept and self-esteem. Accepting the anxious feelings and progressing to the goal of higher education despite adversity along the way, will likely lead to academic success enhancing self-concept and self-esteem. The improved job outcome will also advance self-acceptance.

The psychological flexibility component of ACT, that as I mentioned really should be labeled behavioral flexibility based on the definition of flexibly adapting behavior in the service of valued goals, undoubtedly enhances

Adaptability. Each of the six steps mentioned earlier for "psychological flexibility" operates to improve behavioral flexibility. Generally, by reducing the inhibiting influence of negative emotions and thoughts via acceptance, and encouraging committed action to achieve valued goals despite adversity, ACT can substantially improve adaptive outcomes. This certainly transpires when the focus is repetitive maladaptive behavior that involves cycles of inhibiting emotions and avoidance behavior. A review of ACT studies by Twohig and Levin (2017) summarizing 36 randomized controlled trials found that ACT is more efficacious than waitlist and treatment as usual conditions, and equivalent to CBT, with psychological flexibility emerging as a key mechanism. A study looking at the psychological flexibility component of ACT for chronic pain found that it accounted for 6%–27% of the variance in functioning and depression, even after taking into account pain intensity, with this range of percentages quite high for any psychological variable (Scott et al., 2016). Supporting this outcome, a study by Lin et al. (2018) found that psychological flexibility mediated pre-to-post-treatment changes in pain interference, anxiety, depression, and mental and physical health for chronic pain sufferers. Higher psychological flexibility has been linked to better mental health and lower psychological flexibility to worse mental health (Tyndall et al., 2018). Hence, by improving psychological flexibility, ACT does advance adaptability and mental health.

Summary note

ACT does offer a unique perspective with the acceptance of negative experiences building on mindfulness. By accepting adversity and not engaging in experiential avoidance, along with committed action to achieve valued goals, positive outcomes are more viable. The committed action to achieve valued goals component ensures that activity will be enhanced. Cognitive defusion fosters adaptive dissociation from detrimental cognitive-emotion linkages, thereby advancing psychological defense mechanism functioning. Positive cognitive distortions might be fostered by overcoming experiential avoidance and achieving positive outcomes from committed action. Sublimation is also facilitated by channeling negative energy into constructive actions. Social connectedness can definitely be enhanced provided that this is an area subject to experiential avoidance, with committed actions to achieve the goal of improved social relationships.

Emotion and behavioral regulation is vastly improved by the acceptance component of ACT, with quite solid research evidence, and the benefit appears to be derived mostly from the response side of the equation, as opposed to cognitive therapy acting on the antecedent side. Human-specific cognition in terms of inhibition derived from acceptance, and possibly psychological flexibility as an executive function, might be advanced by ACT. Via overcoming experiential avoidance and committed actions to achieve valued goals, ACT almost certainly can improve self-concept and self-esteem, and from these, self-acceptance. Adaptability is enhanced by the psychological flexibility component of ACT that actually advances behavioral flexibility. From the major components of acceptance, committed action, and behavioral flexibility, ACT does enhance the states and processes for mental health.

References

Beadman, M., Das, R.K., Freeman, T.P., Scragg, P., West, R., Kamboj, S.K., 2015. A comparison of emotion regulation strategies in response to craving cognitions: effects on smoking behaviour, craving, and affect in dependent smokers. Behav. Res. Ther. 69, 29–39.

Bramwell, K., Richardson, T., 2018. Improvements in depression and mental health after acceptance and commitment therapy are related to changes in defusion and values-based action. J. Contemp. Psychother. 48 (1), 9–14.

Burckhardt, R., Manicavasagar, V., Batterham, P.J., Hadzi-Pavlovic, D., 2016. A randomized controlled trial of strong minds: a school-based mental health program combining acceptance and commitment therapy and positive psychology. J. Sch. Psychol. 57, 41–52.

Butryn, M.L., Forman, E., Hoffman, K., Shaw, J., Juarascio, A., 2011. A pilot study of acceptance and commitment therapy for promotion of physical activity. J. Phys. Act. Health 8 (4), 516–522.

Dindo, L., Van Liew, J.R., Arch, J.J., 2017. Acceptance and commitment therapy: a transdiagnostic behavioral intervention for mental health and medical conditions. Neurotherapeutics 14 (3), 546–553.

Forman, E.M., Butryn, M.L., 2015. A new look at the science of weight control: how acceptance and commitment strategies can address the challenge of self-regulation. Appetite 84, 171–180.

Forman, E.M., Butryn, M.L., Manasse, S.M., Crosby, R.D., Goldstein, S.P., Wyckoff, E.P., et al., 2016. Acceptance-based versus standard behavioral treatment for obesity: results from the mind your health randomized controlled trial. Obesity (Silver Spring) 10, 2050–2056.

Hayes, S.C., & Follette, V.M. (2004). Mindfulness and Acceptance: Expanding the Cognitive-Behavioral Tradition. Guilford Press: New York.

Hoffman, S.G., Asmundson, G.J., 2008. Acceptance and mindfulness-based therapy: new wave or old hat?. Psychol. Rev. 28 (1), 1–16.

Ivanova, E., Jensen, D., Cassoff, J., Gu, F., Knauper, B., 2015. Acceptance and commitment therapy improves exercise tolerance in sedentary women. Med. Sci. Sports Exerc. 47 (6), 1251–1258.

Juarascio, A.S., Manasse, S.M., Espel, H.M., Schumacher, L.M., Kerrigan, S., Forman, E.M., 2017. A pilot study of an acceptance-based behavioral treatment for binge eating disorder. Contextual Behav. Sci. 6 (1), 1–7.

Kangasniemi, A.M., Lappalainen, R., Kankaanpaa, A., Tolvanen, A., Tammelin, T., 2015. Towards a physically more active lifestyle based on one's own values: the results of a randomized controlled trial among physically inactive adults. BMC Public Health 15, 260. doi:10.1186/s12889-015-1604-x.

Lin, J., Klatt, L.I., McCracken, L.M., Baumeister, H., 2018. Psychological flexibility mediates the effect of an online-based acceptance and commitment therapy for chronic pain: an investigation of change processes. Pain 159 (4), 663–672.

Moffit, R., Mohr, P., 2015. The efficacy of a self-managed acceptance and commitment therapy intervention DVD for physical activity initiation. Br. J. Health Psychol. 20 (1), 115–119.

Scott, W., Hann, K.E., McCracken, L.M., 2016. A comprehensive examination of changes in psychological flexibility following acceptance and commitment therapy for chronic pain. Contemp. Psychother. 46, 139–148.

Spidel, A., Lecomte, T., Kealy, D., Daignealt, I., 2018. Acceptance and commitment therapy for psychosis and trauma: improvement in psychiatric symptoms, emotion regulation, and treatment compliance following a brief group intervention. Psychol. Psychother. 91 (2), 248–261.

Twohig, M.P., Levin, M.E., 2017. Acceptance and commitment therapy as a treatment for anxiety and depression: a review. Psychiatry Clin. North Am. 40 (4), 751–770.

Tyndall, I., Waldeck, D., Pancani, L., Whelan, R., Roche, B., Pereira, A., 2018. Profiles of psychological flexibility: a latent class analysis of the acceptance and commitment therapy model. Behav. Modif. doi:10.1177/0145445518820036.

Wang, S.M., Lee, H.K., Kweon, Y.S., Lee, C.T., Chae, J.H., Kim, J.J., et al., 2016. Effect of emotion regulation training in patients with panic disorder: evidenced by heart rate variability measures. Gen. Hosp. Psychiatry 40, 68–73.

Young, K.S., LeBaeu, R.T., Niles, A.N., Hsu, K.J., Burkland, L.J., Mesri, B., Saxbe, D., et al., 2019. Neural connectivity during affect labeling predicts treatment response to psychological therapies for social anxiety disorder. J. Affect. Disord. 120, 105–110.

Yovel, I., 2009. Acceptance and commitment therapy and the new generation of cognitive behavioral treatments. Isr. J. Psychiatry Relat. Sci. 46 (4), 304–309.

Zarling, A., Lawrence, E., Marchman, J., 2015. A randomized controlled trial of acceptance and commitment therapy for aggressive behavior. J. Consul Clin. Psychol. 83 (1), 199–212.

Chapter 12

Behavioral therapy

Overview

Historically, behavioral therapy has been concentrated on depression emphasizing how in this condition there is a deficiency of response contingent reinforcement of nondepressed behavior (Hopko et al., 2003). Consistent with behavioral principles, behavior change is primary and cognitive change follows from alterations in behavior (Hopko et al., 2003). In support of this proposition, it has been found that adding automatic thought modification to behavior activation does not improve outcomes, and behavioral activation (BA) therapy is as effective as cognitive therapy for altering negative thinking and dysfunctional attitudes (Jacobson et al., 1996). This is a critical distinction because cognitive therapies, as the name suggests, are based on the premise that thought change is paramount, whereas behavioral therapists view behavior as being more relevant. Confusing issues, thoughts can be viewed as behavior, but let us stick with nonthoughts as behavior. Due to how behavioral therapy has emphasized impaired reinforcement contributing to depression, it has been locked into a focus on depression. However, based on how it can overcome inhibition present with both depression and anxiety, it can be extended to anxiety (Bowins, 2012).

Consistent with how major forms of psychotherapy fracture into variants, behavioral therapy has two main variants—BA and behavioral activation treatment for depression (BATD; Hopko et al., 2003; Jacobson et al., 1996; Lejuez et al., 2001). In the case of BA, depression is seen as arising from low levels of positive reinforcement or high levels of aversive control (Jacobson et al., 1996). BATD is based on matching theory stating that depressive relative to nondepressive behavior is directly proportional to the reinforcement obtained for these two categories of behavior (Lejuez et al., 2001). BA tends to be more diverse in terms of strategies, applying mental rehearsal, periodic distraction, mindfulness training, and skills training, an approach that proponents of BATD do not see as being core to behavioral therapy (Hopko et al., 2003; Jacobson et al., 1996; Lejuez et al., 2001).

Enhancement of states and processes for mental health

With the premise of behavioral therapy in mind we will now see how and why it works, with a focus on advancing the states and processes for mental health. Regarding **Activity**, behavioral therapy achieves this by its very nature; if activity

States and Processes for Mental Health. DOI: 10.1016/C2020-0-00574-8

is not improved then it is not working for the given individual. In line with the principles of behavioral therapy, the given activity should increase reinforcement for nondepressed behavior, and what this entails is activity that is positive to the individual. I practice behavioral therapy applying both formal and informal versions, and always allow the client to identify activities that are positive in some fashion. If the person does not find tennis appealing then this is not an activity that will be included. However, if the person finds tennis to be appealing but is fearful of trying it, then it is on the list.

Another principle is to set up a hierarchy of positive activities from least to most challenging, and start with the least challenging. This graded approach is also applied within activities, such as for a person who wants to play tennis but is somewhat fearful. It would be setting the person up for failure to have them play a game right away. Instead, the individual might start by borrowing a racket and bouncing a tennis ball off the wall of a local school, then signing up for beginner lessons, then starting to play with others of limited ability. The graded steps help to build confidence and secure reinforcement. The more diverse the activities, usually the more effective behavioral therapy is, and I consider physical, social, cognitive, nature, art/hobby, and music forms as possibilities, depending on the interests of the person. Although behavioral therapists focus on reinforcement as yielding the benefit, as we learned in the Activity chapter, the high behavioral activation state (BAS) and low behavioral inhibition state (BIS) profile of being active aligns with the requirements of our evolution in hunting–gathering groups, and hence this profile is natural for us, thereby fostering mental health. Of course, a high BAS and low BIS profile is also highly consistent with reinforcement. An interesting study looking at the role of activation with behavioral therapy (BA) randomly assigned 14 depressed people to behavioral therapy and seven to treatment as usual (Santos et al., 2017). Activation preceded or co-occurred with improvements in depression for 79% of the BA participants, but none of the treatment as usual people.

Improvements in **Psychological Defense Mechanisms** with behavioral therapy are far less straightforward and are less probable, with one crucial exception—absorption. As we covered, absorption in positive foci is likely the most common form of dissociative defense, applied by everyone (see the Psychological defense mechanism chapter). When you immerse yourself in a Netflix show that is absorption, as is learning how to play tennis. Absorption in positive foci draws a person away from negative thoughts, such as occurs with worrying, replacing negative thoughts and the feelings that follow with more positive ones. Since behavioral therapy increases activities that are positive to the person, it translates into absorption in positive foci, ramping up the absorption defense, and its contribution to mental health. Even though with behavioral therapy the emphasis is on behavior, I have noted many times over that when a client engages in positive activities, negative thoughts are replaced by positive ones. Although less probable, it is feasible that as a person improves in confidence from engagement in various activities, positive cognitive distortions applied to oneself can increase. For example, "I must be physically capable as I can now play tennis." These self-referential positive perspectives might further advance mental health.

Social connectedness can definitely improve from behavioral therapy, provided that the activity has a social component. This is one reason why I emphasis social activities, or at least activities with a social aspect, when conducting behavioral therapy, as it adds the social connectedness so important given our evolution in hunting–gathering groups, and hence social brains. Loneliness is a major problem in modern society as it erodes mental health, and leaves those impacted vulnerable to stressors, such as if the person becomes physically ill, who will help? Often people in third world countries with intact families and local communities fair better in terms of mental health despite relative poverty, based on social connectedness. Increasing solitary activities with behavioral therapy obviously will not advance social connectedness, and could conceivably worsen it. If a person is quite isolated, even if not indicating that loneliness is an issue, I then suggest positive social activities. An emphasis here is on positive social activities, given that with politics and game playing that seem to represent hobby activities for many people, social contact can be more of a stress. I frequently encounter this scenario with isolated people suggesting volunteer work or group-based activities, only to have the person report that they could not tolerate the politics.

Any possible link between **Regulation** and behavioral therapy appears less probable on the surface, but is actually quite robust. Absorption in positive foci helps regulate negative emotions, as it draws a person away from negative thoughts and the mutually reinforcing cycles between negative thoughts and feelings. For example, an inactive person might worry about not being accepted, or focus on real and perceived rejection generating feelings of sadness, fear, and loneliness, that in turn create an emotional climate conducive to further thoughts perpetuating these emotions. Absorption in a positive social activity counters this mutually reinforcing negative cycle, replacing it with thoughts about being accepted, generating feelings of happiness and security, with such feelings in turn creating an emotional climate conducive to further prosocial thoughts.

The capacity of behavioral therapy to improve emotion regulation is supported by Sloan et al. (2017) who present a relevant and very interesting perspective. They conducted a review of 67 studies measuring changes in emotion regulation and symptoms of psychopathology, with diverse forms of psychotherapy applied to multiple types of psychopathology including anxiety, depression, substance abuse, eating disorders, and personality disorders. The conclusion the researchers came to is that emotion regulation is a transdiagnostic construct improving with psychotherapy regardless of form and type of psychopathology, evidenced by both maladaptive emotion regulation strategy use and overall emotion dysregulation significantly decreasing following treatment in 65 of the 67 studies reviewed (Sloan et al., 2017)! If this is true, and would seem to be supported by the vast majority of studies finding this outcome, then all forms of psychotherapy likely improve emotion regulation, making in a transtherapy process.

A possible way this might work is derived from a research study by Neacsiu et al. (2017), who had 44 anxious and depressed adults with high emotion dysregulation, attempt to downregulate negative distress induced by a disturbing personal memory recall. No instructions were provided regarding conscious emotion regulation strategies, but the participants were successful in downregulating the negative emotions. The researchers believe that even those with emotion regulation difficulties still retain effective strategies that can be employed with a nonspecific prompt (Neacsiu et al., 2017). Any form of psychotherapy could qualify as a nonspecific prompt to activate latent and effective emotion regulation strategies. Supporting the notion of emotion regulation being a major issue, Berking and Wupperman (2012) indicate that emotion regulation impairments are present in widespread forms of psychopathology. Stein (2008) provides evidence for how psychotherapy in general enhances the psychobiology of emotion regulation, including changes to the prefrontal cortex advancing top-down regulation. Hence, emotion regulation is both transtherapy (across specific types of psychotherapy) and transdiagnostic (across various forms of psychopathology).

As pertains to **Human-Specific Cognition**, the role of behavioral therapy is in the less probable range for basic cognition aside from behavioral cognitive training, and motivation. Regarding behavioral cognitive training, there is some evidence that it can improve executive functions. For example, Enriquez-Geppert et al. (2013) in a review of studies provide evidence that this type of intervention can lead to enhanced performance on tasks such as response inhibition, set shifting, memory updating, and dual task performance (multitasking). They go on to suggest that the benefits of behavioral cognitive training might even generalize to untrained tasks (Enriquez-Geppert et al., 2013), although this is a disputed issue. Motivation can definitely be improved by behavioral therapy, based on how reinforcement derived from activities positive to the individual naturally enhances motivation. For instance, if a person wishes to play the piano, and this becomes an activity focused on, then the reward from actually playing a song typically motivates further efforts to learn the piano, or even music more generally. Of course, the activity has to be positive to the person to generate reinforcement and enhance motivation. If an individual has no interest in the piano increased motivation is unlikely. Although less probable, social activity might in some instances improve social cognition, derived from how relatively isolated people often have social cognitive limitations, with the isolation worsening these limitations. By engaging regularly with people, social cognition skills such as facial expression recognition of emotions can improve.

Self-acceptance from behavioral therapy is actually a common scenario, based on improved self-concept and self-esteem derived from activity (see the Activity chapter). When an inactive person becomes active, self-efficacy for the specific type of activity increases. For instance, our tennis and piano players will experience enhanced self-efficacy for tennis and piano playing, respectively. This will further their self-concept pertaining to physical capacity from tennis self-efficacy and music capacity from piano self-efficacy. Self-evaluations based on these capacities enhance self-esteem over time. Perhaps this is a reason why behavioral therapy seems, at least in my experience, to work better when various forms of activity are addressed, compared to a single type. Consider people that you know who are active in various ways, and they almost always seem to have a robust self-concept and self-esteem, provided that they perceive some degree of success or accomplishment with the various activities. One potential drawback of behavioral therapy is that starting an activity and giving up too quickly can reinforce limited self-concept and self-esteem. By having the person select activities that seem interesting, approaching them in a graded way, and emphasizing how there can initially be a learning curve that needs to be persevered through, I have found improved effectiveness from behavioral therapy interventions.

Behavioral therapy is definitely capable of improving **Adaptability** via different processes relevant to engaging in activity and fitting actions to circumstances. Increased constructive activity is fostered by behavioral therapy and this activity can aid in fitting actions to circumstances. For instance, if a person engages in physical activities their confidence and capacity to act in this way, if required by circumstances, is enhanced. Increased social activity can facilitate interpersonal connections and a comfort level, such that if circumstances require engaging people in a cause the person can recruit assistance and feels more confident doing so. Overcoming repetitive maladaptive behavior requires that a person consciously apply the adaptive alternative pattern repeatedly, which is much more likely if the person is active. For example, if an individual tends to be emotionally distant, actively trying to connect to the emotions of others is necessary to overcome the maladaptive pattern and advance relationships.

The most prominent way the behavioral therapy can improve adaptability is by overcoming avoidance. While avoidance of objectively threatening agents is a key survival defense, avoiding that which is not objectively threatening and offers the potential for reward, is very costly (see the Psychological defense mechanism chapter). Avoidant people lose by default, and if such behavior persists and advances poor outcomes invariably follow (Olsson and Dahl, 2012). A key benefit of behavioral therapy is overcoming avoidance. In this regard, a very common mistake that people and even therapists make is assuming that feelings need proceed actions. Hence, an action is engaged in if a positive feeling regarding the activity is in place first. Briefly considering most of your daily activities the fallacy of this assumption becomes apparent: people routinely engage in actions that they just do or have to do without waiting for the right feeling to be present. Doctors do not think, "I'll see the patient once I feel the motivation," for example. The reverse is what really applies and distinguishes behavioral therapy: act and then feel the benefit. Take a person who is fearful of public speaking, a very common scenario. Waiting for a good feeling translates into ongoing avoidance. Instead, the only real way to overcome fear and the amplified (expanded) version, anxiety, is to face and overcome the fear in a graded way. Based on this approach I have had many people join Toastmasters and learn in a safe and noncritical environment how to speak in public. As long as the person engages, almost invariably they report feeling good having become comfortable with public speaking, and their adaptability increases such as taking on assignments and even jobs that require this skill. In addition, their social interactions often improve as they are more confident in telling stories and expressing their perspectives. Hence, by being active in a strategic fashion the avoidance is overcome.

Summary note

Behavioral therapy emphasizes impaired reinforcement occurring with depression, considering the balance of reinforcement that is positive (for nondepressive behavior) relative to that for depression promoting behavior. Although thoughts can change, behavior change is always primary with cognitions following. The goal is to alter behavior such that positive reinforcement is increased, and reinforcement maintaining depression is reduced. Despite this fairly straightforward and restricted focus, it does appear to advance the states and processes for mental health with a high probability for the most part. Activity is self-evident, instilling the high BAS and low BIS consistent with human evolution. Positive activities greatly enhance the absorption form of psychological defense. Social connectedness follows naturally from increased social activity, at least of a positive form. Regulation over emotions is improved by how absorption shifts the focus from negative content and mutually reinforcing cycles of negative thoughts and emotions, to a focus on positive activities and mutually reinforcing cycles of positive thoughts and emotions. Additionally, all forms of psychotherapy might well improve emotion regulation by prompting the expression of latent emotion regulation strategies. Human-specific cognition can advance in regards to executive functions if behavioral cognitive training is applied, and motivation is enhanced from increased activities and reinforcement. Improved self-concept and self-esteem derived from diverse activities enhances self-acceptance. Adaptability increases via enhanced activity and processes helping to better fit actions to circumstances, and most prominently by overcoming avoidance.

References

Berking, M., Wupperman, P., 2012. Emotion regulation and mental health: recent findings, current challenges, and future directions. Curr. Opin. Psychiatry 25 (2), 128–134.

Bowins, B.E., 2012. Augmenting behavioural activation treatment with the behavioural activation and inhibition scales. Behav. Cogn. Psychother. 40 (2), 233–237.

Enriquez-Geppert, S., Huster, R.J., Hermann, C.S., 2013. Boosting brain functions: improving executive functions with behavioral training, neurostimulation, and neurofeedback. Int. J. Psychophysiol. 88 (1), 1–16.

Hopko, D.R., Lejuez, C.W., Ruggiero, K.J., Eifert, G.H., 2003. Contemporary behavioral activation treatments for depression: procedures, principles, and progress. Clin. Psychol. Rev. 23, 699–717.

Jacobson, N.S., Dobson, K.S., Truax, P.A., Addis, M.E., Koerner, K., Gollan, J.K., et al., 1996. A component analysis of cognitive-behavioral treatment for depression. J. Consulting Clin. Psychol. 64, 295–304.

Lejuez, C.W., Hopko, D.R., Hopko, S.D., 2001. A brief behavioral activation treatment for depression. Behav. Modif. 25, 255–286.

Neacsiu, A.D., Smith, M., Fang, C.M., 2017. Challenging assumptions from emotion dysregulation psychological treatments. J. Affect. Disord. 219, 72–79.

Olsson, I., Dahl, A.A., 2012. Avoidant personality problems—their association with somatic and mental health, lifestyle, and social network. A community-based study. Comprehens. Psychiatry 53 (6), 813–821.

Santos, M.M., Rae, J.R., Nagy, G.A., Manbeck, K.E., Hurtado, G.D., West, P., et al., 2017. A client-level session-by-session evaluation of behavioral activations mechanism of action. J. Behav. Ther. Exp. Psychiatry 54, 93–100.

Sloan, E., Hall, K., Moulding, R., Bryce, S., Mildred, H., Staiger, P.K., 2017. Emotion regulation as a transdiagnostic treatment construct across anxiety, depression, substance abuse, eating and borderline personality disorders: a systematic review. Clin. Psychol. Rev. 57, 141–163.

Stein, D.J., 2008. Emotional regulation: implications for the psychobiology of psychotherapy. CNS Spectr. 13 (3), 195–198.

Chapter 13

Cognitive therapy

Overview

The term is typically cognitive behavioral therapy (CBT) but in practice it is almost exclusively cognitive in focus (Coffman et al., 2007), and since we are trying to determine how the various types of psychotherapy work, it would not be correct to combine forms. Furthermore, if we consider cognitive behavioral, is it the cognitive or behavioral component that advances mental health? Most studies that investigate CBT actually are covering cognitive therapy, unless focused on a specific type of mental illness such as obsessive–compulsive disorder where the standard CBT intervention is behavioral, in this instance, exposure and response prevention. Hence, we will concentrate on how the cognitive component of CBT might improve the states and processes for mental health.

Cognitive therapy is based on the premise that thoughts influence and trigger emotions and behavior (Beck, 1976, 1991). Strict cognitive perspectives might not even consider emotions, but more modern cognitive therapy does address emotions. The thought–emotion linkage aligns with cognitive activating appraisals triggering emotions that we considered in the Activity chapter, for example, "That was such a setback," triggering sadness based on the loss aspect. Likewise, "I know I'll be punished," triggering fear from the threat inherent in this scenario. Depressed and anxiety cognition is characterized by negative cognitive distortions both internally and externally focused (Beck, 1976, 1991). Internal refers to self-referential thoughts as with, "I really screwed that up." Underlying many of these negative automatic thoughts are themes or schemas, for example, "I lack the social skills needed to be successful," and "Everyone is smarter than me." These themes lead to the repetition of negative automatic thoughts consistent with them. Hence, cognitive therapy typically focuses on both negative automatic thoughts and underlying schema.

Cognitive therapy involves various tasks or "homework" assignments, and almost always monitoring, as, for example, daily thought records. Cognitive restructuring or reappraisal is a key component, reframing the negative automatic thoughts into more positive variants. For example, "I know I will be punished," to "I actually do not know what will transpire, and if I prepare well things will go fine." Negative schemas are also identified and reframed, largely by reappraising the negative automatic thoughts reinforcing them, but also directly. An example, of the latter might be, "I lack the social skills to be successful,"

States and Processes for Mental Health. DOI: 10.1016/C2020-0-00574-8

to, "I can and do demonstrate good social skills, such as at work with customers, and can build on these." Various other tasks might be applied but monitoring negative automatic thoughts and cognitive reappraisal, along with altering underlying schema, are central. One subtype—schema therapy—focuses on this aspect, but will be subsumed under cognitive therapy.

Enhancement of states and processes for mental health

Consistent with a focus on psychopathology, CBT is typically thought to work by correcting dysfunctional cognitions and the underlying schema associated with mental illness. However, it is viable that the cognitive focus, much as the behavioral aspect, might advance the states and processes for mental health. For **Activity** the obvious, although indirect way, is by reframing thoughts and underlying schema that hinder or block activity. If a person holds the underlying theme "I always seem to fail," and more specific negative thoughts flowing from this schema like, "I won't be able to learn music," then it follows that activity of various forms, and certainly in this instance music, will be limited. I find that by reframing specific negative thoughts, actions flow. For example, "I can't sing because I'm not good at it." Going over how in most traditional societies singing skill is not required, and most people just sing gradually becoming better, helps a person reframe their perspective to see that it is okay to sing without any real talent. The person might start with low-volume singing in private to a song they like, and gradually progress to a choir. Another common example this time for physical activity is, "I'm really uncoordinated so I cannot do sports." Reframing this to, "You have the coordination to walk as I noted when you entered the office, and walking is being physically active," helps ramp up this form of activity. The person will often start to walk beyond what is required and eventually progress to more challenging hikes, learning that they do have the coordination necessary to be physically active. This same process of reframing negative perspectives hindering or blocking actions applies to all forms of activity.

Psychological Defense Mechanisms are greatly strengthened by cognitive therapy. In the Psychological defense mechanism chapter, we covered how positive cognitive distortions appear to be one of our major defense mechanism templates (Bowins, 2004). Mental health is characterized by a positivity bias, while depression and anxiety involves a negativity bias (Beck, 1976, 1991; Beck and Clark, 1997). By replacing negative cognitive distortions with positive ones, psychological defense is greatly strengthened, thereby conferring the capacity to face adversity without incurring excessive negative emotions. For instance, negative self-referential thoughts occur with depression and anxiety, as with "I can't handle pressure." By reframing these thoughts and the underlying schema, such as "I'm a weak person," an individual will start to believe in their strengths and capacities leading to thoughts like, "Yes, I can manage that assignment because I do have the capacity it requires." It is by applying positive cognitive distortions that a person is more able to cope and be resilient to adversity. Cognitive therapy is also capable of shifting immature classical defense mechanisms to more mature ones, even in short-term therapy, based on a study by Johansen et al. (2011), who randomized 50 participants with personality disorders to either 40 sessions of cognitive or dynamic therapy, finding that even 2 years later defense mechanism functioning remained improved with both forms of psychotherapy.

Cognitive therapy can definitely improve **Social Connectedness**, again via altering negative automatic thoughts and underlying schema eroding social capacity. An occurrence noted by myself and I suspect virtually every therapist who provides cognitive therapy, is that isolation and negative social thoughts go hand in hand. Isolated people commonly express thoughts such as "Everyone's out for their own good," "People always take advantage of me," "No one every wants to remain my friend." It might seem to be something of a chicken and egg scenario, but is actually more of a mutually reinforcing scenario, whereby negative social thoughts foster isolation, and isolation activates social threat–related ideas. Isolation likely fosters such thoughts because during our evolution in hunting-gathering groups isolation was probably a relatively rare occurrence, and often arose from ostracism in response to an individual infringing on the values of the group, such as, for example, hoarding a kill. In this context, isolation would be a threat due to all the predators about, reprisals from offended same-group members, and attacks by other-group members perceiving the new person to be a threat. While a few moments of peace from the group might have been desired, true isolation was rarely a good thing.

Demonstrating how relevant negative social cognitions are for social isolation, and how cognitive therapy can enhance social connectedness, is a meta-analysis of loneliness intervention studies published between 1970 and 2009 analyzing 20 high quality ones, conducted by Masi et al. (2011). Interventions for loneliness included improving social skills, increasing social support, enhancing opportunities for social contact, and altering negative social perceptions via CBT. Although each type of intervention had a positive impact on loneliness, the most effective was altering maladaptive cognitions. This outcome is understandable because by replacing socially isolating thoughts with prosocial thoughts, people start to engage with others and see that it can be very positive and uplifting to be socially connected, leading to further prosocial thoughts, and then more effort.

The topic of **Regulation** and cognitive therapy can be extremely complex at least at a neurological level, but is actually very straightforward in other regards. In the paper, Cognitive Regulatory Control Therapies (Bowins, 2013), I present the perspective that cognitive behavioral and related techniques actually work largely be enhancing regulatory control. One key way that this transpires is by improving the positive cognitive distortion psychological defense mechanisms template, enhancing both bottom-up and top-down emotion regulation; the former by reducing negative emotions and hence limiting limbic system activity, and the latter by establishing cognitive control over emotions. Relevant to this impact, threat- and loss-relevant cognitions generating fear and sadness, respectively, are shifted to those consistent with more positive outcomes. Given the amplification effect of human intelligence on emotional information processing (see the Activity and Psychological defense mechanism chapters), we are vulnerable to amplified negative emotions that need to be regulated. Adjusting cognitive activating appraisals triggering negative emotions and altering thoughts maintaining these emotions, does help with emotion regulation.

Cognitive therapy can also assist with some of the specific emotion regulation strategies identified by Gratz and Roemer (2004), discussed in the Regulation chapter: by recording thoughts and emotional responses as part of cognitive therapy, a person becomes more aware of emotional responses and gains clarity. For example, the thought "Why bother trying, things never work out," is identified as triggering sadness, helping the person become aware of and clear about how loss themes induce this emotion. Reappraisal, a key cognitive therapy technique, in itself greatly assists in regulating emotions by replacing negative cognitive activating appraisals for emotions, such as threat, loss, and violation, with positive cognitive activating appraisals.

An interesting application of cognitive therapy pertinent to regulation is for psychosis. A hallmark of the cognitive approach to psychosis is normalization, with psychotic manifestations viewed as the extreme end of a normal continuum, and the purpose of therapy is to bring the cognitive distortions back to a more moderate level (Kingdon and Turkington, 1994; Landa et al., 2006). Cognitive techniques consist of having the person provide evidence for their beliefs, generating alternative explanations, and testing the various options (Beck et al., 2009; Kuller and Bjorgvinsson, 2010; Landa et al., 2006). For example, a person might claim, "My neighbors are following me." Likely the only "evidence" is that when the person goes outside one of the neighbors is also out, and sometimes seems to go in the same direction, which is weak. Alternative hypotheses might include, "I go out during the day when people are normally out," "I usually walk south to the stores, and my neighbors likely are doing the same." The therapist never directly challenges the psychotic belief, instead treating it as one hypothesis. The more alternatives that the person can generate the more diluted the psychotic one becomes. To test the paranoid hypothesis, the person might go out at variable times including late at night and early morning, discovering they are alone. Also, vary the direction to see if anyone follows. I practice this approach with motivated and insightful psychotic individuals, and have found it to be surprisingly effective, enabling the individual to regulate extreme cognitive distortions. Another more advanced application of cognitive therapy for psychosis applies to the content of auditory hallucinations. Frequently the content is actually expressing self-referential perspectives, such as "You're worthless," "You deserve to be tortured." For insightful individuals, I have applied this perspective with the outcome that they now understand the meaning, and by reframing self-referential negative perspectives the content can actually be less threatening!

The best evidence for how cognitive therapy regulates is provided by the impact at a neural level. In the Regulation chapter, we learned how depression and anxiety appear to involve impaired top-down regulation of excessive limbic system activity, and how the balance between emotion intensity and higher cortical regulation capacity is relevant, such that when the former exceeds the latter emotions escalate to levels consistent with depression and anxiety (Heatherton and Wagner, 2011). While this pattern of findings for depression and anxiety is quite robust, the impact of cognitive and for that matter other forms of psychotherapy is not quite as clear, and very complex. There are multiple issues involved such as whether active emotion processing is occurring, the type of neuroimaging investigation, what specific brain regions are focused on, and whether a control group is included. Interested readers might see the informative review article by Chalah and Ayache (2018) who cover many of the issues. They conclude that despite the inconsistencies and limited well controlled results, CBT does seem to exert at least an antidepressant effect by modulating emotion and cognitive networks involved in emotion generation and control (Chalah and Ayache, 2018).

Other research studies support the conclusion by Chalah and Ayache (2018). For example, Shou et al. (2017) had 17 people with depression and 18 with Post-Traumatic Stress Disorder (PTSD) complete 12 manualized sessions of CBT, and also undergo MRI scans before and after treatment, with a control group included. Enhanced connectivity between the frontoparietal network and amygdala transpired for the depressed and PTSD participants compared to the controls. Since the frontoparietal network is involved in control and regulation, they interpreted the results as CBT working by increasing cognitive control over affective processes impaired in both depression and PTSD (Shou et al., 2017). Goldin (2009) found that patients with social anxiety who complete CBT demonstrate greater prefrontal cortex (PFC) responses and reduced amygdala activation, interpreted as top-down regulation of limbic system activity. Focusing on psychosis, Mason et al. (2017) found that over 8 years of receiving CBT interventions, increased dorsolateral PFC and amygdala connectivity predicted long-term improvements in psychotic symptoms.

Regarding neural regulation, there is the definite possibility that psychotherapy by its very nature might improve neural connectivity associated with healthy regulation. In the Behavioral therapy chapter, I presented the work of Sloan et al. (2017) suggesting that emotion regulation is a transtherapy benefit, regardless of form and type of psychopathology. I proposed that this might transpire by psychotherapy prompting the activation of latent emotion regulation strategies, based on the research of Neacsiu et al. (2017), who found that even those with emotion regulation difficulties still retain effective strategies that can be employed with a nonspecific prompt. The neural component of this process conceivably being that activation of higher cortical regions unfolding naturally with psychotherapy, prompts neural regulation of dysfunctional emotional and cognitive activity, possibly via engagement of the latent emotion regulation strategies.

Human Specific Cognition has a lower probability of improving from cognitive therapy, with the exceptions of cognitive flexibility and motivation. The entire process of monitoring thoughts, seeing how they influence emotions and behavior, reframing negative perspectives, and evaluating the outcome instills flexibility of cognition, thereby enhancing this executive function (Nagata et al., 2018; Oishi et al., 2018). It is also feasible that other executive functions might be improved from the cognitive work involved in reappraisal and other strategies. Motivation can be advanced by altering demotivating thoughts: the negative thoughts so typical of depression and anxiety favor behavioral withdrawal and inhibition, and it is very difficult to feel motivated when withdrawn and inhibited. If cognitive reappraisal alters thoughts such that a person can see the benefits of approach behavior, motivation will be enhanced.

As pertains to **Self-Acceptance**, cognitive therapy can certainly be beneficial, largely based on how self-efficacy and self-esteem involve self-enhancing cognitive distortions (see the Self-acceptance chapter). Self-efficacy and self-concept represent perspectives and self-esteem evaluations that are subject to distortions. When a person experiences depression or anxiety, self-referential perspectives and evaluations are almost always negative, impairing self-concept and self-esteem, thereby detracting from self-acceptance. A person is likely to view their capacity in specific areas as lesser than what is warranted, generating negative self-efficacy. For instance, "I'm not as good as the other workers when it comes to managing customers." These negative self-efficacy perspectives in turn produces a negative self-concept. Evaluations of oneself based on these perspectives will be negative resulting in lower self-esteem. Cognitive therapy can shift the negative perspectives and evaluations in a positive direction, thereby enhancing self-concept and self-esteem, and ultimately self-acceptance. This is consistent with how cognitive therapy has emphasized negative perspectives in reference to the self as contributing to mental illness (Beck, 1976, 1991).

Adaptability typically improves with cognitive therapy primarily by enhanced cognitive flexibility. Perspectives can be very narrow and fixed when a person suffers from depression and anxiety, becoming entrenched over time. Indeed, this is one of the challenges of psychotherapy—to promote the flexibility necessary for getting people out of the ruts they are stuck in. Cognitive therapy directly targets the cognitions that reinforce inflexible behavior. Consequently, it assists in adapting behavior to current circumstances. Research has shown that cognitive flexibility increases with cognitive therapy (Nagata et al., 2018; Oishi et al., 2018).

Avoidance behavior is one of the major impediments to adaptability, and cognitive therapy usually addresses the cognitions that maintain such behavior, generating more approach behavior. For example, "There is no way that management will consider me for a promotion," maintaining avoidance to, "If

I identify the skills required to advance and address them, I might well be promoted," favoring approach. Reframing negative cognitions also plays a significant role in altering repetitive maladaptive behavior, by eliminating thoughts that maintain the ongoing dysfunctional actions. Take the thought, "People never have my best interests in mind," maintain distancing. Altering this to, "If I show that I care, then others will care about me," helps in overcoming the distancing by eliminating blocks to closeness. In terms of neural plasticity, the enhanced cognitive flexibility appears to foster alterations in neural connectivity consistent with mental health (Chalah and Ayache, 2018).

Summary note

Cognitive therapy as the name suggests focuses on thoughts. Conscious or unconscious thoughts trigger emotions aligning with the notion of cognitive activating appraisals specific to a given universal emotions: loss-sadness, threat or danger-fear, violation or damage-anger, for instance. Underscoring more specific thoughts are themes referred to as schema, from which negative automatic thoughts follow. Psychopathology such as depression and anxiety entail negative cognitive distortions. The focus of cognitive therapy is to alter the negative automatic thoughts and underlying schema through techniques such as cognitive reappraisal, to foster positive emotions and hence positive cognitive distortions.

This very popular form of psychotherapy does advance the states and processes for mental health. Although cognitive therapy is focused on thoughts, it can indirectly improve activity by altering cognitions that hinder or block activity of various forms. Psychological defense mechanisms in terms of positive cognitive distortions is vastly ramped up by shifting negative cognitive distortions to positive ones, and cognitive therapy appears to produce lasting improvements in classical defense mechanisms. Social connectedness is advanced when negative automatic thoughts and underlying schema consistent with social isolation, are replaced by prosocial cognitions, and this has been shown to be the most effective strategy for overcoming social isolation. A key way that cognitive therapy works is by enhancing regulation over negative emotions and even psychotic cognitions, such that cognitive and related psychotherapy strategies might best be referred to as cognitive regulatory control therapies. It is feasible that psychotherapy of any form actually improves the neural connectivity involved in healthy regulation, helping to explain the trans-therapy regulation benefit. Human-specific cognition with regard to cognitive flexibility and motivation can improve, the latter if thoughts limiting or blocking it are altered. By shifting negative perspectives and evaluations of oneself relevant to self-concept and self-esteem, respectively, to positive variants cognitive therapy typically enhances self-acceptance. Adaptability advances with cognitive therapy via increased cognitive flexibility better enabling a person to fit actions to circumstances, approach rather than avoid, and replacing repetitive maladaptive behavior with more adaptive actions. The impressive capacity of cognitive therapy to advance the states and processes for mental health, likely accounts for its tremendous success and popularity.

References

Beck, A., 1976. Cognitive Therapy And The Emotional Disorders. Meridian Books, New York.

Beck, A., 1991. Cognitive therapy: a 30-year retrospective. Am. Psychol. 46 (4), 368–375.

Beck, A., Clark, D., 1997. An information processing model of anxiety: automatic and strategic processes. Behav. Res. Ther. 35 (1), 49–58.

Beck, A., Rector, N., Stolar, N., Grant, P., 2009. Schizophrenia: Cognitive Theory, Research, And Therapy. Guilford, New York, NY.

Bowins, B.E., 2004. Psychological defense mechanisms: a new perspective. Am. J. Psychoanal. 64, 1–26.

Bowins, B.E., 2013. Cognitive Regulatory Control Therapies. Am. J. Psychother. 67 (3), 215–236.

Chalah, M.A., Ayache, S.S., 2018. Disentangling the neural basis of cognitive behavioral therapy in psychiatric disorders: a focus on depression. Brain Sci. 8 (8). doi:10.3390/brainsci8080150.

Coffman, S.J., Martell, C.R., Dimidjian, S., Gallop, R., Hollon, S.D., 2007. Extreme nonresponse in cognitive therapy: can behavioral activation succeed where cognitive therapy fails? J. Consult. Clin. Psychol. 75 (4), 531–541.

Goldin, P., 2009. Effects of cognitive–behavioral therapy on neural bases of emotion regulation in social anxiety disorder. Biol. Psychiatry 65 (Suppl. 1), 1215–1221.

Gratz, K.L., Roemer, L., 2004. Multidimensional assessment of emotion regulation and dysregulation: development, factor structure, and initial validation of the difficulties in emotion regulation scale. J. Psychopathol. Behav. Assess. 26, 41–54.

Heatherton, T.F., Wagner, D.D., 2011. Cognitive neuroscience of self-regulation failure. Trends Cogn. Sci. 15 (3), 132–139.

Johansen, P.O., Krebs, T.S., Svartberg, M., Stiles, T.C., Holen, A., 2011. Change in defense mechanisms during short-term dynamic and cognitive therapy in patients with cluster C personality disorders. J. Nerv. Ment. Dis. 199 (9), 712–715.

Kingdon, D., Turkington, D., 1994. Cognitive-Behavioural Therapy Of Schizophrenia. Lawrence A. Earlbaum Associates, Hillsdale.

Kuller, A., Bjorgvinsson, T., 2010. Cognitive behavioral therapy with a paranoid schizophrenic patient. Clin. Case Stud. 9 (5), 311–327.

Landa, Y., Silverstein, S., Schwartz, F., Savitz, A., 2006. Group cognitive behavioral therapy for delusions: helping patients improve reality testing. J. Contemp. Psychother. 36 (1), 9–17.

Masi, C.M., Chen, H.Y., Hawkley, L.C., Cacioppo, J.T., 2011. A meta-analysis of interventions to reduce loneliness. Pers. Soc. Psychol. Rev. 15 (3), 216–266.

Mason, L., Peters, E., Williams, S.C., Kumari, V., 2017. Brain connectivity changes occurring following cognitive behavioural therapy for psychosis predict long-term recovery. Transl. Psychiatry 7 (1). doi:10.1038/tp.2016.263.

Nagata, S., Seki, Y., Shibuya, T., Yokoo, M., Murata, T., Hiramatsu, Y., 2018. Does cognitive behavioral therapy alter mental defect and cognitive flexibility in patients with panic disorder?. BMC Res. Notes 11 (1). doi:10.1186/s13104-018-3130-2.

Neacsiu, A.D., Smith, M., Fang, C.M., 2017. Challenging assumptions from emotion dysregulation psychological treatments. J. Affect. Disord. 219, 72–79.

Oishi, S., Takizawa, T., Kamata, N., Miyaji, S., Tanaka, K., Miyaoka, H., 2018. Web-based training program using cognitive behavioral therapy to enhance cognitive flexibility and alleviate psychological distress among schoolteachers: pilot randomized controlled trial. JMIR Res. Protocols 7 (1). doi:10.2196/resprot.8541.

Shou, H, Yang, Z., Satterthwaite, T.D., Cook, P.A., Bruce, S.E., Shinohara, R.T., et al., 2017. Cognitive behavioral therapy increases amygdala connectivity with the cognitive control network in both MDD and PTSD. Neuroimage Clinic 14, 464–470.

Sloan, E., Hall, K., Moulding, R., Bryce, S., Mildred, H., Staiger, P.K., 2017. Emotion regulation as a transdiagnostic treatment construct across anxiety, depression, substance abuse, eating and borderline personality disorders: a systematic review. Clin. Psychol. Rev. 57, 141–163.

Chapter 14

Compassion-focused therapy

Overview

A self-critical nature seems to characterize many people receiving psychotherapy, based on my experience. Indeed, I rarely find strong self-reassurance. It might be the case that with mental illness people become more negative and self-critical, but persistent self-criticisms do erode the mental health foundation, an analogy being a home builder who continually uses a sledge hammer against the foundation of the house. Noting that many people in psychotherapy struggle to generate self-supporting inner voices, Paul Gilbert founded compassion-focused psychotherapy, particularly for those with shame and self-criticism (Gilbert, 2014). Gilbert (2014) takes the perspective that compassion has an evolutionary basis derived from the mammalian affiliative system, evolving in synch with attachment and affiliation. Additional relevant evolutionary systems consist of threat and protection triggering negative emotions, and the seeking and acquiring of resources generating positive emotions. When these systems are out of balance, and the threat and protection one too strong, mental health is compromised with lack of compassion (Gilbert, 2014).

Compassion enables negative emotions to be regulated, necessary given that evolved motivational and emotional systems contribute to negative emotions and destructive behaviors (Gilbert, 2014). Evolved affiliative capacities including empathy, caring, and altruistic behavior applied to others and oneself counter the more negative influences (Gilbert, 2014). Psychopathology is associated with low compassion for oneself and others, while high compassion fosters mental health, a hypothesis supported by Leaviss and Uttley (2015) in a review of compassion-focused studies. An interesting aspect regarding the origin and role of compassion is how it applies to both other people and oneself, having evolved with attachment and affiliation systems.

From the presentation of compassion-focused therapy so far, it follows that the goal is to bolster compassion for both oneself and others. Regarding how this is achieved, in general terms therapy emphasizes, first, sensitivity to suffering, and second, a commitment to alleviating the suffering (Leaviss and Uttley, 2015). This approach is logical because a person has to be aware of their own suffering and that of others to do anything about it, and then commit to relieving it. Steps to alleviate suffering include the following (Leaviss and Uttley, 2015):

- Compassionate reasoning referring to mental processing focused on suffering, such as with shame, and how to rectify it.

States and Processes for Mental Health. DOI: 10.1016/C2020-0-00574-8

- Compassionate behavior involving self-reassurance and self-soothing when applied to oneself.
- Compassionate imagery with visualization of what a compassionate stance for a given circumstance looks like to facilitate its application.
- Compassionate feelings to generate empathy and motivation.
- These steps foster a compassion orientation applied to oneself and others.

Specific strategies vary depending on the version of compassion-focused therapy, but some of the main ones include compassionate thinking about oneself and others, noting self-criticisms and responding with self-reassurance, addressing feelings of shame with compassion, countering avoidance-based coping, appreciating early life attachment problems and engaging in corrective affiliative experiences, solving problems with a focus on compassion, diary writing to facilitate compassionate behavior, and fostering a positive inner voice (Gilbert, 2014; Leaviss and Uttley, 2015; McLean et al., 2018; Sommers-Spijkerman et al., 2018). Regarding versions of this therapeutic approach, at least eight versions have been developed, such as compassion-focused therapy, mindful self-compassion, cultivating compassion training, and cognitively based compassion training (Kirby, 2017). This occurrence highlights the staggering number of psychotherapy types that exist when taking into account specific versions of major forms, and how fast variants can arise, given that this approach only started in 2000 (Gilbert, 2014). Despite the number of specific variants of this form of therapy, research is still in its infancy pertaining to what ingredients work. However, increased self-reassurance, reduced self-criticism, and reduced fear of self-compassion do appear to be crucial, when applied to oneself of course (Clapton et al., 2018; Cuppage et al., 2018; Kelly et al., 2017; Sommers-Spijkerman et al., 2018). The development of self-reassurance (self-soothing) might be a prerequisite for reduced self-criticisms (Sommers-Spijkerman et al., 2018). Considering how common lack of self-compassion is with mental illness, it is not surprising that compassion-focused therapy has been extended to many problems including depression (Diedrich et al., 2017), trauma (Kelly et al., 2017; McLean et al., 2018), eating disorders (Cuppage et al., 2018), intellectual disability (Clapton et al., 2018), dementia (Craig et al., 2018), and personality disorders (Lucre and Corten, 2013). Compassion-focused therapy appears to be expanding rapidly in its application.

Enhancement of states and processes for mental health

Compassion applied to oneself and others is very positive and brings to mind the notion of one good thing leading to another, such as if you help another person that individual might reciprocate and assist you when there is a need. However, in a world and universe ruled by the progression of order to disorder (entropy) these positive scenarios have a way of not working out, such as those who take and do not reciprocate. Hence, despite it being positive and hopeful we cannot just assume that it will be beneficial. Initially, compassion-focused therapy was applied to people who are very self-critical where it does have an intuitive logic, but this therapeutic modality has been rapidly expanded to cover many forms of psychopathology. Based on the premise of this book, we must see if and how it advances the states and processes for mental health, an occurrence that if valid supports its application to diverse conditions.

There does not appear to be any direct and unconditional way that compassion-focused therapy enhances **Activity**. It can indirectly advance activity when self-criticisms hinder efforts, such as a person who is very negative regarding their physical capacities not engaging in physical activity, or a person severely doubting their intellectual capacity refraining from school and other challenging cognitive pursuits. Shifting to self-reassurance and support allows a person to overcome their doubts and take on challenges, with successes backing up the more compassionate perspective.

Psychological Defense Mechanisms are actually very enhanced in terms of both dissociation and positive cognitive distortions (see the Psychological defense mechanism chapter), the former via disconnection from self-critical thoughts distancing a person from the ongoing negativity they subject themselves to (Gilbert, 2014). The emphasis on self-reassurance and support expressed in imagery, thoughts such as the inner voice, and compassion-based problem solving, effectively absorbs a person in positive foci furthering distancing them from negativity. Positive cognitive distortions are increased in a very straightforward fashion: self-critical thoughts clearly represent negative distortions applied to oneself, and by shifting these to self-reassuring thoughts positive perspectives are advanced. When applied to other people critical thoughts also represent negative cognitive distortions, but compassion toward others shifts these to positive cognitive distortions, such as taking the perspective that an angry person is only defending against inner pain.

Social Connectedness can be advanced when compassion is applied to others, as harsh perspectives regarding the behavior of people tend to block a person from forming solid social connections. For example, "Larry did not return my call because he is an inconsiderate jerk," shifted to, "Larry is one busy guy who also struggles with disorganization due to his ADHD, so he almost certainly just forgot to call back." The former motivates distancing from Larry, whereas the latter motivates further attempts to connect. Indirectly, social connectedness can be improved when self-critical perspectives relate to the social environment, such as "I'm so useless around people," a thought that limits efforts to engage socially. Replacing it with, "I'm a decent person and try my best with people," encourages efforts to connect with others, despite any personal limitations.

Regulation in terms of emotion regulation is believed to be enhanced by compassion-focused therapy (Gilbert, 2014; Sommers-Spijkerman et al., 2018). This occurrence naturally follows from the self-reassuring and soothing orientation, and how self-criticisms produce excessive negative emotions, including shame, guilt, regret, sadness, and anxiety. By ending self-criticisms and instilling self-support, negative emotions are soothed and hence regulated.

Analyzing eight client samples with diverse issues, Sirois et al. (2015) found that self-compassion reduced negative emotions and increased positive emotions. Negative emotions toward others can also be regulated when perceptions of violation inducing anger are replaced with understanding and compassion. For instance, "My boss was really short with me today as she is under a great deal of pressure; it can't be easy doing her job." Emotion regulation is then a major way that compassion-focused therapy advances mental health.

There does not seem to be any direct and/or highly probable way that **Human-Specific Cognition** is enhanced. The only options are indirect and lower probability, such as motivation increasing from improved self-support. It is also feasible that compassion applied to others improves social cognition by providing a more balanced understanding of the motives and intentions of others. For instance, "She is angry because of the pressure she is under, and people do seem to displace their frustration and anger onto others."

Self-compassion interventions powerfully advance **Self-Acceptance** given that ongoing self-criticisms erode self-concept and self-esteem. Returning to the analogy of the home builder who wields a sledge hammer against the foundation, a self-critical person weakens the core that supports their self-concept and self-esteem. Self-acceptance is then lacking. By adopting a self-reassuring stance and ending the self-criticisms, self-concept and self-esteem steadily improve, leading to greater self-acceptance. Self-compassion therapy is generally very empowering, and so ideally suited to those who feel disempowered.

Adaptability is not clearly and directly advanced, but might be when confidence improves from greater self-acceptance. This benefit can transpire because with solid confidence a person is willing to try behaviors that they might otherwise not have, and the increased behavioral repertoire can enhance adaptability. For example, if a person is self-critical of their appearance and desirability, attempts to engage a prospective partner are unlikely to unfold when an opportunity arises. However, with a better perspective regarding their appearance and desirability, the opportunity is more likely to be capitalized on.

Summary note

Given how self-critical many people are, and certainly those seeking or needing psychotherapy, it follows that an approach emphasizing compassion can be very helpful. Compassion toward oneself and others does counter the negativity that often exists within a person and in relationships. To achieve compassion the approach emphasizes sensitivity to suffering, self and other, and a commitment to alleviating it. Steps include compassion-oriented reasoning, behavior, imagery, and feelings. Consistent with how basic forms of psychotherapy subdivide, several versions of compassion-focused therapy have arisen despite the approach only starting with the new millennium. Through various techniques clients are made aware of criticisms applied to the self and other, negative feelings related to these negative perspectives, and the likely origins in earlier relationships.

Compassion is actively fostered in terms of feelings, thoughts, and behavior, with the goal of developing a supportive inner voice and understanding toward others.

Although a seemingly straightforward approach—instilling compassion toward oneself and others—several of the states and processes for mental health are advanced, but there is substantial variability in the robustness of this outcome. Activity is only likely to be enhanced when self-criticisms limiting efforts are replaced with perspectives encouraging the person to challenge themselves. Psychological Defense Mechanisms are powerfully advanced in terms of both dissociation and positive cognitive distortions: dissociation by distancing a person from self-criticisms along with absorption in positive messages, and positive cognitive distortions by shifting negative perspectives regarding oneself and others to positive compassion-oriented thoughts. Compassion applied to others can improve social connectedness as critical beliefs toward other people typically result in social distancing, whereas understanding fosters approach. Enhanced emotion regulation is a key force with compassion-focused therapy, because criticisms applied to the self and others result in excessive negative emotions that are difficult to regulate, whereas compassionate perspectives sooth these negative emotions and foster positive ones. Human-specific cognition is not likely to be improved from a compassion approach, and only will when increased self-support enhances motivation, and elevated understanding of others strengthens social cognition. Self-acceptance is robustly advanced because ongoing self-criticisms erode self-concept and self-esteem, while self-compassion steadily improves these important aspects of psychological functioning. Adaptability is only likely to advance when greater self-acceptance leads to improved confidence, and a person increases their behavioral repertoire accordingly yielding greater behavioral capacity. Despite its simplicity compassion does align with good mental health and is capable of advancing the key aspects of it.

References

Clapton, N.E., Williams, J., Griffith, G.M., Jones, R.S., 2018. 'Finding the person you really are… on the inside': compassion focused therapy for adults with intellectual disabilities. J. Intellect. Disabil. 22 (2), 135–153.

Craig, C., Hiskey, S., Royan, L., Poz, R., Spector, A., 2018. Compassion focused therapy for people with dementia: a feasibility study. Int. J. Geriatr. Psychiatry 33 (12), 1727–1735.

Cuppage, J., Baird, K., Gibson, J., Booth, R., Hevey, D., 2018. Compassion focused therapy: exploring the effectiveness with a transdiagnostic group and potential processes of change. Br. J. Clin. Psychol. 57 (2), 240–254.

Diedrich, A., Burger, J., Kirchner, M., Berking, M., 2017. Adaptive emotion regulation mediates the relationship between self-compassion and depression in individuals with unipolar depression. Psychol. Psychother. 90 (3), 247–263.

Gilbert, P., 2014. The origins and nature of compassion focused therapy. Br. J. Clin. Psychol. 53 (1), 6–41.

Kelly, A.C., Wisniewski, L., Martin-Wagar, C., Hoffman, E., 2017. Group-based compassion-focused therapy as an adjunct to outpatient treatment for eating disorders: a pilot randomized controlled trial. Clin. Psychol. Psychother. 24 (2), 475–487.

Kirby, J.N., 2017. Compassion interventions: the programmes, the evidence, and implications for research and practice. Psychol. Psychother. 90 (3), 432–455.

Leaviss, J., Uttley, L., 2015. Psychotherapeutic benefits of compassion-focused therapy: an early systematic review. Psychol. Med. 45 (5), 927–945.

Lucre, K.M., Corten, N., 2013. An exploration of group compassion-focused therapy for personality disorder. Psychol. Psychother. 86 (4), 387–400.

McLean, L., Steindl, S.R., Bambling, M., 2018. Compassion-focused therapy as an intervention for adult survivors of sexual abuse. J. Child Sex. Abuse 27 (2), 161–175.

Sirois, F.M., Kitner, R., Hirsch, J.K., 2015. Self-compassion, affect, and health-promoting behaviors. Health Psychol. 34 (6), 661–669.

Sommers-Spijkerman, M., Trompetter, H., Schreurs, K., Bohlmeijer, E., 2018. Pathways to improving mental health in compassion-focused therapy: self-reassurance, self-criticisms and affect as mediators of change. Front. Psychol. doi:10.3389/fpsyg.2018.02442.

Chapter 15

Emotion-focused therapy

Overview

Emotions are prominent in mental illness of various forms, and given how we like to set up discrete entities, it was inevitable that someone would create a form of therapy with this focus. Actually, it was two people—Les Greenburg and Sue Johnson—who in the 1980s established emotionally focused couple therapy (Greenberg and Johnson, 1988). Following this early united start Sue Johnson continued developing the approach for couple therapy, while Les Greenberg shifted to individual therapy creating process-experiential therapy (Greenberg, 2004). The name emotion-focused therapy (and also emotionally focused therapy) replaced the earlier title, and is typically applied to all such therapies, including Les Greenburg's newer revised version of couple therapy (Goldman and Greenberg, 2013).

The different names and discrete variants carry over to the structure of emotion-focused therapy, with segmenting of theoretical entities and therapeutic processes into numerous distinct types. For example, Greenberg lists six principles of emotion processing: awareness, expression, regulation, reflection on experience, transformation of emotion by emotions, and corrective emotional experience (Elliot and Greenberg, 2007; Greenberg, 2004, 2010). There are also four emotion responses types (Greenberg, 2004, 2010; Pavio, 2013):

- Primary adaptive—emotions that have a benefit in the current situation, such as fear when there is a real threat, anger with violations, and sadness when a loss occurs (see the Activity and Regulation chapters). These emotions motivate adaptive responses, such as withdrawal when fear is experienced.
- Primary maladaptive—in this scenario emotions are elicited by circumstances but guided by past experiences, such as fear in response to benign events based on being traumatized in the past; in other words, they are not accurately capturing current circumstances and hence are maladaptive.
- Secondary reactive—emotional responses to primary emotions, either adaptive or maladaptive. For instance, when sadness leads to more sadness and fear to intensified fear.
- Instrumental—expressed emotions based on learning the impact they have and applying it, such as contrived shame to escape punishment for a social transgression.

States and Processes for Mental Health. DOI: 10.1016/C2020-0-00574-8

Consistent with the extensive segmenting, emotion-based problems are viewed as arising from: lack of awareness or avoidance of emotions, emotion dysregulation, maladaptive emotion responses, or issues with making meaning of experiences. Carrying this segmenting approach into assessment, Goldman and Greenberg (2015) set up a 14-step case formulation to evaluate emotion-based problems. Then there are various therapeutic tasks including but not exhaustive of empathy (exploration and/or affirmation), alliance (formation and dialogue), experiencing of emotions, meaning-making, emotion expression with reprocessing, and action (Goldman and Greenberg, 2015). Four intervention processes for each session consist of collaborating on a focus, empathy, responding to client issues, and promoting client experiences such as attention to and exploration of meanings (Greenberg, 2010; Pavio, 2013). In couple therapy three motivational systems of attachment, identity, and attraction/liking are focused on (Goldman and Greenberg, 2013).

A comment I have to make at this juncture is that while emotions are very elegant and informative, there is far too much complexity in this approach, and although there are indeed primary emotions, with shades of each and combinations of these primary emotions, more of a continuous picture often emerges, aligning with how multiple individual interpretations and meanings apply. Where the approach is highly powerful based on my experience and research, primary emotions are yoked to specific evolutionary relevant circumstances. For example, rarely does a person with anger management issues make much progress without appreciating how unconscious or conscious perceptions of violation or damage precede and trigger their anger. However, to try and set up straightforward links between all these categories of emotion processes, responses, reasons for emotion-based problems, case formation procedures, and therapeutic tasks with markers appears far too complex, in my opinion. Add in the variants for individual, couple, and family therapy and the complexity escalates. For instance, a 3-stage, 9-step model of attachment restructuring for couples (Greenberg and Johnson, 1988), expanded to 5-stage and 14-step model with Greenberg and Goldman's couple therapy version (Goldman and Greenberg, 2015).

From this enormous complexity, it is challenging to distill key elements of the approach beyond the emotion focus. One such feature is that emotions are adaptive and provide information relevant to a person's circumstances. In some instances, these adaptive responses can be distorted by past life influences and amplified, contributing to mental health problems with a strong emotional component, namely depression and anxiety. People also react emotionally to their emotions, such as fearing and hence avoiding significant emotions. Exploring these emotion themes in therapy, allowing the person to safely experience them (it is a very experiential form of therapy consistent with the term process-experiential therapy), developing awareness of the emotion meaning, and providing a corrective emotional experience leading to more adaptive emotional responses foster healthier individual, couple, and family functioning. In couple and family therapy emotion meaning related to attachment problems is addressed. For example, a person might be expressing anger based on past experiences of not being listened to and/or being taken advantage of, which are emerging in the current relationship. By realizing that this is a different relationship and verbalizing needs, the person has a corrective emotional experience, no longer viewing and reacting to the other person as violating. I will focus on these core elements when looking at how emotion-focused therapy might advance the states and processes for mental health.

Enhancement of states and processes for mental health

Very little research informs regarding whether or not emotion-focused therapy impacts the states and processes for mental health, with the vast majority oriented to establishing efficacy, typically by those practicing this form of therapy, and process-related research. Regarding **Activity**, emotion-focused therapy is unlikely to have a direct effect, but can when emotional blocks to various forms of activity are removed. For instance, a person experiences a primary maladaptive emotional response of fearing, even when there is nothing objective to fear. By having the person learn the informational value of fear and how they are not reacting to real threats, a corrective emotional experience is likely to transpire, recalibrating the fear emotion such that it only arises in response to real dangers. Previously feared and avoided agents can now be approached, such as social relationships, physical pursuits, and other challenges involving activity.

Psychological Defense Mechanisms in terms of positive cognitive distortions can advance from emotion-focused therapy, and likely will with corrective emotional experiences. This outcome transpires by shifting primary maladaptive and secondary reactive emotional responses to positive emotions. To elaborate, negative emotional responses not adaptive to circumstances (primary maladaptive) and the intensification of these (secondary reactive) entail negative thought processes related to the nature of the given emotion/s, as with loss themes for sadness and threat for fear/anxiety. By correcting these negative emotional information processing distortions, positive shifts are likely to transpire fostering positive emotions and thoughts (positive cognitive distortions). The person who previously viewed benign agents as a threat reacting with fear, now sees opportunity for reward generating positive feelings and thoughts, as an example.

Emotions often relate to the social environment and attachment processes, which is a major reason for couple and family forms of emotion-focused therapy. For instance, if a person expects losses based on early life circumstances, then social relationships are perceived as an opportunity for loss and sadness. **Social connectedness** suffers as a result with impaired attachment patterns pertaining to friendships, romances, and family interactions. Focusing on the theme of sadness and loss, and the origins from past experiences, facilitates the corrective emotional experience of not linking social relationships to loss, but instead an opportunity for gain and happiness. The empathic and experiential nature of the therapeutic alliance in emotion-focused therapy also assists in improving the person's attachment capacity, thereby fostering greater social connectedness.

Regulation over emotions is a major strength of emotion-focused therapy, and with such an emphasis on emotions it would be almost unimaginable that it would not improve emotion regulation. This impact is derived from several of the tasks and processes, including awareness, experiencing, reprocessing, meaning-making, and action. To regulate emotions such as fear and anger a person must be aware of the emotion and its meaning or information value. Excessive emotional reactions of a given type are experienced and processed in therapy, with a shift to more appropriate applications of the emotions, as with real threats eliciting fear and actual violations anger. The person acts on these shifts rather than just understanding the process, helping ensure that the corrective emotional experience takes in their life. A way of capturing this emotion regulation gain from emotion-focused therapy is that the signal for negative emotions is cleaned up, reducing noise that makes emotion regulation difficult. For example, if a person reacts to day-to-day irritants as threats, the frequency and intensity of fear/anxiety can be overwhelming. By having it only arise in response to real threats, the signal for fear responses is "cleaned up" advancing regulation.

Exploration of how clients relate to their emotions and shifting maladaptive styles to adaptive ones also assists with emotion regulation. For instance, if a person fears their emotions and tries to suppress them, any negative emotional experience will be very stressful. By having the person experience emotions and appreciate the meaning relative to circumstances, the person gains a sense of control. The very empathic and "affect-tuned" therapeutic alliance also advances regulation over challenging emotions (Greenberg, 2014). Problematic emotions are "soothed" providing a template for regulation, which proponent of this form of therapy believe account for its applicability and success with eating disorders and borderline personality disorder where emotional dysregulation is common (Pos and Greenberg, 2012; Wruk et al., 2015). Hence, emotion-focused therapy does appear to strengthen emotion regulation with the therapeutic alliance providing a template that is internalized by the client.

Human-Specific Cognition is only likely to be improved if social cognition issues are present, given that understanding and working with one's own emotions and that of others is crucial for solid social cognition. Emotion-focused therapy assists in understanding the meaning of emotions relevant to circumstances, and the negative distortions present with a person's emotion processing. For instance, a person who perceives others as violating repeatedly triggering anger, learns that this distortion in emotion information processing involves a faulty perception, whereas if there is an actual violation then the reaction is valid. This type of understanding assists in improving the person's emotional reaction to others, and correctly reading emotions displayed by those interacted with, thereby advancing social cognition.

Self-Acceptance might increase if a person achieves better performance in important domains of their life from improved emotional functioning, or what can be viewed as superior emotional intelligence. For example, if the corrective emotional experiences free a person to approach rather than avoid challenges, then success is more likely. A study of generalized anxiety, applying emotion-focused therapy, found that based on qualitative data the 14 participants experienced better emotional functioning, confidence, and self-acceptance (Timulak et al., 2017).

Emotion-focused therapy can improve **Adaptability** when primary maladaptive emotional responses occur fostering maladaptive behavior. For instance, take the person who perceives that others only mean loss of one form or another, and so withdraws from people and social circumstances. By correcting this distortion and emotionally experiencing the impact of an altered perspective, the individual will respond positively to social circumstances that are likely to produce gains. This represents enhanced adaptability given that the person can distinguish positive from negative signals and respond accordingly.

Summary note

Emotion-focused therapy assists clients in understanding and working with their emotions. In my opinion it is overly complex with far too many discrete theoretical constructs, processes, and therapeutic strategies. However, distilled to the core elements the notion of attending to emotions in therapy is important. Key elements consist of: emotions (at least primary ones) have adaptive value relative to circumstances, emotional responses can be distorted by past experiences, and people do have emotional reactions to their emotions that can be adaptive or maladaptive. Exploring these emotion themes in therapy, having a client experience relevant emotions, and fostering a corrective emotional experience can advance the states and processes for mental health. However, most of the options in this regard are conditional on the corrective emotional experience removing impediments to advancement:

- Activity of various forms can be increased if emotions or the person's reaction to them is blocking such activity.
- Social connectedness is improved when dysfunctional emotional responses impair relationships.
- Human-specific cognition in terms of social cognition advances if emotional understanding and capacity is impaired.
- Self-acceptance increases when functioning improves due to greater emotional intelligence.
- Adaptability advances if a primary maladaptive emotional response contributes to maladaptive behavior.

Psychological defense mechanisms in terms of positive cognitive distortions are likely to improve, based on emotional information processing shifting from negative to positive, fostering positive cognitive distortions. Emotion-focused therapy appears to have the strongest impact on emotion regulation, via assisting clients in understanding emotions relative to circumstances, why maladaptive emotional responses are occurring, emotional reactions to emotions, and providing an impactful corrective emotional experience. The empathic and affect-tuned therapeutic alliance also assists with emotion regulation.

References

Elliot, R., Greenberg, L.S., 2007. The essence of process-experiential/emotion-focused therapy. Am. J. Psychother. 61 (3), 241–254.

Goldman, R.N., Greenberg, L.S., 2013. Working with identity and self-soothing in emotion-focused therapy for couples. Fam. Process 52 (1), 62–82.

Goldman, R.N., Greenberg, L.S., 2015. Case Formulation in Emotion-Focused Therapy: Co-Operating Clinical Maps for Change. American Psychological Association, Washington, DC.

Greenberg, L.S., 2004. Emotion-focused therapy. Clin. Psychol. Psychother. doi:10.1002/cpp.338.

Greenberg, L.S., 2010. Emotion-focused therapy: a clinical synthesis. J. Lifelong Learning Psychiatry 8 (1), 32–42.

Greenberg, L.S., 2014. The therapeutic relationship in emotion-focused therapy. Psychotherapy (Chicago) 51 (3), 350–357.

Greenberg, L.S., Johnson, S., 1988. Emotionally Focused Therapy for Couples. Guildford Press, New York.

Pavio, S.C., 2013. Essential processes in emotion-focused therapy. Psychotherapy (Chicago) 50 (3), 341–345.

Pos, A.E., Greenberg, L.S., 2012. Organizing awareness and increasing emotion regulation: revising chair work in emotion-focused therapy for borderline personality disorder. J. Pers. Disord. 26 (1), 84–107.

Timulak, L., McElvaney, J., Keogh, D., Martin, E., Clare, P., Chepukova, E., et al., 2017. Emotion-focused therapy for generalized anxiety disorder: an exploratory study. Psychotherapy (Chicago) 54 (4), 361–366.

Wruk, S.M., Greenberg, L.S., Dolhanty, J., 2015. Emotion-focused therapy for women with symptoms of bulimia nervosa. Eat. Disord. 23 (3), 253–261.

Chapter 16

Existential psychotherapy

Overview

All other forms of psychotherapy covered have drawn primarily from psychology, but existential psychotherapy is mostly derived from philosophy, establishing it as distinct just from the very origin. While the history of existential philosophy is extensive, the two most influential writers, at least for the psychotherapy application, are Soren Kierkegaard and Friedrich Nietzsche who back in the 1800s formulated key perspectives. Soren Kierkegaard believed that anxiety is inherent in human existence, and people avoid it through means such as religion and science, instead of living with passion and commitment from the inner depth of their existence (Kaufman, 1975). Friedrich Nietzsche proposed that God is dead, and that science and rationality had become the new deity, but less comforting than religious beliefs (Kaufman, 1975). Understanding of life should come from a personal perspective and not from these external influences, and one crucial aspect of this understanding is that people long to become more than they are due to a state of perceived deprivation, referred to as ontological privation (Kaufman, 1975).

Philosophy is renowned for perspectives as opposed to absolute realities. Consistent with the notion of perspectives there are multiple ideas both contributing to the development of existential psychotherapy and shaping the actual therapeutic approach. However, the contributions of Kierkegaard and Nietzsche do resonate throughout these. At the core is the notion that human existence does entail anxiety, derived from the threat inherent in conflicts between the demands of reality and our preference for alternative options, focused on the themes of death, aloneness, meaninglessness, and freedom and responsibility (Frankel, 2002; Frankl, 1997; Yalom, 1980). The conflict arises because each of these themes has stress and challenges associated with them that we would prefer not to have to encounter: the reality of death conflicting with the desire to continue living, how we essentially live our own life contrasting with the need to be with others, the absence of absolute meaning to life when we want some purpose, not wishing to have the pressure of responsibility but that comes with freedom. These conflicts produce existential anxiety that many people avoid, the avoidance producing negative consequences, whereas facing the anxiety leads to a more successful life (Frankel, 2002; Frankl, 1997; Yalom, 1980). For instance, mentally blocking the notion of death, instead of facing it and

States and Processes for Mental Health. DOI: 10.1016/C2020-0-00574-8

consequently living life fully based on the reality of mortality. There is also the related notion of how people need to make their own meaning in life, and not seek external solutions, while taking responsibility for these choices (Frankel, 2002; Frankl, 1997; Yalom, 1980). These choices remade over the course of life provide meaning and contribute to a person's identity.

From a perspective of mental health, failure to manage the conflicts generating existential anxiety results in mental illness including depression, anxiety, guilt/shame, addictions, and others such as worse outcomes with trauma (Frankel, 2002; Frankl, 1997; Yalom, 1980). Given the fundamental nature of the conflicts underlying existential anxiety, it is impossible to not experience them, at least without the detrimental trade-off associated with avoidance. For instance, a person might opt to be controlled by another to avoid freedom and responsibility, but that control is often harmful and always limiting. The beliefs of a cult leader might be fully internalized to avoid the reality of death and the search for individual meaning, but at what cost? In terms of the actual therapy, given that everyone experiences these conflicts and existential anxiety, the therapist is an active participant and engages authentically, not acting as an "expert" or being a blank slate (Frankel, 2002; Frankl, 1997; Yalom, 1980). The client explores ways to manage the conflicts and existential anxiety, with the steps taken providing enhanced self-awareness and meaning to their life, that is based on personal values and not derived from an external prescription. What all this translates into is a person leading a life that is authentic to them, and accepting the anxiety that naturally goes with the core conflicts, although significantly diminished from the psychotherapy work pertaining to these conflicts (Frankel, 2002; Frankl, 1997; Yalom, 1980).

In line with the philosophy foundation and resulting variety of perspectives, there are many variants of existential therapy including meaning (meaning-centered) therapy, logotherapy, Daseinasnalysis, other variants applied to psychoanalysis, existential positive psychology and psychotherapy (not equivalent to positive psychotherapy per se), and existential-humanistic therapy. Existential psychotherapy is sometimes critiqued for only being suited to highly intelligent people, but this is a complete misconception as everyone experiences existential anxiety derived from the threat inherent in the core conflicts, with the central therapeutic issue consisting of facing these sources of anxiety to achieve some resolution of the conflicts and live life authentically (Frankel, 2002; Frankl, 1997; Yalom, 1980). The capacity to process complex philosophical perspectives is definitely not required, just the willingness to approach and not avoid the conflicts. Indeed, it could even be argued that an excessive emphasis on complex philosophical perspectives might even be a way of avoiding the anxiety.

Enhancement of states and processes for mental health

Existential psychotherapy is hypothesized to work by having the client manage existential anxiety and the underlying conflicts that produce mental illness manifestations, with the end result being authentic ongoing change in the person's life. This aligns with **Activity**, and although there is no direct way that it is enhanced, approach over avoidance typically does translate into activity of various forms. For instance, the person who avoids the notion of death is likely leading an unfulfilled life, compared to accepting the inevitability of death and responding by activities that enrich their life. Likewise, accepting that freedom does bring anxiety due to the range of choices and responsibility, and making the most of the potential to improve life will almost certainly lead to greater activity of some form.

Avoiding core existential conflicts and anxiety limits a person. When a person accepts anxiety as part of life and works with the core conflicts, positive changes are made that at least have the potential to induce positive cognitive distortions and absorption in positive foci, thereby advancing the **Psychological Defense Mechanism** templates of positive cognitive distortions and dissociation, respectively. This impact is indirect and perhaps not that robust, but is quite probable given how successful existential psychotherapy does produce positive changes with authentic meaning to the individual.

Social connectedness might be advanced when a person resolves the conflict between aloneness and the need to be with others, by helping to better define boundaries and what a person can realistically expect in relationships—the person cannot expect others to relieve the reality that we are really independent beings living separate lives, something quite obvious when unwanted change occurs such as terminal illness, but people can provide companionship and support along the way. This is an indirect effect and less probable.

Regulation of emotions can be both directly and strongly advanced because existential anxiety is part of human existence and attempts to avoid it, first, fail to reduce anxiety and might even increase it as is typical with avoidance, and second, any attempt to avoid limits the person often producing negative emotions, such as persevering with dismal circumstances. By facing and accepting that anxiety arising from the core conflicts is inevitable but yet can be managed, existential anxiety is directly reduced, and the personally meaningful life changes made often lead to outcomes favoring positive emotions over negative emotions. Applied to chronic mental health conditions, an existential model can improve motivation and reduce distressing negative emotions such as shame, hopelessness, and suicidality (Johnson, 1997), and instill meaning and hope (Huguelet, 2014).

There does not appear to be any direct or highly probable way that **Human-Specific Cognition** can advance from existential approaches, other than motivation indirectly improving when a person works with freedom to make meaningful changes, accepting the responsibility for setbacks. Fear of taking ownership of life can greatly limit positive motivation, and from my experience is a major reason why people get stuck in negative ruts, while taking ownership is very empowering and motivating although with some risk. Another way of framing this occurrence is that when a person is guided by fear and avoidance, as with the core conflicts and existential anxiety that is avoided, the motivation is very negative. Shifting to positive reward-based motivation is far more constructive and inspiring.

Self-Acceptance is robustly advanced from the entire process of existential psychotherapy. Self-awareness is increased and certainly pertaining to how the person is impacted by anxiety derived from the core conflicts, which most people are only vaguely aware of. Accepting that some existential anxiety is unavoidable and managing the conflicts results in a person identifying what constitutes an authentic and meaningful life to them. For instance, the person might become aware that the pursuit of wealth is pointless (to them), and what really counts is creativity of some form, shifting their career and hobby pursuits to align with this insight. From these changes, self-perspectives (self-concept) and self-evaluations (self-esteem) will gradually progress contributing to enhanced self-acceptance.

Leading life on the basis of fear and avoidance rarely entails adaptive behavior. By freeing oneself of this negative motivation and making changes that fit with a person's nature, it follows that more constructive behavior will transpire, enhancing **Adaptability**. For instance, the person who just pursues wealth without really valuing it, will miss opportunities for creative expression that fit well with their values and provide a meaningful existence. Shifting to a focus on creative expression while potentially less lucrative will yield behavior that fits and generates authentic meaning. At the very least, by facing anxiety arising from the core conflicts, a person is better able to adapt to the negative realities of life.

Summary note

Despite differences between people, we all share existential anxiety arising from the threat inherent in the core conflicts of death, aloneness, meaninglessness, and freedom and responsibility. The conflict arises from the stress and challenges of these issues and how we prefer alternative options. Failure to manage the core conflicts producing existential anxiety results in psychopathology of various forms. Avoidance in response to the core conflicts and existential anxiety limits life, whereas accepting the inevitability of some anxiety arising from these conflicts, facing the fear, and managing the conflicts, results in less existential anxiety and psychopathology. Shifting to an authentic and meaningful life is in itself capable of overcoming much of the anxiety.

Regarding the states and processes for mental health, regulation of emotions and self-acceptance are robustly advanced. Negative emotions are worsened by avoiding sources of anxiety, unless objectively threatening, and avoidance of existential anxiety and the core conflicts favors negative affectivity. Facing the anxiety and managing the core conflicts directly regulates negative emotions, and the more authentic and meaningful life changes that follow produce positive outcomes and emotional reactions. This combination favors positive emotions over negative emotions advancing emotion regulation. By becoming more self-aware of how existential anxiety has guided or misguided life, and making ongoing changes that produce an authentic and meaningful life, self-concept and self-esteem supporting self-acceptance are powerfully enhanced.

The impact of existential psychotherapy on the other states and processes for mental health is indirect, less powerful, or less probable. Activity is indirectly advanced by shifting from a life strongly influenced by anxiety from the core conflicts, to one of approach and change that is meaningful, usually increasing constructive activity. This shift will also quite likely entail positive pursuits that can induce positive cognitive distortions and dissociative absorption, furthering psychological defense mechanisms, but the impact is indirect and perhaps limited. Reduction of the conflict between aloneness and the desire to be with others can improve social connectedness, by better defining boundaries and expectations of what others can do—people cannot eliminate the reality that we move through life on our own, but can provide companionship and support along the way. Human-specific cognition is only likely to improve in terms of motivation, and this transpires by replacing negative motivation linked to avoidance with positive motivation, based upon working with freedom to make meaningful changes and accepting the responsibility for decisions (taking ownership). When a person is guided by fear and avoidance, behavior is rarely adaptive, whereas removing oneself from this negative motivation and making changes that are meaningful to the person can increase adaptability. Additionally, the negative anxiety-provoking realities of life can be faced and adapted to. So even though existential anxiety is hypothesized to work by remedying the core conflicts and existential anxiety producing psychopathology, it actually advances the states and processes for mental health, and in a very robust fashion for emotion regulation and self-acceptance.

References

Frankel, B., 2002. Existential issues in group psychotherapy. Int. J. Group Psychother. 52 (2), 215–231.

Frankl, V., 1997. Man's Search For Meaning. Pocket, New York.

Huguelet, P., 2014. The contribution of existential phenomenology in the recovery-oriented care of patients with severe mental disorders. J. Med. Philos. 39 (4), 346–367.

Johnson, D.R., 1997. An existential model of group therapy for chronic mental conditions. Int. J. Group Psychother. 47 (2), 227–250.

Kaufman, W. (1975). Existentialism from Dostoevsky to Satre (Revised and Expanded Edition). New York: Penguin Publishing Group.

Yalom, I., 1980. Existential Psychotherapy. Basic Books, New York.

Chapter 17

Gestalt therapy

Overview

Gestalt means whole, and the primary originator of this form of therapy, Frederick (Fritz) Perls, based it on the perspective that people are whole entities (Brownwell, 2010; Perls, 1969; Perls et al., 1951). The notion of wholeness focuses on experience and how it is organized into a coherent pattern, with good mental health creating complete Gestalts and healthy responses. For example, the perception of snow and cold along with the physiological sensation of coldness is integrated into seeking warmth. With mental illness such as neuroticism, there can be failure to integrate experiences resulting in incomplete Gestalts that result in inadequate responses, such as by creating blind spots. For instance, a person who is abused might not integrate the experience and then does not react to abusive treatment later in life. A goal of therapy is to transform incomplete Gestalts to complete ones, allowing the person to progress and grow (Brownwell, 2010; Perls, 1969; Perls et al., 1951).

Due to how the person's experience has not been properly processed, integrating incomplete Gestalts requires a focus on the experience of the person, emphasizing first, awareness in the present moment, and second, feeling the experience and not just talking about it (Brownwell, 2010; Perls, 1969; Perls et al., 1951). Past experiences are brought into the present moment instead of being discussed as a distant event. All aspects of the experience are to be actively expressed. A major aspect of experience that needs to be processed and expressed are emotions, with the notion that if they remain unexpressed psychological and somatic problems arise. Therapy then encourages the expression of emotions and other aspects of experience with techniques such as role playing, with one unique form the empty chair (chairwork), whereby the person addresses their own self or a significant other in the empty chair. There is the notion of experimenting to overcome experiential avoidance and foster integration of experience, providing a flexible component to therapy in contrast to a manualized approach (Brownwell, 2010; Perls, 1969; Perls et al., 1951).

A major goal of Gestalt therapy is the development of self-awareness, and from this self-actualization (Brownwell, 2010; Perls, 1969; Perls et al., 1951). Self-awareness involves the whole of experience, and not just the prominent focus. A distinction is made between figure and ground, drawing on perception from Gestalt psychology, referring to a continuum from the prominent focus to

States and Processes for Mental Health. DOI: 10.1016/C2020-0-00574-8

the background. We tend to focus on the figure such as a source of pain until this is resolved. Coherent self-awareness is impeded by excessive focus on the figure, as with a person only concentrating on their role as a parent, and not experiences in other areas. Therapy assists the person in including the background in self-awareness providing a wholeness to experience (Brownwell, 2010; Perls, 1969; Perls et al., 1951).

The discussion to this point makes it appear that Gestalt therapy is only about the self, but it does address interactions with others. These interactions are viewed as a contact boundary, that is healthy when it is flexible and a person correctly distinguishes self from others, but unhealthy when there is failure to distinguish self from others, providing for an inflexible form of relating (Brownwell, 2010; Perls, 1969; Perls et al., 1951). Identification and alienation are relevant to this contact boundary, identification referring to identifying with aspects of our true self, and correctly distinguishing what belongs to others. Alienation arises when there are deficits in seeing faults in our own self, viewing these as being in another person. Consequently, the person relates in an inflexible fashion to others, for example, not being aware of one's own anger, seeing it in others and then withdrawing. Full experiential awareness from therapy enables a person to correctly identify what arises from the self and others, fostering flexible behavior at the contact boundary (Brownwell, 2010; Perls, 1969; Perls et al., 1951). Improved relationships, actively worked on therapy as with role playing, and full self-awareness helping a person achieve individual goals and self-actualize, are the desired outcome of Gestalt therapy.

Enhancement of states and processes for mental health

Activity indirectly follows from Gestalt therapy, based on the focus on self-awareness and from this growth and self-actualization: it is impossible to self-actualize without engaging in constructive activity. Integrating incomplete Gestalts that block constructive actions facilitates this shift to personal growth and self-actualization. As an example, a person with self-doubts regarding competency fails at several jobs, repeating the doubts and inadequate behavior. Gestalt therapy brings these doubts and related negative feelings into current experience and awareness, having the person express them. The person then has a chance to see how detrimental and negative this is while expressing strengths. From this very active work in therapy, the incomplete Gestalt related to self-doubts and competency is transformed into a complete Gestalt, leading to successful work efforts.

Psychological Defense Mechanism gains from Gestalt therapy take the form of resolving dissociation which is central to Gestalt therapy, although not framed in this fashion. Incomplete Gestalts are really referring to dissociated elements of experience, blocking a healthy integration consistent with constructive responses. Typically, the impetus for this dissociation is psychological defense, such as a person who has been abused defensively dissociating aspects of the overall experience (Bowins, 2012). By becoming aware of these dissociated aspects of the experience and expressing them, integration is facilitated by Gestalt therapy. The notion of figure and ground also ties into dissociation, because excessive focus on the figure, such as abuse elements, effectively dissociates a person from the background of their life. By learning how to include the background in awareness figure merges with the background. Resolving contact boundary issues can also improve psychological defenses, because viewing aspects of the self in others represent projection, an immature classical defense. When the person learns to accurately identify self from others this immature defense ceases to be applied.

Gestalt therapy improves **Social Connectedness** from the contact boundary aspect. When a person cannot identify true aspects of the self, alienation occurs consisting of viewing one's own faults in others, and reacting to them in a repetitive negative and inflexible fashion. Clearly this does not facilitate connectedness to others. Through the full experiential awareness derived from Gestalt therapy, a person learns to distinguish what arises from the self and from others. This new understanding encourages much more flexible behavior at the contact boundary, with the person responding to true aspects of others and not the negative aspects of oneself projected onto people. For example, if the person fails to identify their own selfishness seeing it as arising from others, it will be hard to connect with people given the inflexible perspective that they will not care. By becoming aware that the selfishness is actually their own, others can now be seen as caring affording the option of social connectedness. Of course, this only applies when a person has relationship difficulties.

Regulation over emotions and thoughts occurs in various ways, some unconscious and automatic, others much more conscious and active. An example of the latter is via awareness in the moment as transpires with Gestalt therapy. Experiential awareness is a key focus with past events brought into present awareness and actively expressed. For example, if a person's parents were neglectful, instead of discussing it as some distant occurrence, the person brings the anger, sadness, and related thoughts into the present, perhaps addressing the parent in the empty chair. This experiential awareness in the moment and active expression gives a person control over the negative experience that previously was part of an unregulated incomplete Gestalt. Integrating the experience in the present moment facilitates this control as it provides for a wholeness to the experience, including the synthesis of figure and ground aspects.

Any impact of Gestalt therapy on **Human-Specific Cognition** is of lower probability, and if anything will take the form of enhanced motivation derived from the focus on personal growth and self-actualization. In addition, transforming incomplete Gestalts to complete ones and shifting rigid behavior at the contact boundary to more flexible social actions improves personal growth and likely motivation from successes. Conceivably by enhancing experiential awareness in the moment, even of past experiences brought into the present, attention might be improved.

Self-acceptance is fostered by Gestalt therapy from its emphasis on the wholeness of self-awareness as the basis of personal growth and self-actualization. An important component of this comprehensive self-awareness is resolving figure and ground instead of the common focus on disturbing foreground figures. For example, people often focus on disturbing events in their life, such as job stress and ignore the much more extensive and overall positive background. By seeing the negative figure as only one aspect and merging it into the overall more positive background, positive perspectives (self-concept) and self-evaluations (self-esteem) are fostered. Additionally, Gestalt therapy actively attempts to remove blocks limiting progress to growth and self-actualization, such as by transforming incomplete Gestalts to complete ones. For instance, a person who fails to integrate bullying experiences in youth might view people in general as being rejecting. By moving this past experience into present awareness and expressing the hurt, such as to the therapist role playing as the bully, the fragmented experience can be integrated facilitating more flexible responses to people and from this, better social outcomes advancing self-acceptance.

Adaptability is compromised when a person responds in a negative repetitious way to circumstances, as occurs with dissociated aspects of experience characterizing incomplete Gestalts. For instance, a person who has incurred abuse might not see the abuse potential in another person because of the disconnection, repeatedly becoming immersed in relationships that turn out to be abusive. Likewise, problems at the contact boundary based on not distinguishing what arises from the self and others, and projecting negative qualities of the self onto others, represent inflexible social behavior with detrimental outcomes. Gestalt therapy indirectly transforms these inflexible behaviors into flexible adaptive responses, by fusing the dissociated aspects of experience into complete Gestalts and reworking identification issues to improve behavior at the contact boundary.

Summary note

Consistent with the psychology it is derived from, Gestalt therapy emphasizes wholeness to experience. Healthy functioning follows from integrated experiences referred to as complete Gestalts, whereas nonintegrated experiences or incomplete Gestalts result in unhealthy states. Full experiential awareness in the present moment is required to transform incomplete Gestalts to complete Gestalts, with expression of emotions and thoughts paramount. Inflexible and maladaptive interactions with others are viewed as contact boundary problems, due to impaired identification of what arises from the self and others, and reacting to others as if they are the source of negativity. Full experiential awareness enables a person to correctly identify characteristics of the self and others, and respond in a more flexible and adaptive way to people.

Gestalt therapy advances the states and processes for mental health, although with variable potency and directness. The focus on comprehensive self-awareness and from this personal growth and self-actualization indirectly translates into activity of various forms. Psychological defense mechanism functioning is addressed in regards to dissociated experiences: while it is adaptive to defensively dissociate the given traumatic experience in the moment of occurrence, the ongoing impact with incomplete Gestalts is maladaptive, and by fusing the dissociated experience into complete Gestalts more healthy functioning transpires. Projection of negative aspects of the self onto others ceases with accurate identification of self and others at the contact boundary, further improving psychological defense mechanism functioning. By addressing contact boundary problems involving repetitive negative responses to people based on impaired identification, Gestalt therapy also improves social connectedness. Regulation of emotions and thoughts is advanced by full experiential awareness and expression in the present, providing control over aspects of experience that are poorly regulated. Improvements in human-specific cognition are lower probability and likely restricted to enhanced motivation derived from personal growth and self-actualization. Self-acceptance is advanced by the emphasis on full self-awareness, and in particular blending figure and ground to remove the common focus on negative aspects of experience that dominate the foreground (figure), thereby providing an overall more positive self-perspective and self-evaluation. Removal of blocks to personal growth and self-actualization also improves self-acceptance. Nonfused aspects of experience and inflexible social behavior due to impaired identification greatly reduce adaptability. By transforming incomplete Gestalts to complete ones and resolving contact boundary issues by accurate identification, Gestalt therapy can indirectly advance adaptability.

References

Bowins, B.E., 2012. Therapeutic dissociation: compartmentalization & absorption. Counsel. Psychol. Q. 25 (1), 307–317.

Brownwell, P., 2010. Gestalt Therapy: A Guide to Contemporary Practice. Springer, New York.

Perls, F., 1969. In and Out of the Garbage Pail. Real People Press, Lafayette, CA.

Perls, F., Hefferline, R., Goodman, P., 1951. Gestalt Therapy: Excitement and Growth in the Human Personality. Julian, New York.

Chapter 18

Interpersonal psychotherapy

Overview

Depression occurs in a context as opposed to a random event, and often this context is social in nature. Appreciating this occurrence, Gerald Klerman and Myrna Weissman developed interpersonal therapy for depression originating back in the 1970s (Markowitz and Weissman, 2004, 2012). As with several other forms of psychotherapy initially targeted at depression, it has been extended to additional mental health problems including anxiety, eating disorders, bipolar disorder, and addiction. The approach is humanistic taking the perspective that depression (or other mental health problems) is not the person's fault but an illness, and that mood and life situations are related (Markowitz and Weissman, 2004, 2012). Four categories of interpersonal scenarios are focused on (Markowitz and Weissman, 2004, 2012):

- Complicated bereavement (unresolved grief) following a distressing major loss.
- Role disputes involving a struggle with a significant person/s.
- Role transition where there is a major change such as starting or ending a marriage.
- Interpersonal skills deficits commonly resulting in isolation.

These four interpersonal scenarios quite comprehensively cover the range of relationship issues contributing to depression and other mental health problems.

As pertains to the delivery of interpersonal psychotherapy, it can be individual or group as with the other forms of psychotherapy we have looked at, and it is typically short term over 16 weeks. During the beginning phase (1–3 sessions), the therapist evaluates the problem and the interpersonal context, including the scenario/s that apply (Markowitz and Weissman, 2004, 2012). The client's relationship capacity is also assessed, with a focus on current relationships. The middle phase (4–14 weeks) is the actual treatment part during which the client works on improving the applicable interpersonal scenario/s, and learning to assert the solutions to achieve success (Markowitz and Weissman, 2004, 2012). The final sessions (15–16) focus on managing the loss associated with therapy ending, given that it is an interpersonal issue, and reviewing the progress made (Markowitz and Weissman, 2004, 2012). Booster sessions a month apart following the main intervention are quite commonly applied. Various techniques including role play

States and Processes for Mental Health. DOI: 10.1016/C2020-0-00574-8

and interpersonal skills training are often part of the treatment process. A goal is to have the client understand mood fluctuations in reference to their interpersonal context, and address the changes producing negative mood states (Markowitz and Weissman, 2004, 2012). Interpersonal psychotherapy draws on theoretical approaches, namely, attachment theory emphasizing how insecure attachments relate to mental health issues, and interpersonal theory focusing on how maladaptive communication patterns result in relationship difficulties (Bartholomew and Horowitz, 1991; Kiesler and Watkins, 1989; Markowitz and Weissman, 2004, 2012). Hence, interpersonal psychotherapy aims to improve attachment patterns and communication to foster healthier social relationships.

Enhancement of states and processes for mental health

Of the various forms of activity, social **Activity** is the one that will logically be advanced by interpersonal psychotherapy, and this transpires in two ways. First, as the term interpersonal suggests both the quantity and quality of social activity are typically increased. This is certainly the case when interpersonal skills deficits resulting in some degree of isolation apply. Addressing these deficits improve the quantity and quality of social interactions. Increased social activity can also transpire when role disputes and role transitions are the focus, because these interpersonal scenarios commonly lead people to withdraw or avoid relationships. For example, rather than experiencing friction with work colleagues a person has lunch alone away from the work setting. Fearing a transition from home into university, a person might avoid developing friendships that could make the shift much easier. The second way that interpersonal psychotherapy increases social activity is by the very active nature of the intervention compressed into a short time frame (Brakemeier and Frase, 2012; Markowitz and Weissman, 2004). The client must be active regarding interpersonal relationships which will increase social activity one way or another. Interestingly, physical activity might well be improved in the elderly by enhancing interpersonal strategies, according to McMahon et al. (2017) who randomly assigned 102 community living elderly people to either an interpersonal behavioral change plus evidence-based physical activity protocol, or just a physical activity group. Those receiving the interpersonal behavior change engaged in significantly more physical activity even at 6-months postintervention, than did the physical activity controls. Hence, interpersonal psychotherapy activity benefits appear to extend to physical activity!

Improvements in **Psychological Defense Mechanisms** likely ensues from better social skills and interventions for complicated bereavement, role disputes, and role transitions, as this therapeutic approach will produce much more positive beliefs pertaining to one's impact on the social environment. These beliefs qualify as positive cognitive distortions protecting against depression, anxiety, and stress: difficulties in interpersonal domains producing depression (and anxiety), entail negative cognitive distortions, and by addressing the interpersonal problems a shift from negative to positive social perspectives is highly probable, even though interpersonal psychotherapy is not focused on beliefs per se.

Social connectedness follows from successful interpersonal psychotherapy, at least when role disputes and interpersonal skills deficits are the focus: insecure attachment problems align with these interpersonal issues, and by having the person learn how to resolve role disputes and approach relationships with a better skill set, more secure attachment transpires—enhanced social connectedness. In some instances, resolving complicated bereavement and role transitions can lead to better social connectedness, such as when failure to resolve grief pertaining to a divorce prevents a person from moving on to a new romance, and when avoidance of threatening role transitions leaves a person isolated. Regarding the latter scenario, Reay et al. (2012) summarize evidence for how group interpersonal psychotherapy helps mothers suffering from postpartum depression remedy the role transitions, conflicts, losses, and social isolation they often experience that trigger depression.

Regulation over emotions is advanced by interpersonal psychotherapy given how complicated bereavement, role disputes, difficult role transitions, and interpersonal skills deficits unleash a slew of negative emotions, based on our nature as a social species. Solitary animals are not encumbered by these concerns aside from role transitions such as shifting from mother's care to making it on their own. For better or worse, mostly better, we rely on the interpersonal environment and this reliance translates into negative emotions such as sadness and fear, the root emotions of depression and anxiety, respectively, when relationships are not going well. Based on a review of emotion regulation as pertains to depression and interpersonal relationships, Marroquin (2011) indicates that emotion regulation related to depression is responsive to interpersonal influences, and such influences are very much a part of interpersonal psychotherapy. Focusing on interpersonal therapy for eating disorders, Rieger et al. (2010) identify negative social evaluations being a contributing factor to eating disorders pathology, including affect regulation, and present how the re-interpretation of these negative social evaluations during interpersonal psychotherapy produces improvements in symptoms, in part by enhanced regulation over negative affect. With a subtype of interpersonal psychotherapy—metacognition interpersonal psychotherapy—emotion–cognition integration furthering emotion regulation transpires with relevant client metaphors (Gelo and Mergenthaler, 2012). Beyond these specific ways that interpersonal psychotherapy improves emotion regulation there is the transtherapy improvement in emotion regulation occurring with all psychotherapies (see the Behavioral therapy chapter).

The social cognition component of **Human-Specific Cognition** is likely to improve from interpersonal psychotherapy, at least when interpersonal skills deficits are an issue. Such deficits are an indication that social cognition is lacking, and by addressing these issues interpersonal therapy improves various aspects of social cognition, such as gaining insight into how the client approaches interactions and reacts to others, the typical way that others respond to them based on their behavior, and biases in interpreting the intentions of others. For example, a client approaches relationships and responds to others with distrust, and others respond by distancing themselves due to the hesitancy sensed in the client. Until this pattern becomes evident from interpersonal therapy, the person repeats it endlessly. Role playing different approaches expressing trust demonstrates how alternative more positive responses from others can occur. Even deficient facial expression recognition can be remedied in therapy when the person responds to the facial expression of the therapist incorrectly, such as curiosity interpreted as anger. Resolving role disputes can also improve social cognition in some circumstances. For instance, learning to compromise and reciprocate instead of insisting on everything desired. Motivation for social actions, and even other scenarios, might improve from the active aspect of interpersonal psychotherapy which includes having the person make changes in their behavior, such as for example, grieving the loss of their marriage and moving on to other relationship opportunities.

Enhanced **Self-Acceptance** will not directly ensue from interpersonal psychotherapy, but indirectly this psychological benefit will if social behavior and outcomes improve, given that we base much of our self-concept, self-esteem, and hence self-acceptance on what transpires in the social environment. By resolving complicated grieving, role disputes, role transitions, and interpersonal skills deficits, and encouraging actions based on these changes, social outcomes shift in a positive direction. These social gains will enhance a person's social self-concept, and when re-evaluating themselves self-esteem should increase. By resolving role transition issues, other aspects of self-concept can improve, such as the student who successfully manages moving away from home and engaging with their university program.

Adaptability will be enhanced from improvements in interpersonal deficits and role transitions. Regarding the latter, when people struggle with role transitions there is frequently an inflexibility issue, such as avoiding rather than facing fears. Addressing the reason for the problematic role transition usually helps resolve the underlying issue, in this instance having the person approach rather than avoid. Altering these underlying sources of inflexible behavior enhances adaptability. In addition, improving social skills can clearly advance social flexibility. In select instances, resolving role disputes can also foster adaptability to the social environment. For instance, if the problem is failure to compromise then learning the value of this approach and applying it will greatly enhance adapting to social relationships where compromise is usually crucial.

Summary note

By focusing on complicated bereavement, role disputes, role transitions, and interpersonal skills deficits, interpersonal psychotherapy even at face value can improve functioning in the social sphere. The active nature of this time-limited approach encourages real change. Linkage of mood to the social context provides insight into why affective responses transpire, providing a way of influencing these mood fluctuations. Aspects of mental health relevant to the social environment are clearly advanced, and in some instances more general aspects are also enhanced. Regarding activity, both the quantity and quality of social activity typically improve, and the active nature of the approach ensures that benefits are applied. Better social skills and interventions for complicated bereavement, role disputes, and role transitions foster positive cognitive distortions pertaining to the social environment, thereby advancing psychological defense mechanisms. Insecure attachment problems often underlie impaired interpersonal functioning, and by improving key components of social behavior, interpersonal psychotherapy fosters better attachment and hence social connectedness.

Complicated bereavement, role disputes, challenging role transitions, and interpersonal skills deficits yield negative emotions, and improvements in these scenarios from interpersonal psychotherapy assist in emotion regulation. Given our nature as a social species, impaired relationships hinder emotion regulation while robust relationships assist with it. Human-specific cognition in terms of social cognition is likely to improve when interpersonal skills deficits are an issue. The active nature of the therapeutic approach might also enhance motivation. Self-acceptance can indirectly improve based on how we base much of our self-concept and self-esteem on what transpires in the social environment: by improving social functioning better social outcomes occur resulting in improved self-concept, self-esteem, and hence self-acceptance. Resolving interpersonal deficits and issues underlying role transition that produce inflexible behavior improves adaptability. Interpersonal psychotherapy is ultimately able to advance the states and processes for mental health, due to our nature as a social species ensuring the importance of the social environment to mental health.

References

Bartholomew, K., Horowitz, L.M., 1991. Attachment styles among young adults: a test of a four-category model. J. Personality Social Psychol. 61 (2), 226–244.

Brakemeier, E.L., Frase, L., 2012. Interpersonal psychotherapy (IPT) in major depressive disorder. Eur. Arch. Psychiatry Clin. Neurosci. 262 (Suppl. 2), 117–121.

Gelo, O.C., Mergenthaler, E., 2012. Unconventional metaphors and emotional-cognitive regulation in a metacognitive interpersonal therapy. Psychother. Res. 22 (2), 159–175.

Kiesler, D.J., Watkins, L.M., 1989. Interpersonal complementarity and the therapeutic alliance: a study of relationship in psychotherapy. Psychotherapy 26 (2), 183–194.

Markowitz, J.C., Weissman, M.M., 2004. Interpersonal psychotherapy: principles and applications. World Psychiatry 3 (3), 136–139.

Markowitz, J.C., Weissman, M.M., 2012. Interpersonal psychotherapy: past, present and future. Clin. Psychol. Psychother. 19 (2), 99–105.

Marroquin, B., 2011. Interpersonal emotion regulation as a mechanism of social support in depression. Clin. Psychol. Rev. 31 (8), 1276–1290.

McMahon, S.K., Lewis, B., Oakes, J.M., Wyman, J.F., Guan, W., Rothman, A.J., 2017. Assessing the effects of interpersonal and intrapersonal behavior change strategies on physical activity in older adults: a factorial experiment. Ann. Behav. Med. 51 (3), 376–390.

Reay, R.E., Mulcahy, R., Wilkinson, R.B., Owen, C., Shadbolt, B., Raphael, B., 2012. The development and consent of an interpersonal psychotherapy group for postnatal depression. Int. J. Group Psychother. 62 (2), 221–251.

Rieger, E., Van Buren, D.J., Bishop, M., Tanofsky-Kraff, M., Welch, R., Wilfley, D.E., 2010. An eating disorder-specific model of interpersonal psychotherapy (IPT-ED): causal pathways and treatment implications. Clin. Psychol. Rev. 30 (4), 400–410.

Chapter 19

Mindfulness-based therapy

Overview

In researching a topic, the typical pattern is increasing clarity with more progress, but in the case of mindfulness the more articles read the less clear I became, due to how there are so many takes on what it actually involves. Some themes do repeat although by various names, including attention, awareness, being present, acceptance, experience without judgment, nonreactivity, self-compassion (Baer, 2009; Coffey et al., 2010; Van Dam et al., 2018; White, 2014). With so many diverse terms applied mindfulness must represent a spectrum of approaches, rather than something more focused such as behavioral activation or thought change. In a revealing article pertaining to "mind the hype," Van Dam et al. (2018) point to how mindfulness has really become a fad based on both researcher and media involvement, with research glossing over variations. Consistent with this scenario, the research literature is characterized by mostly cross-sectional studies lacking active control conditions, an occurrence that will artificially accentuate its effectiveness (Van Dam et al., 2018). Interestingly, although almost everything has been thrown into the pot, it has been commented that key ingredients of Buddhist philosophy from which it is derived have been neglected, such as deconstruction of the self and nonself (Samuel, 2015).

Making matters even more convoluted, there are numerous "types" of mindfulness-based psychotherapeutic interventions including but not exclusive of: mindfulness-based stress reduction, mindfulness-based cognitive therapy, mindfulness-based relationship enhancement, mindfulness-based relapse prevention, mindfulness-based eating approaches, Integrative Body–Mind Training, and basic meditation. Furthermore, a given type can have multiple components such as meditation, yoga, body scans, stretching, thought change, and a host of options for how attention is to be directed. No wonder further reading resulted in less clarity!

Taking it back to its roots, mindfulness is meditation at a core level. All forms of meditation pertain to how attention is directed in the present moment with awareness a key aspect (Waelde, 2004). The term, present moment is crucial to consider and yokes to the notion of time. We perceive time as past, present, and future—the psychological arrow of time. Having an interest in the notion of time and it being an important theoretical construct, some of my work has focused on time and the relationship to consciousness, expressed in a

States and Processes for Mental Health. DOI: 10.1016/C2020-0-00574-8

paper hypothesizing that consciousness evolved on the basis of time distinctions (Bowins, 2017). I propose that the future represents potentialities only varying in probability, the present actualization of potentialities, and the past actualized potentialities in a "quantum actualization record." For example, in the next few minutes there are various options pertaining to what you might do. Some are more probable, as with reading on or getting a coffee, and others less probable such as spontaneously brake-dancing. It is said in physics that anything that is not impossible (based on the laws of the universe) is possible, but vary in probability. The present moment from milliseconds to at most a few seconds involves actualization of potentialities; this is hypothesized to occur at a quantum level involving a constellation of micro quantum wave functions collapsing to yield the macro form (Bowins, 2017). Let us say that you go with the less probable brake-dancing option instead of reading on. No matter how you wish or try to change it, the "record" will show that you started to brake-dance. This occurrence becomes part of the past in what I believe is a permanent record.

Considering evolution, the present moment is all-important because it is within that very brief stretch that fitness enhancing or diminishing behavior is engaged in. If you miss a predator, then it is game over, and likewise, if you miss the interest of a prospective partner you lose out. What distinguishes consciousness from unconsciousness is awareness and the ensuing motivation in the present moment, as attention and very sophisticated information processing actually transpires unconsciously (Bowins, 2018). Conscious awareness appears to have evolved to minimize the actualization of maladaptive potentialities and maximize the actualization of adaptive potentialities in the present moment (Bowins, 2017). Awareness of a predator motivates a rapid survival response. Likewise, awareness of an opportunity motivates actions to capitalize on it. In contrast to what is often thought, conscious awareness likely characterizes animal species from reptiles to primates consistent with its hypothesized evolutionary value (Butler, 2012; Butler et al., 2005; Fabbro et al., 2015; Tannenbaum, 2001). Awareness of the present moment and the ensuing motivation enables rapid shifts in behavior to optimize evolutionary fitness outcomes.

Time distinctions, conscious awareness, and actualization of potentialities in the present moment, ties in very well to Buddhist teachings. Siddhartha Gautama as the originator of Buddhism accepted many tenants of Hinduism, but diverged by rejecting the notion of a soul or atman that is reborn, based on a critical observation and belief: there is no permanence to anything, only a sequence of one moment of appearance leading to the next (Harvey, 2012). Essentially, the only thing that is permanent is change! He believed that human suffering originates from seeking permanence when none exists, or in other words attachment and longing (Harvey, 2012). Nirvana occurs when a person is free of attachment and longing. This perspective aligns with the notion of the present moment being a very brief time period during which potential occurrences are actualized and pass quickly into a past that we cannot access, other than via memories, whereby a mental representation is introduced into the present moment. Based on these aligned concepts there is a logic to not seeking permanence and accepting that everything is indeed fleeting. Both also emphasize the importance of the present moment and conscious awareness of it. Of crucial significance is what an organism is aware of in the present moment.

Most animal species with limited, but not insignificant, intelligence relative to humans, likely have a cleaner signal for conscious awareness emphasizing evolutionary fitness relevant occurrences, such as the approach of a predator or opportunity for a meal. Human intelligence and the ensuing complexity of thought processes, often muddies the signal with many negative thoughts and experiences intruding into conscious awareness, a very common scenario with depression and anxiety related to how human intelligence amplifies emotions by making the cognitive activating appraisals underlying them more intensive, extensive, and repetitive (Bowins, 2004). Muddying the waters of conscious awareness further, we cling to these experiences in a misguided attempt to seek permanence. From a therapeutic standpoint, cleaning up the signal such that negativity not relevant to immediate evolutionary fitness considerations is removed, makes a great deal of sense. Based on Buddhist teachings the benefit is even greater if we do not attach to whatever is in the present moment, and instead observe and accept it without reacting and judging, unless of course the awareness has evolutionary fitness implications such as the approach of a real tiger. Hence, the replacing of negative conscious awareness with a more peaceful experience is at the core of mindfulness. I believe that all forms of meditation and yoga, via various strategies, actually work by eliminating or at least reducing negativity in conscious awareness. Hence, when we now look at how mindfulness might advance the states and processes for mental health, I will frame it as meditation (and yoga) to go against the grain and counter the fad aspect.

Enhancement of states and processes for mental health

Given my focus on meditation and not just the mindfulness, I will point out how meditation, including yoga, might advance the states and processes for mental health, but the presentation will be somewhat slanted to mindfulness based on the research literature. Regarding **Activity**, the passive nature of meditation would actually seem to counter it, but by freeing oneself of negative awareness in the moment, unless that negative awareness requires actions to preserve or advance evolutionary fitness, many outcomes are possible. Focusing on mindfulness-based approaches for physical activity, Schneider et al. (2018) conducted a systematic review of 40 such studies. They found that mindfulness interventions emphasizing psychological factors relevant to physical activity, do appear to produce a benefit, but many of the studies are cross-sectional and so correlation, preventing a firm conclusion regarding direction: it is possible that those with high levels of physical activity have better mental health, and hence respond better to mindfulness targeted to psychological factors pertinent to physical activity.

Countering the findings of the Schneider et al. (2018) review is a workplace study by Van Berkel et al. (2014), randomly assigning 259 workers to either a mindfulness training intervention or a control group only receiving information on existing lifestyle behavior. Outcome measures were taken at baseline, 6, and 12 months, and included physical activity based on accelerometers, and also fruit consumption as an indicator of healthy eating. No differences emerged between the experimental and control groups at 6 or 12 months (Van Berkel et al., 2014). A finding with mindfulness research is that due to how the literature is saturated with cross-sectional studies having a high risk of bias, mindfulness outcomes appear to be unrealistically positive, and often not confirmed by well-designed experimental studies containing an active control condition, as opposed to a waiting list group for instance (Van Dam et al., 2018).

One way that meditation likely advances activity of diverse forms is by countering the negative awareness occurring with stress, anxiety, and depression, given that such content favors inhibition, withdrawal, and avoidance. For example, worry equally present with stress, anxiety, and depression but labeled rumination in this condition (Olatunji et al., 2010), makes it very difficult to engage in positive activities advancing mental health. However, at least based on research evidence, the probability of increased activity from meditation is not in the high range.

Meditation actually appears to operate largely through **Psychological Defense Mechanisms**, or more specifically absorption. In the Psychological defense mechanism chapter, we covered how dissociation is a major template with absorption the most common and adaptive form applied by everyone. What it entails is immersion in a positive focus drawing a person away from the negative thoughts and emotions characterizing depression, anxiety, and even worry without formal mental illness. The absorption focus can be unlimited provided that it is positive to the individual. If a person cannot stand rap music immersion in a rap music video is not likely to work well, but if the individual loves the blues then watching a video with this theme will foster absorption.

Absorption in a positive focus naturally transpires with meditation and yoga of all forms (Bowins, 2012). Consider the mindfulness themes mentioned at the start of this chapter—attention, awareness, being present, acceptance, experience without judgment, nonreactivity, self-compassion—and note how they are all compatible with immersion in positivity. As mentioned in the Psychological defense mechanism chapter, meditation involves absorption in repeated vocalizations, breathing, other bodily sensations, peaceful thoughts, images, or external stimuli producing a trance like state, dissociating the person from distressing reality allowing pleasing mental images or fantasies to dominate conscious awareness (Castillo, 2003). Furthermore, there is typically active instruction in how to redirect attention away from distressing cognitions, emotions, and memories, maximizing the more positive or neutral stimulus focus consistent with the particular form of meditation (Waelde, 2004).

Divisions of meditation into types have been proposed with arguably the most straightforward, concentrative, and mindful, the former occurring when there is an object of meditation such as the traditional "Om" representing the primordial vibration of creation from Hinduism (Waelde, 2004). Mindfulness emphasizes awareness of the present moment (Waelde, 2004). Like with so many distinctions, this typing only goes so far as there are many overlapping components applied to the numerous forms of meditation, limiting the applicability of neat classifications. However, immersion in a chant, for instance, does involve an object or focus. Likewise, awareness of mental states with acceptance and compassion, and without judgment and reactivity, fosters peaceful absorption in the present moment. Both remove a person from negative conscious awareness, and certainly that associated with mental illness, replacing it with a positive conscious awareness fostering mental health. Yoga in the form of stretching and breathing exercises involves absorption in the physical activity. More aerobic varieties of Yoga, and vigorous exercise generally, also generate absorption with the added advantage of released endogenous opioids that likely enhance the dissociative state (Bowins, 2012). One advantage of subsuming meditation (and yoga) under absorption, assuming that it is true, is bringing a unifying framework to a very disparate and confusing area, as evidenced by the pronounced lack of clarity for even just mindfulness.

Social Connectivity on the surface seems unrelated to meditation and mindfulness, and any possibility will likely be in the lower probability category. A potential option is that by diminishing negative awareness in the present moment and fostering positive awareness, a person is more open to social engagement and connections. Conceivably this might even extend to nature connectedness, as emerged from an interesting study by Apsey and Proeve (2017) who divided 115 undergraduates into mindfulness meditation, loving-kindness meditation, and progressive muscle relaxation groups, each receiving Internet presentations of the given intervention. Afterward, they tested participants social and nature connectedness. Both forms of meditation produced equal and enhanced perceived social and nature connectedness compared to progressive muscle relaxation (Apsey and Proeve, 2017). This study is limited in a number of ways including 75% females, undergraduate students only, and small numbers in each group, hence replication with a broader population is necessary before the results can be considered valid. A qualitative study applied to real life circumstances examined the connection between homeless women and their young children, finding that mindfulness training improved the parent–child relationship (Alhusen et al., 2017). Obvious limitations of research in this area require more controlled investigations. However, results from the two studies suggest the possibility that mindfulness training can improve social connectedness.

Mindfulness and meditation more generally is believed to enhance **Regulation**. Various components of regulation have been linked to mindfulness including, emotion regulation, self-regulation, and self-control (Leyland et al.,

2018a; Tang et al., 2016). Many of the research studies incorporate neuroimaging, hence the psychological and neural aspects of regulation and mindfulness will be covered together. In a review of 27 studies, Leyland et al. (2018a) concluded that mindfulness is superior to comparison groups for regulating negative affect, and this appears to transpire directly as opposed to via a mediating psychological change. Comparing smokers and nonsmokers, Tang et al. (2016) found that for both groups enhanced self-control occurred following Integrative Body–Mind Training, with increased activation of the anterior cingulate cortex (ACC) and medial prefrontal cortex (mPFC), suggesting top-down regulation. Focusing on anxiety, Zeidan et al. (2014) discovered that mindfulness training relative to just attending to breathing, reduced anxiety and this improvement was associated with increased activation of the ACC, ventromedial PFC, and anterior insula. Countering the negative result for attention to breathing, Doll et al. (2016) trained healthy individuals in this technique and then exposed them to aversive pictures. Attention to breathing regulated the aversive emotions with a neural activation pattern consistent with top-down regulation: left dorsolateral PFC and fronto-parietal activation, and reduced amygdala activation. Resting state amygdala activity appears to be increased with stress, anxiety, and depression, and mindfulness training can reduce it (Taren et al., 2015; Way et al., 2010). Supporting the notion of a common neural pathway for regulation (see the Cognitive therapy chapter), Opialla et al. (2015) compared healthy participants receiving either mindfulness or cognitive reappraisal training, discovering that both interventions recruited overlapping brain regions involved in neural regulation, with the medial PFC and amygdala central.

Among the various issues connected with mindfulness research is the distinction between short-term and long-term practitioners. Chiesa et al. (2013) in a review suggest that for the former top-down regulation applies, whereas with long-term practitioners, bottom-up regulation involving reduced resting limbic system reactivity transpires. Focusing on long-term mindfulness meditation practitioners, Laneri et al. (2017) discovered increased anterior ACC, mPFC, and anterior insula activation compared to a control group, when processing social pain for another person. This pattern of neural activation supports top-down processing for experienced mindfulness meditation practitioners. Comparing Vipassana meditators having a mean of 8 years, 2 hour/day experience to matched control participants, Holzel et al. (2007) found greater rostral ACC and dorsal medial PFC activity with meditation focused on breathing. Hence, experience with meditation appears to influence the degree of regulation and associated neural activation/connectivity, but the pattern seems consistent with increased top-down regulation.

The potential of mindfulness, or meditation more broadly, to advance **Human-Specific Cognition**, only appears to be probable for executive functioning given how it promotes focused attention and mental control. Lin et al. (2018) found that trait mindfulness is related to less interference on accuracy and reaction time tasks, consistent with enhanced attention. In a review of earlier studies, Chiesa et al. (2011) discovered support for improved attention, and possibly working memory, but comment that there are a mix of outcomes and studies have methodological limitations. Additional studies have identified enhanced attention (Fabbio and Towey, 2018; Moore and Malinowski, 2009). In another review, Gallant (2016) uncovered evidence supporting increased inhibition with mindfulness, understandable given how a person gains more control over what is experienced in the present moment. Cognitive flexibility appears to improve with the evidence covered under Adaptability (see below). Attempts have been made to improve executive functions in older adults applying mindfulness with mixed outcomes. Smart and Segalowitz (2017) found that compared to an active control condition, older adults experienced improved performance monitoring with a mindfulness intervention. However, a review of randomized controlled trials by Berk et al. (2017) did not find any cognitive improvement from mindfulness-based interventions applied to older adults. Leyland et al. (2018b) tested the impact of mindfulness training on executive functions in young children, discovering that it did not impact on these capacities. Hence, while specific executive functions, namely, attention, inhibition, and cognitive flexibility, might well improve with mindfulness at least in adults, a broader impact appears doubtful.

Social cognition and mindfulness has been examined but with mixed results. For instance, Schonert-Reichl et al. (2015) compared children in a social and emotional learning program involving mindfulness to those in a regular social responsibility program, finding that prosocial behavior including empathy and perspective taking, improved more in the former group. However, focusing on adults, Melloni et al. (2013) did not uncover any social cognitive benefit from mindfulness meditation compared to a control group. More research needs to be conducted to determine what if any benefits meditation has on social cognition.

Self-Acceptance and mindfulness do not seem to have a clear link on the surface, but might due to how mindfulness helps a person be more accepting of what is experienced in the present moment, without judgment and reactivity. Negative awareness involves a slew of adverse thoughts and emotions frequently reinforcing one another, and many of these are typically self-referential. For example, "Did I really screw up with that job interview," triggering negative emotions leading to more self-depreciating thoughts, and so on. Mindfulness encourages a person to passively observe such thoughts and accept them without reacting. This accepting stance opens the door to more self-enhancing thoughts and perceptions that can flow during awareness of the present moment. Noting that the impact of mindfulness on self-concept is still in its infancy, Crescentini and Capruso (2015) reviewed existing studies relevant to this linkage, finding that it can shape self-concept in a healthier direction. Applying a cross-sectional design to 301 university students, Xu et al. (2016) found that self-acceptance mediates the relationship between mindfulness and wellbeing. So, mindfulness quite likely improves self-acceptance.

The capacity of mindfulness to advance **Adaptability** likely transpires via increased cognitive flexibility. People often get trapped into negative thought processes, both internally and externally focused, not showing flexibility in the processing of new information. This occurrence certainly applies to various forms of mental illness, such as overly anxious people repeatedly perceiving threats that either do not exist or are vastly amplified. By countering this negative awareness, mindfulness and likely any form of meditation can restore cognitive flexibility. Even just inhibiting one stream of thought and shifting to another more positive focus with absorption, fosters cognitive flexibility. Providing experimental support, Fabbio and Towey (2018) compared 18 long-term meditation practitioners to a matched control group who had never practiced meditation, measuring attention, visual search abilities, working memory, interference task performance, and information processing styles. They found that the experienced meditators showed greater cognitive flexibility, as well as attention and working memory. Likewise comparing experienced meditators to meditation-naive controls, Moore and Malinowski (2009) uncovered enhanced attention and cognitive flexibility in the meditation group, based on interference and concentration/endurance tests. Hypothesizing that cognitive inflexibility occurs with anxiety, Lee and Orsillo (2014), randomly assigned 66 anxious participants to either a mindful-breathing, music-assisted relaxation, or thought wandering condition, testing task-switching capacity. They discovered improved cognitive flexibility in both the mindful-breathing and relaxation groups compared to the thought wandering condition. Via enhanced cognitive flexibility meditation improves adaptability: the cognitive component of adaptability is being able to flexibly shift thoughts, plans, and strategies, based on incoming information. Given the cognitive fixation inherent in many forms of mental illness this change is very challenging limiting adaptability, but cognitive flexibility is restored by meditation.

Summary note

Meditation of all forms, including mindfulness, appears to replace negative awareness in the present moment so prominent in mental illness, with positive awareness. This shift in the content of awareness counters the inhibition, withdrawal, and avoidance that occurs with depression, anxiety, and even stress. Activity of various forms is then more likely to ensue, although the literature is limited in its support at this point. The absorption form of dissociation places psychological defense mechanisms in a central role with mindfulness and meditation generally, given that all variants of meditation likely operate via absorption in positive awareness, removing a person from negative awareness. Enhanced social connectedness from mindfulness is in the lower probability range, but with the shift from negative to positive awareness removing or reducing inhibition, withdrawal, and avoidance, more constructive social contact might transpire.

Meditation definitely appears to ramp up regulation of various forms with quite an impressive body of research support. This research also demonstrates that for the most part top-down neural regulation is involved, consistent with the notion of a general effect of psychotherapy on emotion regulation (see the Behavioral therapy chapter), with neural processes facilitating this benefit (see the Cognitive therapy chapter). The executive functioning component of human-specific cognition is improved by mindfulness, at least for attention, inhibition, and cognitive flexibility. Preliminary evidence suggests some benefit for social cognition, but this is lower probability. Once again by replacing negative awareness with positive awareness, and in particular that pertaining to self-referential thoughts, self-concept and hence self-acceptance can improve from mindfulness. The cognitive flexibility that seems to transpire with meditation, perhaps by shifting attention away from negative awareness to positive content, advances adaptability. Overall then it certainly appears that mindfulness and meditation in general advances some of the states and processes for mental health, with a strong impact for psychological defenses mechanisms (dissociative absorption), emotion regulation, and select aspects of human-specific cognition.

References

Alhusen, J.L., Norris-Shortle, C., Cosgrove, K., Marks, L., 2017. "I'm opening my arms rather than pushing away:" perceived benefits of a mindfulness-based intervention among homeless women and young children. Infant Mental Health J. 38 (3), 434–442.

Apsey, D.J., Proeve, M., 2017. Mindfulness and loving-kindness meditation. Psychol. Rep. 120 (1), 102–117.

Baer, R.A., 2009. Self-focused attention and mechanisms of change in mindfulness-based treatment. Cognit. Behav. Ther. 38 (Suppl. 1), 15–20.

Berk, L., Van Boxtel, M., Van Os, J., 2017. Can mindfulness-based interventions influence cognitive functioning in older adults? A review and consideration for future research. Aging Mental Health 21 (11), 1113–1120.

Bowins, B.E., 2004. Psychological defense mechanisms: a new perspective. Am. J. Psychoanal. 64, 1–26.

Bowins, B.E., 2012. Therapeutic dissociation: compartmentalization & absorption. Counsel. Psychol. Q. 25 (1), 307–317.

Bowins, B.E., 2017. Consciousness & time: a time-based model of the evolution of consciousness. J. Behav. Brain Sci. 7 (1), 9–20.

Bowins, B.E., 2018. The rational unconscious: implications for mental illness & psychotherapy. Am. J. Psychother. 71, 28–38.

Butler, A.B., 2012. Hallmarks of consciousness. Adv. Exp. Med. Biol. 739, 291–309.

Butler, A.B., Manger, P.R., Lindahl, B.I., Arhem, P., 2005. Evolution of the neural basis of consciousness: a bird-mammal comparison. Bioessays 27 (9), 923–936.

Castillo, R.J., 2003. Trance, functional psychosis, and culture. Psychiatry 66 (1), 9–21.

Chiesa, A., Calati, R., Serretti, A., 2011. Does mindfulness training improve cognitive abilities? A systematic review of neuropsychological findings. Clin. Psychol. Rev. 31 (3), 449–464.

Chiesa, A., Serretti, A., Jakobsen, J.C., 2013. Mindfulness: top-down or bottom-up emotion regulation strategy?. Clin. Psychol. Rev. 33 (1), 82–96.

Coffey, K.A., Hartman, M., Fredrickson, B.L., 2010. Deconstructing mindfulness and constructing mental health: understanding mindfulness and its mechanism of action. Mindfulness 1 (4), 235–253.

Crescentini, C., Capruso, V., 2015. Mindfulness meditation and explicit and implicit indicators of personality and self-concept changes. Front. Psychol. doi:10.3389/fpsyg.2015.00044.

Doll, A., Holzel, B.K., Mulej-Bratac, S., Boucard, C.C., Xie, X., Wohlschlager, A.M., et al., 2016. Mindful attention to breath regulates emotions via increased amygdala-prefrontal cortex connectivity. Neuroimage 134, 305–313.

Fabbio, R.A., Towey, G.E., 2018. Long-term meditation: the relationship between cognitive processes, thinking styles and mindfulness. Cogn. Processes 19 (1), 73–85.

Fabbro, F., Aglioti, S.M., Bergamasco, M., Clarici, A., Panksepp, J., 2015. Evolutionary aspects of self and world consciousness in vertebrates. Front. Hum. Neurosci. 26 (9). doi:10.3389/fnhum.2015.00157.

Gallant, S.N., 2016. Mindfulness meditation practice and executive functioning: breaking down the benefit. Consciousness Cognit., 116–130. doi:10.1016/j.concog.2016.01.005.

Harvey, P., 2012. An Introduction to Buddhism: Teachings, History, and Practices. Cambridge University Press, Cambridge.

Holzel, B.K., Ott, U., Hempel, H., Hackl, A., Wolf, K., Stark, R., et al., 2007. Differential engagement of anterior cingulate and adjacent medial frontal cortex in adept mediators and non-mediators. Neurosci. Lett. 421 (1), 16–21.

Laneri, D., Krach, S., Paulus, F.M., Kanske, P., Schuster, V., Sommer, J., et al., 2017. Mindfulness meditation regulates anterior insula activity during empathy for social pain. Hum. Brain Map. 38 (8), 4034–4046.

Lee, J.K., Orsillo, S.M., 2014. Investigating cognitive flexibility as a potential mechanism of mindfulness in generalized anxiety disorder. J. Behav. Ther. Exp. Psychiatry 45 (1), 208–216.

Leyland, A., Emerson, L.M., Rowse, G., 2018b. Testing for the effect of a mindfulness induction on child executive functions. Mindfulness 9 (6), 1807–1815.

Leyland, A., Rowse, G., Emerson, L.M., 2018a. Experimental effects of mindfulness inductions on self-regulation: systematic review and meta-analysis. Emotion. doi:10.1037/emo0000425.

Lin, Y., Fisher, M.E., Moser, J.S., 2018. Clarifying the relationship between mindfulness and executive attention: a combined behavioral and neurophysiological study. Social Cogn. Affect. Neurosci. doi:10.1093/scan.nsy113.

Melloni, M., Sedeno, L., Couto, B., Reynoso, M., Gelormini, C., Favaloro, R., et al., 2013. Preliminary evidence about the effects of meditation on interoceptive sensitivity and social cognition. Behav. Brain Funct. doi:10.1186/1744-9081-9-47.

Moore, A., Malinowski, P., 2009. Meditation, mindfulness and cognitive flexibility. Consciousness Cognit. 18 (1), 176–186.

Olatunji, B.O., Broman-Fulks, J.J., Bergman, S.M., Green, B.A., Zlomke, K.R., 2010. A taxometric investigation of the latent structure of worry: dimensionality and associations with depression, anxiety, and stress. Behav. Ther. 41 (2), 212–228.

Opialla, S., Lutz, J., Scherpiet, S., Hittmeyer, A., Jancke, L., Rufer, M., et al., 2015. Neural circuits of emotion regulation: a comparison of mindfulness-based and cognitive reappraisal strategies. Eur. Arch. Psychiatry Clin. Neurosci. 265 (1), 45–55.

Samuel, G., 2015. The contemporary mindfulness movement and the question of nonself. Transcult. Psychiatry 52 (4), 485–500.

Schneider, J., Malinowski, P., Watson, P.M., Lattimore, P., 2018. The role of mindfulness in physical activity: a systematic review. Obes. Res. doi:10.1111/obr.12795.

Schonert-Reichl, K.A., Oberle, E., Lawlor, M.S., Abbott, D., Thomson, K., Oberlander, T.F., et al., 2015. Enhancing cognitive and social-emotional development through a simple-to-administer mindfulness-based school program for elementary school children: a randomized controlled trial. Dev. Psychol. 51 (1), 52–66.

Smart, C.M., Segalowitz, S.J., 2017. Respond, don't react: the influence of mindfulness training on performance monitoring in older adults. Cogn. Affect. Behav. Neurosci. 17 (6), 1151–1163.

Tang, Y.Y., Tang, R., Posner, M.I., 2016. Mindfulness meditation improves emotion regulation and reduces drug abuse. Drug Alcohol Depend., S13–S18. doi:10.1016/j.drugalcdep.2015.11.041.

Tannenbaum, A.S., 2001. The sense of consciousness. J. Theor. Biol. 211 (4), 377–391.

Taren, A.A., Gianaros, P.J., Greco, C.M., Lindsay, E.K., Fairgrieve, A., Brown, K.W., et al., 2015. Mindfulness meditation training alters stress-related amygdala resting state functional connectivity: a randomized controlled trial. Social Cogn. Affect. Neurosci. 10 (12), 1758–1768.

Van Berkel, J., Boot, C.R., Proper, K.I., Bongers, P.M., Van Der Beek, A.J., 2014. Effectiveness of a worksite mindfulness-based multi-component intervention on lifestyle behaviors. Int. J. Nutr. Phys. Activity 11, 9. doi:10.1186/1479-5868-11-9.

Van Dam, N.T., Van Vugt, M.K., Vago, D.R., Schmalzl, L., Saron, C.D., Olendzki, A., et al., 2018. Mind the hype: a critical evaluation and prescriptive agenda for research on mindfulness and meditation. Perspect. Psychol. Sci. 13 (1), 36–61.

Waelde, L.C., 2004. Dissociation and meditation. J. Trauma Dissoc. 5 (2), 147–162.

Way, B.M., Creswell, J.D., Eisenberger, N.I., Lieberman, M.D., 2010. Dispositional mindfulness and depressive symptomatology: correlations with limbic and self-referential neural activity during rest. Emotion 10 (1), 12–24.

White, L., 2014. Mindfulness in nursing: an evolutionary concept analysis. J. Adv. Nurs. 70 (2), 282–294.

Xu, W., Oei, T.P., Liu, X., Wang, X., Ding, C., 2016. The moderating and mediating roles of self-acceptance and tolerance to others in the relationship between mindfulness and subjective well-being. Health Psychol. 21 (7), 1446–1456.

Zeidan, F., Martucci, K.T., Kraft, R.A., McHaffie, J.G., Coghill, R.C., 2014. Neural correlates of mindfulness meditation-related anxiety relief. Social Cogn. Affect. Neurosci. 9 (6), 751–759.

Chapter 20

Narrative therapy

Overview

We tend to think of storytellers as having a special talent enabling them to speak elegantly or write fiction, but we all generate stories about our own life referred to as narratives. Often these narratives are repeated and expressed to others, and in the process refined. Back in the 1980s, it occurred to a couple of New Zealand therapists, Michael White and David Epston, that this concept lent itself to psychotherapy, ushering in narrative therapy (White and Epston, 1990). At a more informal level, psychotherapists of different theoretical orientations routinely listen to the explanations clients generate to explain various occurrences. The relevance of narratives in mental illness actually goes way back to Freud, who claimed that neurosis creates gaps in autobiographical narratives (Habermas, 2006).

The notion of a story implies something not objective or real, as the term fiction versus nonfiction captures. Subjectivity is a hallmark of narrative therapy, representing a postmodernist perspective that there is no objective reality, only subjectivity with reality socially constructed (White and Epston, 1990). In the process of producing and telling a story, or if you like a fiction, about one's life, the person is including psychologically relevant content pertaining to experience, meaning, and the way that they process information. Representing linguistic creations, narratives have features including a structure and time sequence that can be informative (Gale et al., 2003). From a mental health perspective narratives that are positive, organized with an internally and externally coherent structure counter mental illness, whereas negative, disorganized narratives lacking coherence are problematic (Gale et al., 2003; White and Epston, 1990). Internal coherence refers to consistency within the given story regarding some aspect of one's life, whereas external coherency pertains to alignment with other self-relevant stories. For example, a story about career is characterized by success while a story about social involvements entails failure, demonstrating external lack of coherence.

Beyond the general emotional tone and coherency of a narrative there are key aspects that can be addressed and remedied, one being whether a person portrays agency: the stories a person generates often indicate the control and influence they perceive over others and their own life (Polkinghorne, 1996). Agentic (agent) narratives indicate a perception of influence and capacity to impact on

States and Processes for Mental Health. DOI: 10.1016/C2020-0-00574-8

others and situations, while victim narratives express an ineffectual perspective (Polkinghorne, 1996). The degree of complexity is also relevant, with "thin" narratives frequently prescribed by others and limiting, such as "lazy" (White and Epston, 1990). More embellished narratives are usually healthier as they are multilayered with a balance of perspectives, such as, "When it comes to physical labor I've never been that motivated, but really enjoy solving problems, and have made a career of it." Narratives also vary in dominance relative to other narratives, with negative dominant ones being highly detrimental and positive dominant ones very beneficial (White and Epston, 1990). The various aspects of narratives reveal how they can and do impact on identity and self-concept: narratives that are positive, organized, coherent, indicating agency with a depth to them are clearly going to foster a better self-concept and identity (Gale et al., 2003; Polkinghorne, 1996; White and Epston, 1990).

In regards to narrative therapy, the role of a therapist is to listen with respect, empathy, and nonjudgment to the stories generated, paying particular attention to the experience and meaning (Zimmerman and Dickerson, 1994). The goal as a "co-author" is to foster the reformulation and generation of narratives that are positive, organized, coherent, "thick," with a theme of agency (Gale et al., 2003; Polkinghorne, 1996; White and Epston, 1990). Certain techniques and approaches are conducive to the client generating alternative stories with these healthy characteristics. At a basic level the client is encouraged to tell about themselves in a nonblaming manner, and the therapist provides feedback assisting in the client generating positive alternatives. A key approach is externalization: people often see a problem as characterizing them, such as I'm a loser instead of I've had losses, and narrative therapists assist the client in externalizing the problem, "The person is not the problem, the problem is the problem" (White and Epston, 1990). Externalization is consistent with how it is easier to change something that does not characterize you than alter a fundamental aspect of the self. As a caveat, externalization does not mean disowning the problem, as it is crucial to take ownership of issues.

Deconstruction is also applied to assist in breaking complex problems into manageable components, and identifying the fundamental aspects (White and Epston, 1990). For example, the person might see relationships as a total mess, but what aspects are there to this and which is most influential? Another approach, known as unique outcomes, pays attention to the threads that narratives weave in a person's life and the context of these, assisting the person in selecting dominant narratives that weave a positive thread. For instance, "I'm a conscientious person who does get things done," with this thread fostering positive self-perspectives in various areas. Narrative therapy also includes more specific approaches, such as formally "mapping" how problematic stories influence crucial areas of functioning, such as family, romances, work, and school.

Narrative therapy has been applied extensively within the context of family therapy, as not only individuals but social units generate narratives. For example, a family might produce the narrative that one member is the source of problems and the rest suffer as a result. The application of narrative therapy to individual therapy has tended to be more focused on trauma and health related conditions, such as, for example, how a person with cancer processes the illness. Interestingly, it has been noted that narratives in the form of testimony regarding atrocities occurs in many cultures with potential value in processing the traumatic experience (Weine and Laub, 1995). Although concentrated on more select areas, narrative therapy is relevant to many mental and physical health issues, given that we all are storytellers in our own lives and the narratives have powerful psychological import.

Enhancement of states and processes for mental health

Narratives are thought and language oriented, and so would not on the surface seem to impact **Activity**, but they actually have quite a significant impact. Self-generated narratives that do not emphasis agency aligning with the powerless of trauma, and even the impact of mental illness generally, inhibit activity. Why bother acting if one's actions will not have any influence? By generating alternative stories emphasizing agency, narrative therapy can move a person to activity. For example, people who have been sexually traumatized commonly have a narrative of being vulnerable and not in control in any potentially romantic context, frequently avoiding such engagements, or allowing further abuse. By shifting the narrative to appreciate the capacity to actually have an impact on a partner, a person feels empowered enough to engage and guide the relationship in a more constructive direction. Beyond abuse scenarios, any narrative that is limiting will favor inactivity. For example, the "thin" narrative derived from others that you are "lazy" is clearly not conducive to being active. Generating an alternative narrative seeing that Attention Deficit Disorder (ADD) made it difficult to focus, and now that it is treated more effective efforts can be made, entails a sense of power and agency. By fostering "thick" and dominant narratives with a theme of agency, narrative therapy weaves threads consistent with activity that extend to diverse areas of a person's life. Research has revealed that certain types of narratives block physical activity, and identifying and removing these limiting stories is a way to foster such activity (Buman et al., 2009).

An additional way that activity and narratives are related is applying activity to help generate positive narratives. For example, Caddick et al. (2015) had combat veterans suffering from Post-Traumatic Stress Disorder (PTSD) engage in surfing and generate stories around this very active experience. The researchers found that the narratives generated helped the participants process the trauma and gain a sense of respite. Likewise, by engaging in structured social activity more positive narratives pertaining to the social environment can ensue with mental health benefits. Based on my book, Activity for Mental Health (Bowins, 2020), activity of various types yields positive narratives emphasizing empowerment, social connectedness, motivation, and self-actualization, highly consistent with good mental health.

Narrative therapy has a powerful impact on **Psychological Defense Mechanism** functioning in regards to positive cognitive distortions, dissociation, and grieving. By generating positive alternative narratives to negative themed ones, positive cognitive distortions protecting against depression, anxiety, and stress are vastly ramped up. For example, instead of narratives with a theme of being at the mercy of others, and only succeeding if allowed, a person shifts to themes of being able to guide actions to produce successes. If these positive and agentic narratives are dominant and weave a coherent thread in a person's life, the impact of the positive spin can be profound. A key notion of narrative therapy—subjectivity—is very consistent with cognitive distortions, as reality is extremely difficult to accurately characterize, and with psychological functioning it is really about the spins or distortions we place on events (Beck, 1991; Beck and Clark, 1997; Bowins, 2004; Bowins, 2006).

Adaptive dissociation is fostered by a key approach of narrative therapy—externalization. By having a client separate the problem from their own self, psychological distance (dissociation) is achieved, better enabling the problem to be addressed and rectified, or in some instances compartmentalized. Returning to the ADD example, instead of, "I'm lazy," a quality of the self, "I have ADHD," a condition independent of the self. It is much harder to treat or compartmentalize a central aspect of the self than a condition such as ADHD.

Trauma and PTSD is a common mental illness scenario where narrative therapy has been applied. In the Psychological defense mechanism chapter, we considered the grieving process to be an evolved defense helping us manage loss and by extension trauma, given that loss of some form invariably occurs with trauma. In contrast to PTSD where dissociated elements of the traumatic experience repeat without fusion, grieving helps to fuse the various cognitive and emotional aspects of the trauma. The grieving process appears to do this by generating a coherent narrative of the events. For instance, "She had to leave home and move far away as she has the migration gene like her mother, and genetics are too powerful." For a person experiencing trauma, narrative therapy directly assists in producing a story or stories that fuse aspects of the trauma in a coherent fashion. For example, "Given the odds that were against my troop it is a miracle that I survived at all, and must have been God's will to have someone live through it." As the Caddick et al. (2015) study of surfing for PTSD shows narratives can help process trauma.

Social Connectedness is advanced by narrative therapy both generally and more specifically. Generally, via the collaborative nature of the positive narrative generation process with the client and therapist co-authoring it, providing a template for social connectedness. Specifically, when the negative narrative addressed pertains to the social sphere, limiting or blocking the person's capacity to bond with others. For example, "I'm the last one chosen like with those sports teams during my childhood when everyone was picked before me, and there I am standing alone!" This narrative obviously does not favor social connectedness, whereas the narrative, "I'm intelligent and accomplished academically, and this is respected by like-minded people," does favor forming friendships and romances, at least with people having and appreciating intelligence. It has been suggested that narratives in Western culture tend to focus on the autonomous, independent individual fostering social disconnection, whereas a shift to relational narratives can advance social connections (Fishbane, 2001).

Enhanced **Regulation**, at least in regards to emotions, is achieved by narrative therapy. This impact has been examined for diary writing, a way of generating narratives. Suhr et al. (2017) randomly assigned 89 patients recently discharged from a psychiatric inpatient ward, to either a writing intervention resource diary group or control group receiving no intervention. Self-report questionnaires assessing depression and emotion regulation were filled out before and after 4 weeks of the writing intervention. Participants in the diary writing group had significantly lower depression and increased emotion regulation in terms of reappraisal at the end of the intervention (Suhr et al., 2017). One limitation of the Suhr et al. (2017) study is that the control group received no intervention, and so conceivably just being part of any active group could have improved emotion regulation. Graf et al. (2008) conducted a study not having this limitation, randomly assigning outpatient psychotherapy clients to an expressive writing group or control writing (not expressive). Participants in the written emotional disclosure group had significantly less depression and anxiety than those in the control writing group at the end of the study, suggesting improved emotion regulation, although specific measures of this were not conducted (Graf et al., 2008). Research examining narrative expression pertaining to attachment indicates that the emotional tone and structure of narratives express information processing and affect regulation associated with relationships (Daniel, 2009).

A major approach of narrative therapy—deconstruction—also enhances regulation over emotions and other psychological processes, in that when problems seem convoluted and indecipherable it is very difficult to regulate thoughts and feelings about the issue. However, when the problem is deconstructed into separate components regulation over thoughts and feelings is much easier. This even extends to psychosis (see the Cognitive therapy chapter) where a psychotic narrative such as, "Agents of the FBI are after me having people spy, looking into my house," is very difficult to manage generating threat perceptions and feelings of fear. Deconstructing this to the evidence for these beliefs and alternative options for sounds heard at night, essentially producing a more reasonable narrative, makes the experience much more manageable, with this strategy capable of normalizing psychotic beliefs. France and Uhlin (2006) produced evidence that narrative change in psychosis aligns with recovery.

The strongest form of evidence for emotion regulation is typically neurological. Adenauer et al. (2011) tested 34 refugees experiencing PTSD randomly assigning half to a narrative exposure therapy group and half to a wait list control group, with neuromagnetic oscillatory brain activity in response to aversive pictures measured before and after the intervention. PTSD and depression scores improved in the narrative exposure therapy group, and the neural evidence was consistent with top-down cortical regulation (Adenauer et al., 2011). Hence, it appears that a narrative approach does assist with top-down regulation of emotions.

Human-Specific Cognition in terms of motivation can quite conceivably be advanced by narrative therapy, based on how negative narratives lacking coherence are highly de-motivating, whereas positive coherent narratives strongly motivate. Considering narratives expressed by clients and others I have encountered this seems quite evident. For example, "I've always excelled at school and intellectual pursuits, and so it follows that I will do well in my Masters of Business Administration program," motivates a person to succeed. In contrast, "I struggled with school and teachers never seemed to think I was any good," demotivates for any academic and related job scenario. Altering the latter narrative to, "Where I have excelled is with visual-spatial tasks and things like woodworking," strongly motivates progress to a successful trades career. Of lower probability, the intellectual work of actively generating positive, multilayered, and both internally and externally coherent narratives might ramp up executive functions and other aspects of basic cognition, much as producing a coherent novel likely does for an author.

It logically follows that **Self-Acceptance** will improve from narratives about the self that are positive, multilayered, and coherent. Indeed, it would be unlikely that this impact would not occur. Conversely, narratives that are negative, overly simple and/or not coherent will diminish self-concept, and from this self-acceptance (Gale et al., 2003; Polkinghorne, 1996; White and Epston, 1990). This process has been tested for self-stigma associated with mental illness. Hansson et al. (2017) randomly assigned 106 participants with severe mental illness to narrative enhancement within the context of cognitive therapy or a wait list control group, the results demonstrating that self-stigma decreased and self-esteem increased from the narrative enhancement intervention, compared to being on the wait list. By replacing negative self-referential narratives with positive themed compelling ones, narrative therapy is likely to advance self-acceptance.

Adaptability likely follows from narrative therapy due to how negative narratives, and particularly "thin" ones are very limiting, even contributing to repetitive maladaptive behavior. For instance, "I'm useless," ensures that inadequate efforts or no useful actions ensue with novel challenges, resulting in repeated dysfunction. More extensive and balanced narratives facilitate adjustment to a variety of circumstances as with, "Even though I have my limitations like everyone else, I do have skills and strengths." An interesting study by Ribeiro et al. (2011) investigating how the construction of a new self-narratives contributes to successful psychotherapy, sheds light on their role in enhancing adaptability. These researchers found that "innovative moments" and the themes within them referred to as protonarratives were instrumental in transforming problematic rigid self-narratives into new, more flexible ones. Even the process of generating innovative themes would seem to foster flexibility and adaptability.

Summary note

Storytelling is part of the human experience and we all seem to love fiction, perhaps due to how everyone generates narratives about their own life. Tapping into this universal experience via narrative therapy is then promising even at face value. Consistent with this potential outcome, shifting negative and limited narratives lacking coherence to positive, multilayered, and both internally and externally coherent self-narratives, advances all of the states and processes for mental health. Narratives emphasizing powerlessness and victimization restrict activity of various forms, and replacing them with narratives having themes of power and agency fosters activity. Psychological defense mechanisms in regards to positive cognitive distortions and adaptive dissociation are strongly advanced by narrative therapy, with the key process of externalization fostering adaptive dissociation. Successful grieving facilitating fusion of disconnected elements of traumatic experiences follows from the generation of positive narratives. The collaborative nature of narrative therapy with the client and therapist coauthoring stories about the person is a general way that it advances social connectedness. More specifically, social connectedness is fostered when negative narratives, limiting social contact and bonding, are replaced with narratives consistent with successful social activity.

Regulation, and certainly over emotions, is facilitated by narrative therapy, with research examining written narratives supporting this conjecture. There is some neurological evidence demonstrating top-down regulation over emotions from narratives. The narrative therapy technique of deconstruction also assists in regulation by transforming overly complex scenarios into manageable ones. The motivation aspect of human-specific cognition is advanced by replacing negative narratives that demotivate with positive inspiring ones. Additionally, the cognitive activity involved in generating positive, multilayered, and coherent (internally and externally) stories might ramp up executive functioning. Much as positive characters in fiction almost invariably display self-acceptance, it is understandable that positive self-referential narratives improve self-acceptance. Adaptability is also likely advanced from positive narrative generation, in that negative ones, and particularly "thin" variants, tend to be limiting often contributing to repetitive maladaptive behavior. Innovative moments with positive protonarratives appear to underlie how narrative therapy can advance flexibility and adaptability. It is interesting how a form of psychotherapy that tends to be restricted to certain spheres, actually does seem to be highly consistent with diverse aspects of mental health.

References

Adenauer, H., Catani, C., Gola, H., Keil, J., Ruf, M., Schauer, M., et al., 2011. Narrative exposure therapy for PTSD increases top-down processing of aversive stimuli—evidence from a randomized controlled treatment trial. BMC Neurosci. doi:10.1186/1471-2202-12-127.

Beck, A., 1991. Cognitive therapy: a 30-year retrospective. Am. Psychol. 46 (4), 368–375.

Beck, A., Clark, D., 1997. An information processing model of anxiety: automatic and strategic processes. Behav. Res. Therap. 35 (1), 49–58.

Bowins, B.E., 2004. Psychological defense mechanisms: a new perspective. Am. J. Psychoanal. 64, 1–26.

Bowins, B.E., 2006. How psychiatric treatments can enhance psychological defense mechanisms. Am. J. Psychoanal. 66, 173–194.

Bowins, B.E., 2020. Activity for Mental Health. Academic Press, San Diego.

Buman, M.P., Giacobbi, P.R., Yasova, L.D., McCrae, C.S., 2009. Using the constructive narrative perspective to understand physical activity reasoning schema in sedentary adults. J. Health Psychol. 14 (8), 1174–1183.

Caddick, N., Smith, B., Phoenix, C., 2015. The effects of surfing and the natural environment on the well-being of combat veterans. Qual. Health Rev. 25 (1), 76–86.

Daniel, S.I., 2009. The developmental roots of narrative expression in therapy: contributions from attachment theory and research. Psychotherapy (Chicago) 46 (3), 301–316.

Fishbane, M.D., 2001. Relational narratives of the self. Family Process 40 (3), 273–291.

France, C.M., Uhlin, B.D., 2006. Narrative as an outcome domain in psychosis. Psychol. Psychother. 79 (Pt 1), 53–67.

Gale, D.D., Mitchell, A.M., Garand, L., Wesner, S., 2003. Client narratives: a theoretical perspective. Issues Ment. Health Nurs. 24 (1), 81–89.

Graf, M.C., Gaudiano, B.A., Geller, P.A., 2008. Written emotional disclosure: a controlled study of the benefits of expressive writing homework in outpatient psychotherapy. Psychother. Res. 18 (4), 389–399.

Habermas, T., 2006. Who speaks? Who looks? Who feels? Point of view in autobiographical narratives. Int. J. Psychoanal. 87 (Pt 2), 497–518.

Hansson, L., Lexen, A., Holmen, J., 2017. The effectiveness of narrative enhancement and cognitive therapy: a randomized controlled study of a self-stigma intervention. Soc. Psychiatry Psychiatr. Epidemiol. 52 (11), 1415–1423.

Polkinghorne, D., 1996. Transformative narratives: from victimic to agentic life plots. Am. J. Occup. Ther. 50 (4), 299–305.

Ribeiro, A.P., Bento, T., Salgado, J., Stiles, W.B., Goncalves, M.M., 2011. A dynamic look at narrative change in psychotherapy: a case study tracking innovative moments and protonarratives using state space grids. Psychother. Res. 21 (1), 54–69.

Suhr, M., Risch, A.K., Wilz, G., 2017. Maintaining mental health through positive writing: effects of a resource diary on depression and emotion regulation. J. Clin. Psychol. 73 (12), 1586–1598.

Weine, S., Laub, D., 1995. Narrative constructions of historical realities in testimony with Bosnian survivors of "ethnic cleansing". Psychiatry 58 (3), 246–260.

White, M., Epston, D., 1990. Narrative Means to Therapeutic Ends. W.W. Norton, New York.

Zimmerman, J.L., Dickerson, V.C., 1994. Using narrative metaphor: implications for theory and practice. Family Process 33, 233–245.

Chapter 21

Person-centered therapy

Overview

Forms of psychotherapy focus on various aspects of psychological functioning and are hypothesized to remedy psychopathology via the given focus. The "person" is an obvious focus that forms the basis of an approach developed by Carl Rogers back in the 1940s (Rogers, 1951, 1957, 1986). Several terms have been applied including client-centered, Rogerian, nondirective, and of course person-centered, with either therapy or psychotherapy following the first component of the title. Person-centered therapy appears to be the most common, and best identifies the focus of this approach, so I will apply this term.

The general theme of person-centered therapy is that the client knows themselves best, and it is not the therapist's role to determine what is wrong or provide a solution; the capacities for both are within the person (Rogers, 1951, 1957, 1986). The therapist is to listen and repeat back to assist with clarifying the problem. Hence, the therapist does not make a diagnosis or offer advice. For psychotherapy to be successful Rogers proposed that three components, known as core conditions, are essential (Rogers, 1951, 1957, 1986):

- First, empathy enabling the therapist to develop an empathic understanding of the person's experiences. Real empathy enables the therapist to perceive the internal frame of reference along with the emotions and meanings.
- Second, congruence referring to being genuine allowing the client to experience the therapist as they really are. The therapist then cannot relate behind a professional screen or blank slate.
- Third, unconditional positive regard involving a nonjudgmental and accepting stance regardless of what the client is relating.

The three core conditions to successful psychotherapy pertain to the therapist's stance in relation to the client, highlighting how specific techniques are not emphasized, instead the manner of relating to the client is crucial (Rogers, 1951, 1957, 1986). This "nondirective" approach also aligns with the person knowing themselves best and being the one to determine what is wrong and devise a solution. In addition to the three therapist-oriented components, there are three others involving the client, consisting of (Rogers, 1951, 1957, 1986) the following:

- Therapist-client psychological contact: An alliance must exist between the client and therapist that involves the client forming a relationship.

States and Processes for Mental Health. DOI: 10.1016/C2020-0-00574-8

- Client incongruence: The meaning here is different than for the therapist, referring to discrepancies between the client's self-image and actual experience, or the ideal and experienced self, an occurrence that generates negative emotions. Therapy aims to resolve the discrepancy.
- Client perception: The client perceives the therapist's empathy, genuineness, and unconditional positive regard.

With the therapist and client components in place a safe environment exists for the person to explore their feelings and thoughts. Essentially, the therapist is providing a facilitative environment for self-discovery. Rogers believed that each person has a capacity and desire for personal growth and change, known as the actualizing tendency (Rogers, 1951, 1957, 1986). Within the right therapeutic environment this capacity can be realized, and the therapist's role is to create the right conditions. Rogers extended person-centered therapy to diverse conditions and settings such as political encounter groups and student-centered learning. He passed away in 1987, and demonstrating how the originator and their students can be so crucial in the ongoing application of a given form of therapy, this approach has gradually faded, now mostly occurring as person-centered strategies applied in eclectic therapy.

Enhancement of states and processes for mental health

As the term person-centered suggests, the client is in the driver's seat with this form of therapy and expected to play a prominent role. Although this does not directly link to **Activity**, it follows that if the client engages with the approach and positive change transpires, activity might indirectly increase. This scenario applies when there is incongruence between a person's ideal and experienced self in a way that entails activity. For instance, if a person views themselves as being athletic but is not engaging in any physical activity supporting that perspective, the person might resolve the discrepancy by partaking in sports that are of interest.

Psychological Defense Mechanisms are not likely to change from person-centered therapy in any direct fashion, but positive cognitive distortions indirectly might due to the positive shift in the person's perspective regarding themselves. The core therapist-based conditions of empathy, congruency, and unconditional positive regard can powerfully enhance a person's self-perspective when the individual engages, strives to resolve incongruent perspectives, and experiences the therapist as authentic. Even outside of a psychotherapeutic context, another person providing the core conditions almost invariably will advance a person's self-perspective which entails positive cognitive distortions.

When incongruent perspectives pertaining to oneself relate to the social sphere, person-centered therapy can advance **Social Connectedness**. For instance, a person wishes to be close to others but is quite isolated, not an uncommon scenario in those seeking counseling. Appreciating this discrepancy, the person then resolves it by taking steps to engage with others, supported by the therapist in an unconditional positive way, such that mistakes are okay and to be learned from. The close connection with an authentic therapist also assists with social connectedness providing a template.

Regulation at least over emotions can indirectly advance by resolving lack of congruency between self-image and actual experience, given that this scenario generates negative emotions such as sadness, anger, or fear, when actual outcomes are far less than idealized ones. Emotion regulation might also be enhanced from the highly supportive therapist approach that in some instances can sooth negative emotions. These impacts extend beyond the transtherapy influence on emotion regulation occurring across all forms of psychotherapy covered in the Behavioral therapy chapter.

Improvements in **Human-Specific Cognition** are of lower probability, but increased motivation might occur from two sources. First, the unconditional support provided by the therapist. Second, resolution of cognitive dissonance arising from the discrepancy between actual experience and idealized perspectives: when the person becomes aware of the inconsistency, aversive cognitive dissonance is likely to transpire creating a negative reinforcement scenario, motivating the person to resolve the discrepancy (Draycott and Dabbs, 1998). Negative reinforcement can be potently motivating and cognitive dissonance is a very aversive mental state.

Self-Awareness is powerfully advanced from person-centered therapy, based on how the client is to discover themselves, identify inconsistencies between the actual and ideal self, devise solutions to achieve congruency, and recruit their resources to achieve it. It is an extremely empowering form of psychotherapy with the therapist more of a facilitator (Rogers, 1951, 1957, 1986). From this progression, self-perspectives (self-concept), self-evaluation (self-esteem), and from these self-acceptance is very likely to improve.

The process of person-centered therapy results in both improved understanding of oneself, and greater confidence in recruiting personal resources to achieve success where there are limitations. Through these changes behavior is likely to be more in synch with circumstances, resulting in greater **Adaptability**. Furthermore, when idealized and actual outcomes are incongruent, related behavior is not likely to be adaptive. For example, a person believes that their ability warrants a promotion at work, and then is distressed to incur a "needs improvement" appraisal on a performance review. There is clearly a discrepancy that involves maladaptive behavior relative to the demands of the job. By appreciating this discrepancy and altering job performance more functional behavior will ensue.

Summary note

As the title, person-centered therapy, suggests this form of psychotherapy is very focused on the client, emphasizing their potential for understanding and capacity to improve. The role of the therapist is then one of facilitation derived from the core therapist conditions of empathy, congruency (authenticity), and unconditional positive regard. On the client's side, key aspects consist of making psychological contact with the therapist, addressing incongruence whereby anticipated (ideal) self-image differs from that experienced, and perceiving the therapist's core conditions. Relying on the person's capacity and desire for personal growth and change, known as the actualizing tendency, the therapist helps the client clarify but never directs.

With person-centered therapy, self-acceptance is the only state and process for mental health that is both robustly and directly advanced, due to how this form of therapy is very empowering fostering improved self-concept and self-esteem. Enhancement of the other states and processes characterizing mental health is typically indirect, less probable, or not as strong. The self-directed approach can improve activity when incongruence relates to activity of various types, given that the resolution will usually favor being active. Psychological defense mechanisms in terms of positive cognitive distortions can indirectly advance from the positive self-perspectives, derived from the therapist core conditions, combined with the person's efforts to produce positive change empowered by this form of psychotherapy. Social connectedness is only likely to advance when incongruent perspectives pertain to the social environment, and the resolution leads to better social engagement. Assisting with this outcome is the very positive and authentic relationship with the therapist that serves as a template for social connectedness. Emotion regulation can be indirectly advanced, based on how incongruent self-image and actual experience generates negative emotions that are difficult to contain, and by resolving the incongruent scenario these emotions are settled. Emotions can also be regulated by the very supportive therapist approach capable of soothing negative feelings. Human-specific cognition in terms of motivation might improve from the unconditional therapist support, and also how incongruent cognitions produce cognitive dissonance, motivating behavior to resolve it. Adaptability can advance from greater understanding and confidence, plus how incongruent self-image and experience often entails maladaptive behavior for the given circumstances, and the shift to congruency improves the functionality of behavior. Despite only acting indirectly in some instance, person-centered therapy does advance the states and processes for mental health, and in particular self-acceptance.

References

Draycott, S., Dabbs, A., 1998. Cognitive Dissonance. 1: an overview of the literature and its integration into theory and practice in clinical psychology. Br. J. Clin. Psychol. 37 (3), 341–353.

Rogers, C.R., 1951. Client-Centered Therapy: Its Current Practice, Implications and Theory. Constable, London.

Rogers, C.R., 1957. The necessary and sufficient conditions of therapeutic personality change. J. Consult. Psychol. 21 (2), 95–103.

Rogers, C.R., 1986. Carl Rogers on the development of the person-centered approach. Person-Centered Rev. 1 (3), 257–259.

Chapter 22

Positive psychotherapy

Overview

A key notion of this book is how psychotherapy is typically hypothesized to work by remedying psychopathology, while it actually operates by advancing the states and processes for mental health. In line with this notion is positive psychotherapy oriented to enhancing positivity. Displeased by how psychology in general focuses on the negative, with good mental health the absence of psychological distress, the prominent American psychologist Martin Seligman spearheaded positive psychology at the turn of the millennium. He proposed five pathways to well-being including positive emotions, engagement, relationships, meaning, and achievement (Seligman, 2011). Three domains of functioning consist of (Duckworth et al., 2005):

- Pleasant life linked to positive emotions relevant to the past, present, and future.
- Engaged life drawing on characteristics of the person such as strengths and virtues.
- Meaningful life derived from a sense of belonging and being of service in a positive way.

Happiness follows from success in the five pathways and three life domains, with the goal of shifting mental processes away from the negative (Duckworth et al., 2005; Seligman, 2011). Currently positive psychology is an umbrella term for research into positive psychological processes such as creativity, optimism, resilience, strengths, empathy, compassion, forgiveness, humor, creativity, satisfaction, and of course positive emotions (Schrank et al., 2014).

The foundation provided by positive psychology has greatly influenced the development and research focus of positive psychotherapy. Seligman et al. (2011) applied the principles of positive psychology to positive psychotherapy. However, this form of psychotherapy initially arose earlier in Germany, being developed by Nossrat Peseschkian in the late 1960s influenced by the Baha'i faith, and introduced to the English-speaking world in 1987 with the publication of Positive Psychotherapy, Theory and Practice of a New Method. According to Peseschkian, the main pillars are the principle of hope, principle of balance, and principle of consultation (Peseschkian, 1987). The principle of hope involves finding the meaning or purpose of a disorder or conflict. Mental illness manifestations then have a symbolic function. According to the balance

States and Processes for Mental Health. DOI: 10.1016/C2020-0-00574-8

principle, balance is required in the four key life areas of body/health, achievement, contact/relationships, and purpose/meaning. When there is a lack of balance mental illness manifestations occur, such as psychosomatic ailments if body/health is neglected, stress with limited achievement, depression with poor contact/relationships, and fears when there is lack of meaning in life. The balance principle does repeat the notion of psychopathology being the central focus of psychotherapy, given that lack of balance produces mental illness that is remedied by psychotherapeutic interventions directed at restoring balance. The principle of consultation are intertwined steps for therapy and self-help including observation, inventory, situational encouragement, verbalization, and expansion of goals (Peseschkian, 1987).

Two independent streams feeding into one form of psychotherapy could produce much conflict, but consistent with positivity the merger is quite peaceful. There are differences such as Seligman not denying negative experiences while Peseschkian reframes all negative experiences in a positive light, the difference derived from the more transcultural and Baha'i origins of Peseschkian's version (Peseschkian, 1987; Seligman, 2011). However, they both emphasis a focus on positivity and distancing from the negative, and are oriented to a positive life with balance.

Several psychotherapy techniques and strategies to facilitate positivity have been developed (Duckworth et al., 2005; Peseschkian, 1987; Seligman, 2011; Seligman et al., 2006). A major one being the gratitude journal whereby a client writes about things they are grateful for, focusing on specific occurrences. Reminiscence is related to gratitude journaling and can contribute to it by fostering the recall of positive experiences. Designing a beautiful day encourages a client to envision what will be positive and then engaging in such activities, a process that often requires breaking negative routines. Self-esteem journaling involves listing things a person has done well at. With any such exercises the process has to be repeated and made routine for a solid benefit. Signature strengths involve listing individual strengths and capacities with feedback from the therapist to help with ranking them. Techniques vary depending on the practitioner and subtype of this therapy, such as "meaning therapy" and "strength-based therapy," but all approaches focus on positive features of psychological functioning and enhancing these.

Enhancement of states and processes for mental health

With the emphasis on furthering positivity, it is reasonable to assume that positive psychotherapy will advance the states and processes for mental health. **Activity** is fostered by various principles and processes, prominently engagement and achievement. Positive psychotherapy emphasizes real engagement in life to optimize balance and functioning. Achievement and recognizing successes provides reinforcement that motivates further activity. A meaningful life is important and to achieve this activity is required in positive spheres. Mental activity is enhanced by the extensive and ongoing journaling work. The link between activity and positivity ties into the link between behavioral activation and positive affectivity, in contrast to behavioral inhibition and negative affectivity, presented in the Activity chapter.

Psychological Defense Mechanism functioning in terms of both dissociation and positive cognitive distortions is advanced. Adaptive dissociation is achieved by drawing a person away from negativity into positivity, with the ongoing journaling and related mental activity fostering absorption in positive foci. By shifting negativity to positivity, the negative cognitive distortions integral to depression, anxiety, and other mental health problems are transformed into positive distortions. For example, instead of themes associated with loss and setbacks, themes of hope and achievement are generated.

Both Seligman and Peseschkian view successful relationships as integral to positivity. Hence, both streams encourage positive relationships contributing to **social connectedness**. Furthermore, therapeutic strategies such as the gratitude journal and designing a beautiful day with a focus on balance will include relationships. For instance, clients journal social encounters they are grateful for, and include positive interactions in their beautiful day. Indirectly, social connectedness might be advanced by the more positive presentation of the client, given that negative expressions consistent with depression lead others to withdraw, while balanced positivity draws people closer.

Regulation, at least emotion regulation, is enhanced by positive psychotherapy via the positivity shifts. Mutually reinforcing negative feedback loops between negative cognitions and emotions, commonly amplify negative affect associated with depression and anxiety: thoughts pertaining to negative themes generate negative emotions, creating an emotional climate conducive to further negative thoughts, resulting in intensified negative emotions, and so on and so forth. This amplification effect makes it difficult to regulate negative emotions. Shifting to positive thoughts, such as those implicit with hope, generating positive emotions, counters the negative cognitive-emotion cycles, facilitating regulation over negative emotions.

The motivation aspect of **Human-Specific Cognition** will likely advance from positive psychotherapy, given the motivating nature of it. Motivational programs of various forms rely heavily on positive psychology and psychotherapy principles and strategies. A frequent occurrence I have noted with people attending weekend motivational retreats, is how "revved" they are engaging in positive pursuits for a short period, but the motivation returns to normal levels quite quickly. This short-term effect is a key reason for why positive psychotherapy encourages ongoing journaling and other therapeutic work. While this might be interpreted as a person continually having to push against the onslaught of negativity, a more "positive" interpretation is that thought patterns and related neural circuits oriented to positivity have to be established and repeated to become automatic.

Positive perspectives regarding the self almost certainly enhance self-concept, self-esteem, and hence **self-acceptance**. Self-esteem journaling itself is likely to achieve this outcome. In addition, the optimistic broadened horizons approach will foster better self-perspectives. By encouraging engagement and achievement, real improvements ensue making sure that reality bolsters the perceived gains relevant to the self. A study of positive psychotherapy applied to nursing students with depression, found that those in the experimental group experienced improved self-efficacy relative to those in the control group (Guo et al., 2017). Enhanced self-efficacy contributes to better overall self-concept.

Adaptability can indirectly improve by freeing people from the negative repetitive ruts they often become stuck in, strengthened by negative mutually reinforcing cognitive-emotion cycles, such as with viewing relationships with skepticism and pessimism resulting in inadequate engagement, then failure, triggering sadness-related emotions, and further skepticism and pessimism. Much as with enhanced regulation, positivity shifts with real engagement counters these negative feedback cycles, replacing them with positive ones. By ending negative repetitive behavior and encouraging positive behavior adaptability is strengthened.

Summary note

Positive psychotherapy supported by positive psychology principles represents a unique approach to mental health issues. However, as with the rationale for other forms of psychotherapy, it does emphasis psychopathology in terms of lack of balance in key life areas producing mental illness, and by restoring balance these problems are remedied. It recognizes our predisposition to focus on negativity, and why positivity needs to be addressed. In line with this notion, positive psychotherapy helps foster greater meaning, hope, engagement, achievement, and balance. Therapeutic tasks such as gratitude journaling, designing a beautiful day, and self-esteem journaling are practical strategies that when repeated are capable of enhancing mental health. This positivity approach is consistent with the theme of this book—that psychotherapy works not by addressing psychopathology, but by advancing the states and processes for mental health. It also supports the notion that "happiness" is not primary, instead following from the actualization of states and processes for mental health if it is to be sustainable: positive psychology underlying positive psychotherapy, indicates that happiness follows from success in the key pathways and domains of life.

Each of the states and processes for mental health are advanced by positive psychotherapy. Activity is enhanced by the emphasis on engagement and achievement. The extensive journaling work also increases mental activity. Dissociation and positive cognitive distortion psychological defense mechanism templates are both advanced, adaptive dissociation from the way that positive psychotherapy disconnects a person from the negative by absorbing them in positive foci and pursuits. The negative to positive shift transforms the negative cognitive distortions of depression and anxiety to positive ones. Successful relationships are integral to positive psychotherapy with the therapeutic tasks supporting this progression, leading to improved social connectedness. Mutually reinforcing cycles of negative cognitions and emotions are countered resulting in improved emotion regulation. Positive psychotherapy is highly motivating and as such strengthens the motivational component of human-specific cognition. Journaling and other therapeutic tasks performed ongoing ensure that the motivational benefits persist. Self-acceptance is enhanced by self-esteem journaling alone, but improved self-perspectives follow from the overall optimistic shift, while the engagement and achievement focus produce real gains supporting improved self-acceptance. Adaptability is enhanced when the positivity shifts remove people from negative repetitive ruts they are stuck in. Positive psychotherapy then demonstrates the robustness of a positive focus applied to mental illness and health.

References

Duckworth, A.L., Steen, T., Seligman, M.E., 2005. Positive psychology in clinical practice. Annu. Rev. Clin. Psychol. 1, 629–651.

Guo, Y.F., Zhang, X., Plummer, V., Lam, L., Cross, W., Zhang, J.P., 2017. Positive psychotherapy for depression and self-efficacy in undergraduate nursing students: a randomized, controlled trial. Int. J. Ment. Health Nurs. 26 (4), 375–383.

Peseschkian, N., 1987. Positive Psychotherapy: Theory and Practice of a New Method. Springer, New York.

Schrank, B., Brownell, T., Tylee, A., Slade, M., 2014. Positive psychology: an approach to supporting recovery in mental illness. East Asian Arch. Psychiatry 24 (3), 95–103.

Seligman, M.E., 2011. Flourish: A Visionary New Understanding of Happiness and Well-Being. Free Press, New York, NY.

Seligman, M.E., Rashid, T., Parks, A.C., 2006. Positive psychotherapy. Am. Psychol. 61 (8), 774–788.

Chapter 23

Problem-solving therapy

Overview

As with several forms of psychotherapy, problem-solving therapy was initially formulated to treat depression, but has been extended to other conditions including, anxiety, stress, self-harm, relationship issues, workplace difficulties, and physical health issues. It is a short-term approach that is typically applied in a sequential series of steps (Arean et al., 2010; Bell and D'Zurilla, 2009; Pierce, 2012). Problems are initially identified including patterns that underlie them. For example, the client might have a submissive, aggressive, or passive-aggressive approach to people resulting in issues replaying. The problem is clearly defined for the client, given that what is obvious to the therapist might not be to the person with the issue, particularly considering how we naturally distort things in a self-enhancing fashion. For instance, the client might spin an aggressive approach as only being direct with people. Clarity regarding the problem facilitates the next related steps of coming up with realistic solutions and selecting the most promising option. A couple of viable options for a person who is overly aggressive is to let others take the initiative or be assertive. The first might shift the person to a passive approach resulting in a buildup of frustration and then more aggression, while assertiveness will enable feelings and needs to be expressed effectively, hence this is the most promising option. Developing and implementing an action plan follows from identifying the best approach to the problem. Assertiveness skills might be role played and/or examples given, that can be applied to the person's particular problematic circumstances. Once the action plan is implemented monitoring the results to assess the effectiveness is the last major step. Do the assertive actions yield better outcomes than the more aggressive stance? Through these steps problems are solved generating more positive outcomes. In a meta-analysis of problem-solving therapy for depression Bell and D'Zurilla (2009) found that the approach is most effective when each of these steps is included.

Various strategies are applied in problem-solving therapy, a major one consisting of breaking problems into manageable components (Bell and D'Zurilla, 2009; Pierce, 2012). People suffering from depression, anxiety, and stress in response to problematic circumstances often process the issue as a whole making it overwhelming, and by dissecting it into components it seems less disturbing and more manageable. Interactive problem-solving exercises might be engaged to get the client used to the notion of addressing issues in this way and

States and Processes for Mental Health. DOI: 10.1016/C2020-0-00574-8

feeling empowered. Homework assignments can be part of the process, and also enhancement of communication skills. Demonstrating how people love to generate new variants of a given entity, solution-focused psychotherapy also "exists" but has very limited research data. Even the labels problem-solving and solution-focused strongly suggest they are very similar, or in essence identical. I will stick to problem-solving therapy with it having somewhat more research data.

Enhancement of states and processes for mental health

Problem-solving therapy represents a very active approach to issues, and hence **Activity** relevant to the problem area is advanced. For instance, if the problem involves poor health related to physical inactivity with excessive weight, joint pain, and prediabetes, the solution will include increased physical activity. If the problem concerns avoidance of social relationships, then the solution entails enhanced social activity. In addition, the steps of formulating and implementing an action plan, and also monitoring the effectiveness, ensure greater mental activity.

Adaptive dissociation in the form of compartmentalization can be part of problem-solving therapy advancing **Psychological Defence Mechanisms**, in that overwhelming issues are broken down into more manageable components, effectively placing them in compartments. For instance, "I always seem to fail," is an overwhelming and seemingly insurmountable issue. Dissecting this whole into areas of concerns, such as interpersonal interactions at work and family affairs, places the large-scale problem into a relationship compartment with work and family subcompartments. These subcompartments are much more manageable than, "I always seem to fail." The very positive approach of problem-solving therapy, identifying an issue or issues and coming up with workable solutions, facilitates a positive shift—positive cognitive distortions. Warmerdam et al. (2010) comparing problem-solving therapy to cognitive behavioral therapy found that both are equally effective in shifting dysfunctional attitudes and worry-related thoughts in a positive direction, with both superior to a waitlist control group. Even the specific mature defense mechanism of sublimation is advanced, because the negative emotions and energy associated with the problem is redirected and channeled into positive actions. Positive anticipation might also be enhanced when a client learns to anticipate problems and proactively engage in finding solutions. Further supporting the role of these positive shifts with problem-solving therapy, Bell and D'Zurilla (2009) found in their meta-analysis that the approach is more effective when there is a positive problem orientation, as opposed to just a problem-solving focus.

Social connectedness is only likely to be advanced by problem-solving therapy if the client's issues concern social relationships, and then this outcome can be expected given the very results oriented focus. For instance, with the example of our overly aggressive person, poor relationship quality is likely, and by shifting to an assertive stance the quality of interactions will typically improve, resulting in better social connectedness. Given how important the social environment is to people, problems often relate to the social sphere, with the implemented solution improving the quality of interactions.

Problem-solving therapy can improve **Regulation** when this is a problem area. For instance, the overweight, sedentary, prediabetic person who eats excessive amounts of processed carbohydrates does not demonstrate adequate regulation over eating and health behaviors. The solution will involve strategies that enhance this regulation, such as calorie monitoring and restraint. Emotion regulation can be advanced by problem-solving therapy, based on the results of a study focused on borderline personality disorder clients experiencing emotion dysregulation who completed this form of therapy, with emotion regulation scores increased at the end of treatment and at 6 months (Boccalon et al., 2017). As with the other states and processes for mental health, problem-solving therapy must target the issue, and in the case of borderline personality disorder emotion dysregulation is a common problem. However, as mentioned in the Behavior therapy chapter, all psychotherapies appear to enhance emotion regulation as a transtherapy process.

Human-specific cognition in terms of executive functioning appears to improve from problem-solving therapy, when there is a limitation with it. This therapeutic approach has been applied to elderly people with depression who have executive functioning problems (Alexopoulos et al., 2011; Arean et al., 2010). Improved outcomes relative to supportive therapy were more prominent when the depressed participants experienced greater cognitive impairment, likely because the problem-solving addressed executive functioning issues (Alexopoulos et al., 2011). Several executive functions are activated when a client identifies problems, clarifies them, generates realistic solutions, selects the best option, develops an action plan, implements it, and monitors the outcome: attention, set shifting (cognitive flexibility) by generating various solutions, inhibition pertaining to nonviable options, planning with action plans, and monitoring outcomes. Problem-solving therapy does involve conscious thought that engages executive functions, arguably more than the other forms of psychotherapy covered. If motivation or social cognition are problem areas, then problem-solving therapy will also likely produce improvements via the active steps taken including implementation.

A key way that problem-solving therapy appears to work is by empowering a person who feels overwhelmed by problems. Breaking these problems down into manageable components, devising solutions, and then implementing them transforms a sense of being at the mercy of the problem into empowerment. A sense of empowerment combined with improved outcomes will enhance self-concept, self-esteem, and hence **Self-Acceptance**. For instance, the person with poor health habits who controls their calorie intake, shifts to consuming better quality food, and increases activity losing weight and toning up is likely to feel empowered, with an improved self-perspective (self-concept) and evaluation (self-esteem) the end result.

Enhanced **Adaptability** naturally follows from adopting effective problem-solving strategies. Life involves unique challenges and applying the same dysfunctional approach repeatedly demonstrates inflexibility yielding poor outcomes, hence the need for problem-solving therapy. Taking on problems with tailored strategies departing from repetitive maladaptive behavior entails greater flexibility, and the outcome will almost certainly improve adaptive capacity.

Summary note

As the name suggests, problem-solving therapy is a very active approach to issues that involves the sequential steps of: problem identification, clarification, generating realistic solutions, selecting the best option, developing an action plan, implementing it, and monitoring the outcome. Problems are broken down into manageable components. Given the very active nature of problem-solving therapy, activity relevant to the problem is advanced. Dissecting seemingly overwhelming problems into components facilitates adaptive dissociation in the form of compartmentalization, and hence psychological defense mechanism functioning is improved. Positive cognitive distortions are also facilitated by the positive solution oriented focus, and the mature classical defenses of sublimation and positive anticipation can be enhanced. Due to our nature as a social species major problems frequently have a social component, and by solving the issue social connectedness is typically advanced. Beyond the trans-therapy way that psychotherapy improves emotion regulation, broader regulation capacity is bolstered by problem-solving therapy when various regulation issues are targeted. Human-specific cognition can be enhanced when there is a problem involving it, such as depression in the elderly. The cognitive nature of this approach almost certainly improves several executive functions including attention, set shifting, inhibition, planning, and monitoring, particularly when they are addressed. Effective problem solving empowers a person, and from this greater self-acceptance can follow. Significant problems, usually the sort that bring a person to psychotherapy, often entail an inflexible repetitive approach limiting outcomes. Generating unique solutions that fit with the problem enhances adaptability. Problem-solving therapy even though seemingly very focused, actually has a broad and positive impact on the states and processes for mental health, and this impact is very strong when the problem involves the given state or process.

References

Alexopoulos, G.S., Raue, P.J., Kiosses, D.N., Mackin, R.S., Kanellopoulos, D., McCulloch, C., et al., 2011. Problem-solving therapy and supportive therapy in older adults with major depression and executive dysfunction: effect on disability. Arch. Gen. Psychiatry 68 (1), 33–41.

Arean, P.A., Raue, P., Mackin, R.S., Kanellopoulos, D., McCulloch, C., Alexopoulos, G.S., 2010. Problem-solving therapy and supportive therapy in older adults with major depression and executive dysfunction. Am. J. Psychiatry 167 (11), 1391–1398.

Bell, A.C., D'Zurilla, T.J., 2009. Problem-solving therapy for depression: a meta-analysis. Clinic. Psychol. Rev. doi:10.1016/j.cpr.2009.02.003 doi.org.

Boccalon, S., Alesiani, R., Giarolli, L., Fossati, A., 2017. Systems training for emotional predictability and problem solving program and emotion dysregulation: a pilot study. J. Nerv. Ment. Dis. 205 (3), 213–216.

Pierce, D., 2012. Problem solving therapy–use and effectiveness in general practice. Aust. Fam. Physician 41 (9), 676–679.

Warmerdam, L., Van Straten, A., Jongsma, J., Twisk, J., Cuijpers, P., 2010. Online cognitive behavioral therapy and problem-solving therapy for depressive symptoms: exploring mechanisms of change. J. Behav. Ther. Exp. Psychiatry 41 (1), 64–70.

Chapter 24

Psychoanalytic therapy

Overview

To the best of my knowledge, psychoanalysis is the oldest formal type of psychotherapy, although through the ages at least supportive counselling has been conducted. I use the term, psychoanalytic therapy, due to how many versions of this approach have arisen since its origin with Sigmund Freud. There is psychoanalysis, dynamic therapy, short-term dynamic therapy, transference-focused therapy, dynamic deconstructive psychotherapy, and other versions associated with specific analysts, including Carl Jung, Melanie Klein, Karen Horney, and Alfred Adler. In many ways, this diversity of approaches is not surprising given first, how we love to set up discrete entities, particularly when it gives the originator recognition, and second, how long the psychoanalytic approach has existed despite repeated claims that it is finally dead.

The range of psychoanalytic approaches also arises from the diversity and complexity of concepts subsumed under psychoanalysis. Along with several other approaches, I do apply dynamic therapy as part of eclectic psychotherapy, but I am not a psychoanalyst. Even given my theoretical leanings, I find many of the concepts to be excessively complex and questionable on this basis alone, since from what I have seen, the truth ultimately tends to be quite simple. Given that this is an overview and to adequately cover psychoanalysis would take several chapters, I will focus on core concepts that have proven to be robust.

Arguably, the most impressive contribution Sigmund Freud made was identifying the powerful role that the unconscious mind plays in normal development and mental illness. Freud (1915) believed that consciousness only represents a small portion of mental activity. Indeed, modern neuroscience supports this view with research finding that the energy consumed by unconscious active messaging, occurring during sleep, daydreaming, anesthesia, and other states, is 20 times greater than the energy used to respond consciously (Fox and Raichle, 2007; Zhang and Raichle, 2010). Many aspects of mental life including motivation, and cognitive and emotional information processing appear to be largely unconscious (Morsella et al., 2010). Based on the work of Freud and later contributions, several functions are ascribed to the unconscious including primary process thought, pleasure-unpleasure principle, exemption from contradiction, no doubt or uncertainty, and instinctual impulses/energy (Freud, 1915; Miller, 1997; Power and Brewin, 1991). More rational functions such as secondary process thought, reality principle, rational/logical thought, doubt and

States and Processes for Mental Health. DOI: 10.1016/C2020-0-00574-8

uncertainty, and representations of impulses are conscious (Freud, 1915; Miller, 1997; Power and Brewin, 1991).

According to Freud and later analysts, the conscious and unconscious mind interact, and these interactions and boundary events play a very important role in psychological functioning, with transformation a key concept. Unconscious raw material, including wishes, urges, and conflicts, are transformed into conscious experience (Balestriere, 2007; Freud, 1900; Frosch, 1976; Robbins, 2008). Primary process thoughts are transformed into images (hallucinatory wish fulfillment) and then conscious thoughts during dreams (Balestriere, 2007; Freud, 1900; Robbins, 2008). Conflict also undergoes transformation with dreams a distortion of latent conflict (Frosch, 1976). The motivation for transformation is the frustration encountered when libidinal instincts, manifesting in wishes and urges, encounter reality (Balestriere, 2007; Robbins, 2008), transformation reducing the tension (Robbins, 2008). At times, unconscious events are so powerful that they can overwhelm consciousness censorship and break through, resulting in symptoms such as psychosis and panic (Freud, 1900).

Psychological defense mechanisms (see the Psychological defense mechanism chapter) function to protect sensitive conscious system functioning from intolerable unconscious input, serving as a form of regulation (Freud, 1964). Unconscious material is distorted such that it is more acceptable, as with reaction formation where a person acts opposite to what is felt and believed. For example, a minister strongly preaches the values of celibacy while actually wanting to have sex with multiple partners, the latter libidinal urges unacceptable to his conscious mind. Likewise, projection defensively transfers unacceptable qualities of the self to others.

Psychoanalytic therapy entails listening and interpreting what the client expresses to understand the unconscious aspects, and how these are creating tension with reality. A major technique in this regard is free association, whereby the client talks without distractions. Free association allows wishes, urges, dream content, and other unconscious derivatives to freely emerge in a safe environment. Interpretation of these unconscious events is a corrective experience for the client. Transference and countertransference interpretation are crucial for understanding a client, as the person frequently reacts to the therapist as someone from the past, such as a mother or father. For instance, the client might express that he or she feels the therapist does not really care, transferring feelings regarding an uncaring parent to the therapist. Interpreting counter-transference (the therapist's reactions to the patient based on past relationships) is also important, because it provides insight into aspects of the client. For instance, the therapist might feel manipulated like during a past relationship, but in reviewing the feelings realize that the client is acting in a passive-aggressive fashion. Unconscious resistance in therapy can then be addressed and worked on. Perhaps the client has always felt ineffectual and lacks confidence, assuming that they cannot possibly influence people, resulting in passive-aggressive reactions. Through transference and counter-transference interpretations this theme emerges, providing a corrective emotional experience for the client, including an opportunity to see that another person can be influenced, thereby dispensing with the need for passive-aggressive behavior.

Enhancement of states and processes for mental health

Psychoanalytic approaches tend to be very introspective and not obviously capable of fostering **Activity**, so any benefit in this regard is of lower probability. The only viable option that comes to mind is that by resolving intrapsychic conflict and ambivalence that block actions, greater activity could follow. For example, if a person is blocked regarding career progress due to an intrapsychic conflict and ambivalence, revolving around wishing to succeed but fearful of besting an insecure parent, then by resolving the conflict and the ensuing ambivalence the person advances with career aspirations. Conflicted motives and the ambivalence that typically follows do inhibit actions that would transpire otherwise. A scenario where I have often noted this is during grieving when a person feels conflicted about returning to their normal activities, as it then appears that deceased is now forgotten. Becoming aware of this conflict the person usually realizes that the deceased will not be forgotten by such activity, thereby providing a corrective emotional experience, resulting in normal activity for the person consistent with mental health.

Psychological Defense Mechanisms represent a very robust psychoanalytic concept. Since Freud proposed them and presented their benefit, they have been applied to understand both healthy and unhealthy psychological functioning, and how people cope with stress (Freud, 1964). Psychoanalytically oriented therapists evaluate defense mechanisms utilized by the client based on free association, interactions in therapy, and also reports of stress responses. This assessment provides a chance to address immature defenses. For example, if a client is noted to utilize projective identification, whereby feelings such as anger are elicited in the therapist before identification with the emotion is possible, then the therapist can help the client express negative emotions verbally. Similarly, if the client is engaging in widespread denial, the therapist can explore insecurities, fears, and conflicts motivating this defense. Ultimately the goal is to replace immature defenses with mature ones (Vaillant, 1977; Vaillant, 1994).

Research has demonstrated that psychoanalytic therapy does produce a shift from immature to mature defenses (Perry, 2001; Perry and Bond, 2004; Van Wijk-Herbrink et al., 2011; Vlastelica et al., 2005). A study of 20 patients receiving long-term group analytic treatment (4 years) showed a shift to more mature psychological defense mechanisms (Vlastelica et al., 2005). Perry and Bond (2004) enrolled 21 adults experiencing depression, anxiety, and/or personality disorder in long-term dynamic psychotherapy, covering a mean of 248 weeks over a duration of 5.1 years, with a mean of 176 sessions. Assessment consisted of independent interviews to evaluate progress and a median of eight psychotherapy sessions for application of the Defense Mechanism Rating

Scales, whereby trained observers rate defenses observed. Overall defensive functioning improved with a shift from immature to mature defenses. This change was associated with clinical improvement over the 5 years of dynamic therapy. Perry and Bond (2004) did not include a control group, but even if all longer term psychotherapies produce the same result, it supports the proposition that psychological defense mechanism functioning characterizing mental health is enhanced by psychotherapy. Although defense mechanisms were not assessed, a study by Leuzinger-Bohleber et al. (2019) found equal improvement in depression with long-term psychoanalytic and cognitive behavioral therapy, demonstrating similar efficacy. Johansen et al. (2011) compared dynamic and cognitive therapy over 40 sessions for personality disordered participants, finding that defense mechanism functioning shifted from immature to mature in both groups. Hence, psychotherapy over a somewhat longer course does seem to shift defense mechanism functioning in a healthy direction.

Defensive positive cognitive distortions naturally follow from the shift to mature defense mechanisms, with an obvious example humor: placing a lighter positive spin on negative events is very protective. Acting in an altruistic fashion entails the positive cognitive distortion that by treating others in a positive fashion this will come back to you, karma in a sense. Anticipating problems and preparing in a positive fashion likewise involves a positive spin. One of the key reasons why clients with personality disorders benefit from longer term psychotherapy is the positive cognitive distortion shift that ensues by switching from immature to mature defenses (Bowins, 2006, 2010). Transference interpretation can also induce positive cognitive distortions. For instance, a client expresses, "No manager has ever appreciated me." Interpreting the transference, the therapist presents how the client's mother never appreciated her, and perhaps she is seeing this behavior in other authority figures. From this interpretation, the client shifts her perspective in a positive direction now open to the possibility that managers and other authority figures can and do appreciate her. By shifting classical psychological defense mechanisms from immature to mature, and transference interpretations, psychoanalytic therapies induce positive cognitive distortions, thereby further advancing defense mechanism functioning (Bowins, 2006, 2010).

Social Connectedness is often greatly improved via transference interpretation, such as in the above example, allowing the client to bond better with managers and other authority figures. Approaching relationships in a repetitive negative fashion commonly results in isolation and loneliness. Frequently, the origin of painting people of a certain type, or in general, with the same brushstroke is seeing others as a person or persons from the past. For example, a woman lacking female friends only bonds to men who sometimes end up utilizing the "friendship" for sex. The client's mother was rejecting, resenting having to give up her education and a promising career to care for her daughter conceived by accident. The client then assumes that all females will reject her, avoiding contact that could actually lead to friendships. Working with the transference, the client learns that she has incorrectly assumed this response from all females, when it was only her mother that was rejecting. This insight paves the way to forming close relationships with females. Practicing transference interpretations as part of eclectic psychotherapy, I have found this to be a powerful technique, if the interpretation is solid and the person is ready for such an insight. Clients who are not ready typically reject it demonstrating anger toward the therapist. However, when it works the positive transformation, often with much improved social relationships, can be profound.

Psychoanalytic therapy can enhance **Regulation**, or at least emotion regulation, by improving psychological defense mechanism functioning. Immature defenses when applied outside of childhood ensure dysregulated emotions, with an obvious instance acting out essentially producing a temper tantrum. Projecting negative features onto others also fosters poor control over emotions, particularly when the initiator reacts to the perceived projections. For example, a person projects his feelings of anger and aggressive desires onto others and reacts to these people with intense fear. Idealizing and devaluing those in the person's life creates a rollercoaster of emotions that is difficult to regulate. By shifting the client from immature to mature defenses, emotion regulation is greatly advanced. For instance, suppressing negative feelings in the moment to optimize functioning, as opposed to acting out. Likewise, sublimating negative feelings into positive and constructive pursuits effectively regulates adverse emotions. An additional way that psychoanalytic therapy can advance emotion regulation is through reconstructing negative, often early life, experiences into an understanding that relieves distress and fosters personal growth (Cohen, 1990). A neuroimaging study by Buchheim et al. (2012) compared 17 depressed participants to a matched control group, before and after 15 months of psychodynamic psychotherapy. Results were consistent with enhanced emotion regulation, occurring as depressive symptoms declined and general symptom improved.

Psychoanalytic therapy does not obviously appear to advance **Human-Specific Cognition**, although the extensive cognitive activity involved in this approach might well improve some aspects. This occurrence has been suggested for working memory, based on transference interpretations and the associated stimulation of past memories brought into the present (Levin, 1997). Likewise, actively reconstructing past experiences will ramp up working memory. Insights from psychoanalysis, such as those occurring from transference interpretations, also entail inhibiting a familiar sequence of thoughts, and mentally shifting perspectives. For instance, the well-worn perspective that all women will be rejecting based on the client's mother, is shifted to an appreciation that not all women will be rejecting, only my mother. While there is no objective evidence, it does appear that the very cerebral nature of psychoanalytic therapy can improve various executive functions. Social cognition might improve with insights derived from transference interpretations, and applications of these to actual relationships. For example, observing others reactions to discern true from only perceived rejection, and appreciating how one's own behavior influences the reactions of others.

Self-Acceptance is advanced by psychoanalysis due to how this form of therapy resolves conflicts that tend to fragment experience of the self, thereby fostering self-cohesion (Lichtenberg, 1980). The notion here being that healthy development involves integration of diverse aspects of experience forming a cohesive self-image. When this process falters, such as with trauma, self-image remains fragmented and largely unconscious. Psychoanalytic therapy brings these aspects of the self and related conflicts into conscious awareness, where they can be resolved providing for a cohesive self-image. For instance, a person was bullied in childhood for being different. Instead of fusing notions such as the difference arose from superior talent in regards to creativity, the difference is linked to being inferior and socially rejected, creating a conflict in how the creativity is experienced (I'm creative but am lesser than others for it, for example), that blocks fusion of the creativity into a coherent self-image. Consequently, self-concept, self-esteem, and hence self-acceptance suffers. By bringing the conflict and fragmented aspects of the self into consciousness, the conflict can be resolved (I was only rejected for my creativity because others wished to have it and did not, so it is a desired thing), leading to a coherent self-image and self-acceptance. In general, the introspective nature of psychoanalytic therapy leads to improved understanding and acceptance of the self.

Adaptability is fostered by psychoanalysis based on how repetitious dysfunctional behaviors, repetition compulsions (see the Adaptability chapter), impair flexible adaptations to circumstances. Therapy identifies these patterns from free associations, dream analysis, transference and countertransference interpretations, and reworking conflicts. Moving from insight to improvement, these inflexible patterns are altered facilitating more adaptive responses to circumstances. As an example, a therapist becomes aware of feelings of resentment towards the client, and realizes that this is because the client is not initiating any changes. Addressing this with the client it emerges that any change was punished by his parents who valued routine above all else. Hence, even though appealing and having merit, possible changes from therapy are only to be punished in some form. By becoming aware of the conflict between a desire to do things differently and fear of punishment, and how change outside of the early family environment can lead to good outcomes, the client starts experimenting with more flexible approaches often starting in therapy. The good outcomes that ensue further resolve the conflict, and enhance motivation to approach circumstances in more varied and flexible ways. Psychological flexibility and from this behavioral flexibility is then advanced.

Summary note

Psychoanalytic therapy assists clients in understanding how unconscious material is transformed into conscious entities. Techniques including free association and transference interpretation are employed to provide corrective emotional experiences. Given the very introspective nature of this form of therapy, activity is of lower probability and likely restricted to resolving intrapsychic conflicts and ambivalence that block actions. Psychological defense mechanisms in contrast are vastly ramped up by psychoanalytic therapy, with shifts from largely dysfunctional (in adulthood) immature defenses to much more functional mature defenses. This shift fosters positive cognitive distortions, given the much more positive outlook that ensues from these defenses. Transference interpretations also favor positive cognitive distortions, and play a key role in improving social connectedness related to how negative transference commonly impairs social relationships. The shift from immature to mature psychological defense mechanisms greatly improves emotion regulation, due to how difficult it is to regulate emotions with immature defenses, and how mature ones lend themselves to this function. Aspects of human-specific cognition, including working memory, inhibition, and set shifting, might well be strengthened from transference interpretations, reworking past experiences, and the generally very cerebral nature of psychoanalysis. Transference interpretations might in some instances foster better social cognition. Improved self-acceptance occurs when fragmented aspects of the self are fused into a cohesive self-image. Adaptability is fostered when repetitive maladaptive behavior is corrected via free association, dream analysis, transference and countertransference interpretations, and reworking conflicts. Psychoanalysis is probably the oldest formal type of psychotherapy, with many variations employing different techniques. Despite repeated attempts to declare it "dead" it persists, probably due to how it improves the states and processes for mental health.

References

Balestriere, L., 2007. The work of the psychoanalyst in the field of psychosis. Int. J. Psychoanal. 88, 407–421.

Bowins, B.E., 2006. How psychiatric treatments can enhance psychological defense mechanisms. Am. J. Psychoanal. 66, 173–194.

Bowins, B.E., 2010. Personality disorders: a dimensional defense mechanism approach. Am. J. Psychother. 64 (2), 153–169.

Buchheim, A., Viviani, R., Kessler, H., Kachele, H., Cierpka, M., Roth, G., et al., 2012. Changes in prefrontal-limbic function in major depression after 15 months of long-term psychotherapy. PLoS One. doi:10.1371/journal.pone.0033745.

Cohen, D.J., 1990. Enduring sadness. Early loss, vulnerability, and the shaping of character. Psychoanal. Stud. Child 45, 157–178.

Fox, M.D., Raichle, M.E., 2007. Spontaneous fluctuations in brain activity with functional magnetic resonance imaging. Nat. Rev. Neurosci. 8, 700–711.

Freud, S., 1900. The Interpretation of Dreams, Standard Edition 4/5.

Freud, S., 1915. The Unconscious, Standard Edition 14, 166–215.

Freud, S., 1964. The neuro-psychosis of defense In J. Strachey the Standard Edition of the Complete Psychological Works of Sigmund Freud, vol. 3. Hogarth Press, London, pp. 45–61.

Frosch, J., 1976. Psychoanalytic contributions to the relationship between dreams and psychosis-a critical survey. Int. J. Psychoanal. Psychother. 5, 39–63.

Johansen, P.O., Krebs, T.S., Svartberg, M., Stiles, T.C., Holen, A., 2011. Change in defense mechanisms during short-term dynamic and cognitive therapy in patients with cluster C personality disorders. J. Nerv. Ment. Dis. 199 (9), 712–715.

Leuzinger-Bohleber, M., Hautzinger, M., Fiedler, G., Keller, W., Bahrke, U., Kallenbach, L., 2019. Outcome of psychoanalytic and cognitive-behavioral long-term therapy with chronically depressed patients: a controlled trial with preferential and randomized allocation. Can. J. Psychiatry 64 (1), 45–58.

Levin, F.M., 1997. Integrating some mind and brain views of transference: the phenomena. J. Am. Psychoanal. Assoc. 45 (4), 1121–1151.

Lichtenberg, J.D., 1980–81. Clinical application of the concept of a cohesive sense of self. Int. J. Psychoanal. Psychother. 8, 85–114.

Miller, L., 1997. Freud and consciousness: the first one hundred years of neuropsychodynamics in theory and clinical practice. Semin. Neurol. 17 (2), 171–177.

Morsella, E., Krieger, S.C., Bargh, J.A., 2010. Minimal neuroanatomy for a conscious brain: homing in on the networks constituting consciousness. Neural Netw. 23, 14–15.

Perry, C., 2001. A pilot study of defenses in adults with personality disorders entering psychotherapy. J. Nerv. Ment. Dis. 189, 651–660.

Perry, J.C., Bond, M., 2004. Long-term changes in defense styles with psychodynamic psychotherapy for depressive, anxiety, and personality disorders. Am. J. Psychiatry 161 (9), 1665–1671.

Power, M., Brewin, C.R., 1991. From Freud to cognitive science: a contemporary account of the unconscious. Br. J. Clin. Psychol. 30, 289–310.

Robbins, M., 2008. Primary mental expression: Freud, Klein, and beyond. J. Am. Psychoanal. Assoc. 56 (1), 177–202.

Vaillant, G., 1977. Adaptation to Life. Little, Brown and Company, Boston.

Vaillant, G., 1994. Ego mechanisms of defense and personality psychopathology. J. Abnorm. Psychol. 103 (1), 44–50.

Van Wijk-Herbrink, M., Andrea, H., Verheul, R., 2011. Cognitive coping and defense styles in patients with personality disorders. J. Personal. Disord. 25 (5), 634–644.

Vlastelica, M., Jurcevic, S., Zemunik, T., 2005. Changes of defense mechanisms and personality profile during group analytic treatment. Coll. Anthropol. 29 (2), 551–558.

Zhang, D., Raichle, M.E., 2010. Disease and the brain's dark energy. Nat. Rev. Neurol. 6, 15–18.

Chapter 25

Rational-emotive therapy

Overview

Albert Ellis started this form of therapy back in the 1950s, initially naming it rational-emotive behavior therapy, then rational-emotive therapy, and later returning to the original title (Ellis, 1980, 1991). Interestingly, it focuses on emotions, cognitions, and behavior leading some to consider it a form of cognitive therapy and others a variant of behavior therapy. I will apply the rational-emotive title to remove the direct link to behavior therapy, given that the title rational-emotive behavior therapy seems to diminish the cognitive aspect which is a crucial component, and the term rational-emotive is one of the most distinct there is without adding to it. The basic premise advanced by Ellis is straightforward: emotional reactions to stimuli are mediated by cognitions (Ellis, 1980, 1991). In other words, it is the interpretation of a stimulus that determines the emotional reaction. Currently, this notion seems obvious, but when Ellis was developing this form of therapy it was not consistent with behaviorism, diminishing or eliminating the role of cognitions. The ABC's of rational-emotive therapy consist of (Ellis, 1980, 1991):

- A—Activating Event that triggers an emotional reaction.
- B—Beliefs related to the event.
- C—Consequence referring to an emotional response to the belief.

Hence, the link is A to B to C, and not A to C direct.

As pertains to mental health, cognitions (beliefs) that are rational lead to healthy emotional reactions, whereas irrational ones result in mental illness behavior, including depression and anxiety (Ellis, 1980, 1991). Rational and irrational beliefs are said to differ, in that rational ones are flexible shifting with circumstances in keeping with reality, and hence rationality. Irrational beliefs have an inflexible aspect, expressed as absolutes and demands or musts, such as "I cannot," resulting in ongoing dysfunction (Ellis, 1980, 1991). They also tend to be evaluative or appraisal oriented and not descriptive, aligning with their emotional import (David et al., 2018). From this characterization of irrational beliefs, it follows that a primary goal of psychotherapy is to shift irrational beliefs to rational ones, in order that psychopathology be properly treated (Ellis, 1980, 1991). Given the inflexible and repetitive nature of irrational beliefs underlying mental illness manifestations, it can be very challenging to transform them into rational beliefs, and the therapeutic approach is quite

States and Processes for Mental Health. DOI: 10.1016/C2020-0-00574-8

confrontational and expressive (emotive). Ellis was disturbed by the lack of actual behavioral change he noted with other therapies, and strived to ensure that rational-emotive therapy produces actual change in dysfunctional behavior (Ellis, 1980, 1991; Sacks, 2004). Steps taken include (Ellis, 1980, 1991):

- Identifying the irrational beliefs and thought patterns underlying the mental illness manifestation.
- Challenge the irrational beliefs in an emotive way to reveal how the belief leads to dysfunctional emotional reactions. This step includes direct debates and even confrontation.
- Replace irrational beliefs with rational ones eliciting healthy emotional responses.
- Ensuring that the client gains insight into the process so that irrational beliefs are recognized and shifted, as opposed to a therapist being required ongoing to challenge every one that emerges.
- Even though dispute and confrontation is part of the process, necessary due to how inflexible and automatic irrational beliefs are, therapy is collaborative (Ellis, 1980, 1991).

The key assumption of rational-emotive therapy—irrational beliefs underlie psychopathology—has been tested and challenged. The literature is quite extensive but I will provide a sampling of research investigating this premise. Oltean and David (2018) evaluated 26 studies examining the link between the rationality of beliefs and psychological distress, finding a medium negative association: the less rational the belief the more psychological distress. Focusing on PTSD, Hyland et al. (2014) tested 313 active law enforcement, military, and related emergency service personnel, considering various types of beliefs. Depreciating (irrational) beliefs increased PTSD symptoms, while acceptance (rational) beliefs were protective, moderating the impact of catastrophizing thoughts. An earlier study by Muran et al. (1989) compared irrational thinking between 60 normal university students and 45 new clients for mental health services, testing for various emotional problems. They found that the clinical subjects overall did not have more extensive irrational thinking, but those with high depression, and also greater trait anger and total guilt, did have more irrational beliefs. Testing the notion that attribution (evaluative) beliefs are of greatest concern, Ziegler and Hawley (2001) administered the Survey of Personal Beliefs and the Attributional Style Questionnaire to 180 college students, finding that those scoring higher on a pessimistic explanatory style also scored higher on overall irrational thinking. Relevant to how there are common processes to psychotherapy and treatment generally, Szentagotai et al. (2008) compared rational-emotive therapy, cognitive behavior therapy, and pharmacotherapy in the treatment of major depressive disorder, measuring automatic thoughts, dysfunctional attitudes, and irrational beliefs. Each type of intervention produced changes in the three types of cognitions. Hence, research does tend to support the link between irrational beliefs and mental illness, but addressing these directly might not be necessary.

Enhancement of states and processes for mental health

Even at face value it would seem that replacing persistent irrational beliefs contributing to emotional suffering and ongoing dysfunction, with flexible rational beliefs will advance mental health parameters, but let us see how this likely plays out. Regarding **Activity**, rational-emotive therapy strives for real behavioral change; talking is not enough. Irrational beliefs often have a way of blocking action due to their negative, inflexible, and absolute aspects. For example, "I simply cannot work." If the client persists in this belief then it is a safe assumption that he or she will never work, unless a greater need overrides the resistance, such as threatened starvation. Shifting the irrational thought to, "I actually can work based on prior experience and certain strengths," is likely to translate into efforts to return to the work force. The therapeutic emphasis on actual behavior change increases the likelihood of this occurrence. Most therapists have had the experience of clients seemingly shifting to a rational view but never delivering on real change, a problem that rational-emotive therapy addresses even with confrontation. Activity of diverse forms can be advanced when the irrational belief blocks such actions, and rational beliefs favoring activity are generated and followed through on.

Irrational negative beliefs result in negative emotions, which strengthen the initial belief in a mutually reinforcing fashion, fostering negative cognitive distortions. The persistent nature of these beliefs blocks behavior that could instill more positive feelings. Shifting to positive rational beliefs advances the positive cognitive distortion form of **Psychological Defense Mechanism** yielding positive emotions that reinforce the new belief. For instance, "I can work and the social and monetary rewards will help me a lot." Even though the term "rational" might seem inconsistent with "distortions," as presented in the Psychological defense mechanism chapter reality is very elusive to capture accurately, and when thoughts link to emotions where neutral does not apply (+1 and −1 do not = 0, both coexisting), there is a negative or positive distortion. Even classical psychological defense mechanisms appear to advance from rational-emotive therapy, based on a study by Kachman and Mazer (1990), who examined this form of therapy applied to a mental health program for adolescents, with pretest and post-test measures of defense mechanisms, showing that even in 12 sessions a shift to more mature defense mechanisms transpired.

Social Connectedness can improve from rational-emotive therapy related to how Irrational thoughts commonly pertain to the social environment, once again due to human evolution in hunting-gathering groups, and hence the importance of the social environment. An example of an irrational social thought is, "People never accept me." The absolute nature of the belief blocks attempts to socialize or respond positively to other people. If this inflexible irrational belief is shifted to, "I can get along with some people, particularly when they share my dark sense of humor," the client will be much more likely to try and establish good social relationships, and respond positively to the efforts of others, thereby advancing social connectedness.

Regulation of emotions and behavior can transpire indirectly with rational-emotive therapy, based on the persistent negative emotions and behavior that follows from irrational and inflexible negative beliefs: emotional and behavioral reactions, such as fear of people and confrontation, often persist if the irrational beliefs remain in place. By shifting to more rational beliefs negative emotions are diminished and dysfunctional behavior countered, providing enhanced control over them. Furthering the impact on emotion regulation is the transtherapy influence for this important aspect of psychological functioning, discussed in the Behavioral therapy chapter.

Improvements in **Human-Specific Cognition** are of lesser probability and indirect, only occurring when the shift from irrational to rational beliefs enhances motivation and/or social activity, the latter providing an opportunity to improve social cognition. For example, the person who holds the belief that others will never accept her blocking social interactions, now believes that she can be liked and certainly by those sharing her dark sense of humor, resulting in increased social interactions that give her a better sense of her role in relationships and the intentions of other people (improved social cognition).

Self-Acceptance can advance from rational-emotive therapy based on how irrational thoughts are often depreciating to the self, such as a person believing that no one will accept them based on some perceived negative quality. Shifting to a more rational belief that is flexible, such as, "People who are okay with my limitations and value my strengths will want to be with me," enhances self-perspectives (self-concept), self-evaluation (self-esteem), and from these changes self-acceptance. The Hyland et al. (2014) study reviewed above demonstrates how for PTSD rational acceptance related beliefs instilled by rational-emotive therapy counter depreciating beliefs, improving PTSD symptoms.

Adaptability is powerfully advanced due to the ongoing inflexible and maladaptive behavior that commonly follows from irrational beliefs, and certainly the ones that are identified and targeted in therapy. Rational beliefs, on the other hand, are more flexible shifting with circumstances. For instance, "I have a lot to contribute to conversations provided I know something about the topic," as opposed to, "I never have anything useful to contribute." By robustly shifting irrational beliefs favoring inflexible behavior to rational beliefs fostering flexible actions, adaptability is strongly advanced. The solid efforts to produce real behavioral change ensure that adaptive behavior materializes and persists.

Summary note

The core belief of rational-emotive therapy—emotional reactions to stimuli are mediated by cognitions—is very straightforward and robust. Rational beliefs are more in line with the demands of reality, and so tend to be functional, whereas irrational ones produce emotional and behavioral dysfunction. Given that the requirements for functional behavior shifts, rational beliefs change with circumstances. Irrational beliefs tend be evaluative with absolute qualities, impairing responses. Due to the highly rigid nature of irrational beliefs therapy must challenge these thoughts to instill rational beliefs, and ensure actual behavior change consistent with the revised beliefs.

Regarding the states and processes for mental health, improvements are highly likely with some and indirect, conditional, and/or lower probability with others. When irrational beliefs block activity based on their negative and absolute nature, shifting to rational beliefs can result in increased activity, particularly given the active nature of rational-emotive therapy striving for real behavioral change. The positive cognitive distortion form of psychological defense mechanism is advanced, based on how mutually reinforcing irrational beliefs and negative emotions foster negative cognitive distortions, with the shift to rational beliefs favoring positive cognitive distortions. Social connectedness can be enhanced when the irrational beliefs pertain to the social environment, a common scenario, as such thoughts impair good social relationships. Rational thoughts that shift flexibly with social circumstances will improve relationships. Regulation of emotions and behavior can indirectly advance, due to how the persistent and repetitive negative emotions and behavior following from irrational beliefs are difficult to regulate, but are largely eliminated with successful therapy.

Human-specific cognition is less likely to improve and only indirectly when rational beliefs fostered by therapy improve motivation, and increased social activity transpires affording opportunities to improve social cognition. Irrational thoughts with their evaluative aspect are often self-depreciating, and by ending these and shifting to positive rational beliefs self-acceptance can advance. A key notion of rational-emotive therapy is how irrational beliefs are rigid and inflexible repeating when not warranted by circumstances, whereas rational beliefs change with various settings and occurrences. From this, it clearly follows that by replacing irrational beliefs with rational ones, adaptability will be greatly enhanced. Although focused on one form of belief underlying psychopathology—irrational—and the resulting emotions and behavior, rational-emotive therapy does have the capacity to advance the states and processes for mental health, although some of these mechanisms of action are limited.

References

David, D., Cotet, C., Matu, S., Mogoase, C., Stefan, S., 2018. 50 years of rational-emotive and cognitive behavioral therapy: a systematic review and meta-analysis. J. Clin. Psychol. 74 (3), 304–318.

Ellis, A., 1980. Rational-emotive therapy and cognitive behavior therapy: similarities and differences. Cogn. Ther. Res. 4 (4), 325–340.

Ellis, A., 1991. The revised ABC's of rational-emotive therapy (RET). J. Ration. Emot. Ther. 9 (3), 139–172.

Hyland, P., Shevlin, M., Adamson, G., Boduszek, D., 2014. The moderating role of rational beliefs in the relationship between irrational beliefs and posttraumatic stress symptomology. Behav. Cogn. Psychother. 42 (3), 312–326.

Kachman, D.J., Mazer, G.E., 1990. Effects of rational emotive education on the rationality, neuroticism and defense mechanisms of adolescents. Adolescence 25 (7), 131–144.

Oltean, H.R., David, D.O., 2018. A meta-analysis of the relationship between rational beliefs and psychological distress. J. Clin. Psychol. 74 (6), 883–895.

Muran, J.C., Kassinove, H., Ross, S., Muran, E., 1989. Irrational thinking and negative emotionality in college students and applicants for mental health services. J. Clin. Psychol. 45 (2), 188–193.

Sacks, S.B., 2004. Rational emotive behavior therapy: disputing irrational philosophies. J. Psychosoc. Nurs. Ment. Health Serv. 42 (5), 22–31.

Szentagotai, A., David, D., Lupu, V., Cosman, D., 2008. Rational emotive behavior therapy versus cognitive therapy versus pharmacotherapy in the treatment of major depressive disorder: mechanisms of change analysis. Psychotherapy (Chicago) 45 (4), 523–538.

Ziegler, D.J., Hawley, J.L., 2001. Relation of irrational thinking and the pessimistic explanatory style. Psychol. Rep. 88 (2), 483–488.

Chapter 26

Nonspecific factors

Overview

The forms of psychotherapy covered purport to treat mental illness by way of specific strategies and approaches, such as transference interpretation for psychoanalytic therapy and altering negative thoughts with cognitive therapy. The theme of this book is how instead of specific psychotherapeutic approaches working by remedying psychopathology, they are actually improving the states and processes for mental health. Potentially helping to shed light on how psychotherapy actually works, is the notion of nonspecific psychotherapy factors fostering good mental health outcomes. The term "nonspecific factors" is most appropriate, because although the individual factors have some specificity, they act across various specific approaches. The alternative name, common factors, is less appropriate because a specific approach can be common, particularly given how fads often dominate in the mental health sphere.

Consistent with positive cognitive distortions characterizing mental health, psychotherapist tends to view the specific factors of their given approach as being most potent, but nonspecific factors are powerful. Cuijpers et al. (2012) examined 31 studies of nondirective supportive psychotherapy for depression that compared it to control groups, other forms of psychotherapy, or medication. Nondirective supportive psychotherapy seemed to be less effective than the comparison form, but when they controlled for researcher allegiance differences in effectiveness vanished. Extra-therapeutic factors, such as being on a waiting list and treatment as usual, were found to account for 33.3% of overall improvement, nonspecific psychotherapy factors 49.6%, and specific factors of the psychotherapy approaches only 17.1%! Even if this study somehow found too high contributions for nonspecific factors and too low for specific factors (as a psychotherapist I might well be engaging in a positive cognitive distortion here), the role of nonspecific factors is far from insignificant. Backing up the role of nonspecific factors, Palpacuer et al. (2017) conducted a systematic review and meta-analysis of psychotherapy studies for depression covering diverse approaches. Psychotherapy had a significant impact on depression, but after controlling for nonspecific factors including number of treatment sessions, length of treatment, and therapeutic alliance, psychotherapies were no longer significant. Any informed coverage of psychotherapy must then consider nonspecific factors.

States and Processes for Mental Health. DOI: 10.1016/C2020-0-00574-8

Now that we have established the importance of nonspecific factors, what do they consist of (yes, this might be viewed as specific)? As indicated by the Palpacuer et al. (2017) study, basic features such as number of treatment sessions and length of treatment can be included, as well as any other similar component, such as amount of time devoted to treatment. Even intuitively it seems feasible that the more sessions and time spent the greater the likelihood of improvement, at least to a point. Beyond quantity, quality weighs in and in this regard one of the most potent nonspecific factors is the therapeutic alliance (Daniels and Wearden, 2011; Tschacher et al., 2014; Yager and Feinstein, 2017). From my experience and that of other psychotherapists I have spoken to throughout the years, good psychotherapy outcomes are heavily influenced by the quality of the relationship between the client and therapist. When the alliance is really solid, great outcomes often ensue, but rarely do when the alliance is poor, with the client frequently ending therapy prematurely or not progressing well. Indeed, I have come to believe that successful psychotherapists have a capacity to form solid therapeutic alliances. Research backs up this perspective demonstrating that the therapeutic alliance is associated with positive psychotherapy outcomes for diverse conditions: self-harm and suicidal behavior (Dunster-Page et al., 2017), trauma (Ellis et al., 2018), psychosis and schizophrenic spectrum issues (Browne et al., 2019; Shatttock et al., 2018), eating disorders (Graves et al., 2017), depression and anxiety (Pihlaja et al., 2017; Wehmann et al., 2020).

The reason for why the quality of the client–therapist relationship is so prominent, probably resides in how the therapeutic alliance is pivotal for other relationship components, including trust, openness, caring, support, degree of engagement, positive regard and affirmation, collaboration, congruence, overcoming any cultural differences, and agreement over direction (Daniels and Wearden, 2011; Tschacher et al., 2014; Yager and Feinstein, 2017). The therapeutic alliance serves as a "vehicle" for the delivery of these positive relationship factors (Catty, 2004). When people resonate with each other, all such aspects of interacting are advanced, and in a mutually reinforcing fashion: the alliance fosters these components and when they are solid the alliance is strengthened. Ultimately, our evolution in hunting-gathering groups and consequently "social brain" enables positive interpersonal relationships to advance mental health (see the Social connectedness chapter).

Psychological functioning, independent of social relationships, is also advanced with all forms of psychotherapy, and in this regard, the most powerful ingredient is likely hope. Having optimism for good outcomes in the future is a positive cognitive distortion integral to healthy psychological functioning, as Tiger (1979) pointed out in his book Optimism: The Biology of Hope. Without the positive bias of hope despair sets in with depression and anxiety close companions (Dembo and Clemens, 2013). To some extent, hope follows from a good therapeutic alliance and perceiving that another person is supportive and cares. However, it largely ensues from other humanistic psychological influences integral to all psychotherapies, including a rationale for suffering, making sense of the world, ways to resolve or improve the problem, motivation for constructive activity (engagement), a sense of mastery or at least impact on the suffering, and establishing workable expectations (Wampold, 2012). These positive psychological nonspecific factors produce mental health gains on their own, while also fostering the potent benefit of hope.

Nonspecific psychotherapy factors also encompass therapist-based ones with many cited: empathy, caring, reliable, honest, respectful, trustworthy, confident, warm, interested, flexible, open, authentic, psychologically minded, communication, collaboration, rapport building, alliance focus, boundary setting, cultural sensitivity, self-disclosure, and responsiveness (Ackerman and Hilsenroth, 2003; Bachar, 1998; Datta-Barua and Hauser, 2018; Farber et al., 2005; Glass, 2003; Greben, 1977; Goldstein and Suzuki, 2015; Priebe et al., 2011; Spencer et al., 2019; Sue, 1998). Empathy, referring to the capacity to feel the emotional state of another person, stands out as most potent, because it enables the therapist to understand and work with the experience of clients, and facilitates the application of the other therapist-based nonspecific factors. On a continuum of empathy from psychopathic lacking empathy to highly empathic, psychotherapists occupy the higher end; there is little motivation to go into such an occupation if you do not empathize with the experiences of others, and you are unlikely to do well. Research supports the robust role of empathy, such as Elliot et al. (2018) finding that empathy generally accounts for 9% of the variance in psychotherapy outcomes with a moderate effect size, based on a review of 82 studies. The results held across various theoretical perspectives and presenting problems. Empathy contributes significantly to psychotherapy outcomes for various mental illnesses including depression (McClintock et al., 2018), anxiety (Hara et al., 2017), and alcohol abuse (Moyers et al., 2016). Empathy facilitates the application of therapist-based nonspecific factors with psychotherapists varying in these capacities, helping to explain why they do have differing levels of success with clients (Miller and Moyers, 2015). Empathy also fosters the therapeutic alliance, as evidenced by a meta-analysis of 53 studies finding that perceptions of therapist empathy and genuineness were significantly associated with the therapeutic alliance, and that empathy and genuineness overlapped when rated by the same person (Nienhuis et al., 2018).

The social, psychological, and psychotherapist nonspecific factors undoubtedly interact to amplify their benefit. In this regard, therapist empathy is crucial as it favors a good therapeutic alliance with the ensuing benefits, and contributes to the therapist understanding the client well enough to advance the psychological aspects, thereby generating hope. With a good therapeutic alliance, the therapist is more motivated to work with the client and apply empathy. From the client's perspective, a solid therapeutic alliance will foster greater openness to the psychological benefits. If the client experiences hope and the other psychological nonspecific benefits, then the therapeutic alliance will be advanced allowing the therapist factors to be more effectual.

Acting at a more general level, a couple features of the healing process represent nonspecific factors: natural healing and regression to the mean (Chiesa, 2011). Regarding the former, even without treatment many mental illness issues, and certainly depression and anxiety, naturally demonstrate improvement. Regression to the mean refers to how extreme variants of any scenario tend to correct to the mean, in this instance meaning that extremes of mental illness will shift to more average levels, even without intervention.

An additional category of nonspecific factors is the placebo effect, distinct from the other nonspecific factors by its very general nature extending to virtually all treatments. For example, the placebo response to antidepressants is estimated to be at least 31% and rises 7% per decade (Rutherford and Roose, 2013). It is not just positive therapeutic responses that occur, but negative responses blocking or hindering improvement, referred to as the nocebo effect. The variable positive and negative impacts arise from the apparent origin: conscious- and unconscious-shaped expectancies and resulting beliefs (Chavarria et al., 2017; Enck et al., 2017; Frisaldi et al., 2015; Rutherford and Roose, 2013). If a person expects that cognitive psychotherapy will work, then it likely will. Conversely, if a person believes that it will not have any positive impact then it is less likely to be beneficial, although such a belief usually results in a person not continuing.

Placebo-induced expectancies are shaped by influences such as classical conditioning, instructions and explanations, and social/cultural learning (Chavarria et al., 2017; Enck et al., 2017; Frisaldi et al., 2015; Rutherford and Roose, 2013). Classical conditioning is mostly an unconscious route to shaping expectancies: a conditioned stimulus such as a pill or white lab coat is repeatedly paired with the unconditioned stimulus of a health intervention, that yields the unconditioned response of a health improvement, and then the conditioned stimulus starts to produce the conditioned response of improved health. The entire process typically occurs unconsciously, but shapes expectancies and beliefs. For example, most people naturally expect a pill to be beneficial, and believe that a doctor often symbolized by a white lab coat will help improve health. The instructions and explanations that a psychotherapist provides relevant to the form or forms of psychotherapy they intend to apply are a conscious influence shaping expectancies and beliefs. For example, cognitive therapists explaining how thoughts are instrumental in feelings and emotional responses, and by altering thoughts in a positive direction, positive feeling states and emotional responses ensue. If the rationale processed largely consciously is acceptable, then expectancies and resulting beliefs pertaining to cognitive therapy are positive. Social and cultural influences can operate both unconsciously and consciously to shape expectancies. For instance, in many traditional cultures the role of shaman or natural healer is established through experience and delivered information since childhood, guiding the expectation that such a practitioner and their interventions will improve health.

Even if classical conditioning, instructions and explanations, and social/cultural learning shape expectancies and related beliefs, the impact on health outcomes would be nil without a solid link to physiological responses. Indeed, there is neuroimaging evidence that intentional content, such as that derived from placebo-based expectancies, significantly influences brain functioning at various levels including molecular, cellular, neural connectivity, and brain plasticity (Beauregard, 2009). Neurochemicals appear to be the mediating variables, with placebos demonstrated to alter neurotransmitters, including dopamine and serotonin, and endorphins (Dodd et al., 2017; Haour, 2005; Holmes et al., 2016). How the placebo effect and wider intentional content does this has yet to be fully explained, but the explanation undoubtedly captures the power of the mind–body connection.

Placebo effects and the other nonspecific factors relevant to psychotherapy play a powerful role in psychotherapy outcomes, and even though therapists and researchers wish to believe that it is the special sauce they provide (a positive cognitive distortion), these more general influences should not be ignored. The notion of psychotherapy operating not by remedying mental illness through specific techniques, but by advancing the states and processes for mental health, aligns extremely well with nonspecific factors including the placebo effect: nonspecific factors tap into natural healing processes advancing mentally healthy states and processes! Now we will look at how this might transpire.

Enhancement of states and processes for mental health

How the social, psychological, and psychotherapist nonspecific factors interact is relevant to advancing the states and processes for mental health, in that these interactions will amplify benefits. Add in the placebo effect and any benefits will really be furthered. Hence, if a given impact on the states and processes for mental health seems limited it in and of itself, it might well become highly significant through interactive effects.

Activity would not appear to be advanced by nonspecific factors with the exception of social activity. The therapeutic alliance is crucial to psychotherapy effectiveness and the therapeutic relationship constitutes social activity. Many people who attend for psychotherapy are relatively isolated, either as a contributing influence on mental illness or a consequence, such as depression that is more likely with loneliness, and how when depressed a person withdraws while others pull back. Within this relatively isolated context, the therapeutic relationship might be their only real social activity or a very significant component. It is also feasible that with hope and the contributing psychological influences, such as a sense of mastery, a person will be more active generally.

The key psychological nonspecific factor of hope is probably one of the most potent forms of positive cognitive distortion there is, and consequently **Psychological Defense Mechanisms** are strongly advanced. With hope, multiple positive outcomes become viable that previously seemed unattainable. Conversely, lack of hope is a perspective yielding few if any positive outcomes. Based on interactive influences, with hope a person will be more active, and the activity is likely to generate positive outcomes augmenting hope. For example, a person suffering from joint problems who previously was active becomes depressed, partly or largely based on perceiving no chance of ongoing activity. By becoming hopeful that activity can occur, the person starts walking and being active, seeing that it actually relieves the stiffness, and this instills more hope, and so on and so forth.

Social Connectedness is very advanced by the quality aspect of the therapeutic alliance. Many social interactions are characterized by limited depth of interactive content, which restricts the sense of social connectedness. For example, a male client of mine has several "friends" mostly in the context of nights out after work, but to "engage" he had to learn about hockey, although not interested, as conversations went nowhere otherwise at least during hockey season; in Canada, hockey is of much higher status than God to many people. To have "friends" he had to engage in superficial conversation. Trust, openness, caring, compassion, support, understanding, consistency, high engagement, positive regard and affirmation, relevant feedback, and collaboration, are not common features in most relationships, typically only occurring with good friendships, but these features do characterize robust client–therapist relationships, thereby fostering social connectedness and serving as a template for similar connections with other people. Therapist empathy facilitates these quality aspects of the client–therapist relationship, and so contributes greatly to social connectedness.

Conditions that lead people into psychotherapy frequently entail **Regulation** limitations, such as that over emotions. For instance, depression and anxiety are characterized by impaired regulation of the root emotions of sadness and fear, respectively (Bowins, 2004). As presented in the Behavioral therapy chapter, emotion regulation is likely a transtherapy process improving with psychotherapy regardless of the form and subtype (Neacsiu et al., 2017; Sloan et al., 2017). This occurrence strongly suggests that nonspecific factors play a significant role. There are several ways that this could occur, including generally activating regulation as part of the natural healing they induce, since regulation is such a prominent characteristic of mental health. More specifically, psychotherapist factors ensuing from empathy including compassion, understanding, support, consistency, and relevant feedback, appear to be capable of levelling out extremes of emotions and behavior, and provide a template for regulation that the client internalizes. This impact is very obvious for personality disordered clients who lack internal regulation, and initially rely on external regulation from the therapist until they internalize the process. Interactions between therapist factors and the therapeutic alliance can amplify regulation benefits: therapist features that advance regulation also foster a solid therapeutic alliance based on how they increase trust in the therapist, and a superior therapeutic alliance increases the chances that the pro-regulation therapist features will be internalized. A key way that emotion regulation is enhanced by nonspecific factors appears to be interpersonal synchrony transpiring with a solid therapeutic alliance, acting via emotional sharing and common understanding (Koole and Tschacher, 2016).

Human-Specific Cognition can be improved by nonspecific psychotherapy factors, and certainly motivation which follows from the some of the psychological features including, making sense of the world, motivation for constructive activity (engagement), a sense of mastery or at least impact on the suffering, and establishing workable expectations, that all feed into hope. Motivation follows from hope, and de-motivation occurs with lack of hope. Social cognition can improve from features of the therapeutic alliance (trust, openness, caring, support, degree of engagement, positive regard and affirmation, collaboration, overcoming any cultural differences, and agreement over direction) and therapist factors (empathy, compassion, understanding, support, consistency, and relevant feedback), based on how they characterize social cognition. Where I have clearly noted this occurrence is with clients who are lacking in social skills, who shortly start demonstrating the social behaviors I have modeled, often reporting improved social interactions.

Self-Acceptance is advanced from nonspecific factors, and in particular the social acceptance that is implicit with a good therapeutic alliance. We are a social species and high-quality social contact contributes to positive self-concept and self-esteem, with improved self-acceptance. The psychological influences also contribute, such as with hope a person is likely to view their actions more favorably. Making sense of the world, mastery, and reasonable expectations relevant to the self, will also foster self-acceptance. For example, if a person has excessively high expectations for their success, self-criticisms follow from performance not matching expectations. Adjusting expectations allows their achievements to be perceived as gains yielding contentment, improved self-concept, and enhanced self-evaluation (self-esteem).

Research indicates that intentional content such as the placebo effect influences brain functioning at various levels including molecular, cellular, neural connectivity, and brain plasticity (Beauregard, 2009). By improving brain plasticity, the placebo effect alone likely improves **Adaptability**, given that more flexible behavior follows from enhanced neural plasticity. Additionally, several psychological nonspecific factors including making sense of the world, ways to resolve or improve the problem, motivation for constructive activity (engagement), a sense of mastery, and establishing workable expectations, would seem to foster more adaptable behavior, at least as relates to the client's issues. Social adaptability might be improved from the therapeutic alliance based on features such as collaboration, overcoming any cultural differences, and agreement over direction, that foster more flexible social behavior. The therapeutic setting is typically a safe forum for people to experiment with ideas, behaviors, and social engagement. The outcome of these experiments commonly leads to changes outside of therapy with a theme of enhanced adaptability; in fact, if no changes in these parameters occur outside of therapy, then the success of psychotherapy is questionable.

Summary note

The term nonspecific factors is appropriate because although they have some specificity, they operate across various specific psychotherapy approaches. Nonspecific psychotherapy factors contribute to a substantial portion of the variance in outcomes, demonstrating their power. They take the form of basic aspects of therapy provision, therapeutic alliance, psychological influences, therapist features, and the placebo effect. By tapping into natural healing processes, these nonspecific factors advance mental health, with psychological influences, therapeutic alliance, and therapist features frequently interacting to amplify benefits. Social activity is enhanced by the therapeutic relationship, and hope might foster other forms of activity. The potent positive cognitive distortion of hope is a key psychological influence advancing psychological defense mechanisms. Social connectivity follows from the quality aspect of the client–therapist relationship embodied in the therapeutic alliance.

Nonspecific factors appear to contribute to the transtherapy influence of all forms and subtypes of psychotherapy in improving emotion regulation, partly by activating natural healing processes including regulation. Additionally, interpersonal synchrony associated with the therapeutic alliance and therapist nonspecific factors with empathy pivotal, greatly enhance emotion regulation. Human-specific cognition in regards to motivation is advanced by nonspecific psychological factors, while social cognition might benefit from the therapeutic alliance and therapist factors. Self-acceptance follows from the social acceptance implicit with a good therapeutic alliance, and also from some of the psychological influences such as hope. Neural plasticity induced by nonspecific factors enhances adaptability, with many of the psychological factors fostering more flexible behavior, and the therapeutic alliance greater social flexibility. By recruiting natural healing processes yielding mentally healthy states and processes, nonspecific factors align extremely well with and support the central premise of this book that psychotherapy works by advancing states and processes for mental health.

References

Ackerman, S.J., Hilsenroth, M.J., 2003. A review of therapist characteristics and techniques positively impacting on the therapeutic alliance. Clin. Psychol. Rev. 23 (1), 1–33.

Bachar, E., 1998. Psychotherapy—an active agent: assessing the effectiveness of psychotherapy and its curative factors. Isr. J. Psychiatry Relat. Sci. 35 (2), 128–135.

Beauregard, M., 2009. Effect of mind on brain activity: evidence from neuroimaging studies of psychotherapy and placebo effect. Nord. J. Psychiatry 63 (1), 5–16.

Bowins, B.E., 2004. Psychological defense mechanisms: a new perspective. Am. J. Psychoanal. 64, 1–26.

Browne, J., Nagendra, A., Kurtz, M., Berry, K., Penn, D.L., 2019. The relationship between the therapeutic alliance and client variables in individual treatment for schizophrenic spectrum disorders and early psychosis: narrative review. Clin. Psychol. Rev. 71, 51–62.

Catty, J., 2004. 'The vehicle of success': theoretical and empirical perspectives on the therapeutic alliance in psychotherapy and psychiatry. Psychol. Psychother. 77 (2), 255–272.

Chavarria, V., Vian, J., Pereira, C., Data-Franco, J., Fernandes, B.S., Berk, M., et al., 2017. The placebo and nocebo phenomena: their clinical management and impact on treatment outcomes. Clin. Ther. 39 (3), 477–486.

Chiesa, A., 2011. Improving psychotherapy research: the example of mindfulness based interventions. World J. Methodol. 1 (1), 4–11.

Cuijpers, P., Driessen, E., Hollon, S.D., Van Oppen, P, Barth, J., Andersson, G., 2012. The efficacy of non-directive supportive therapy for adult depression: a meta-analysis. Clin. Psychol. Rev. 32 (4), 280–291.

Daniels, J., Wearden, A.J., 2011. Socialization to the model: the active component in the therapeutic alliance? A preliminary study. Behav. Cogn. Psychother. 39 (2), 221–227.

Datta-Barua, I., Hauser, J., 2018. Four communication skills from psychiatry useful in palliative care and how to teach them. AMA J. Eth. 20 (8), E717–E723.

Dembo, J.S., Clemens, N.A., 2013. The ethics of providing hope in psychotherapy. J. Psychiatr. Pract. 19 (4), 316–322.

Dodd, S., Dean, O.M., Vian, J., Berk, M., 2017. A review of the theoretical and biological understanding of the nocebo and placebo phenomena. Clin. Ther. 39 (3), 469–476.

Dunster-Page, C., Haddock, G., Wainwright, L., Berry, K., 2017. The relationship between therapeutic alliance and patient's suicidal thoughts, self-harming behaviors and suicide attempts: a systematic review. J. Affect. Disord. 223, 165–174.

Elliot, R., Bohart, A.C., Watson, J.C., Murphy, D., 2018. Therapist empathy and client outcome: an updated meta-analysis. Psychotherapy 55 (4), 399–410.

Ellis, A.E., Simiola, V., Brown, L., Courtois, C., Cook, J.M., 2018. The role of evidence-based therapy relationships on treatment outcomes for adults with trauma: a systematic review. J. Trauma Dissociation 19 (2), 185–213.

Enck, P., Klosterhalfen, S., Weimer, K., 2017. Unsolved, forgotten, and ignored features of the placebo response in medicine. Clin. Ther. 39 (3), 458–468.

Farber, B.A., Manevich, I., Metzger, J., Saypol, E., 2005. Choosing psychotherapy as a career; why did we cross that road?. J. Clin. Psychol. 61 (8), 1009–1031.

Frisaldi, E., Piedimonte, A., Benedetti, F., 2015. Placebo and nocebo effects: a complex interplay between psychological factors and neurochemical networks. Am. J. Clin. Hypn. 57 (3), 267–284.

Glass, L.L., 2003. The gray areas of boundary crossings and violations. Am. J. Psychother. 57 (4), 429–444.

Greben, S.E., 1977. On being therapeutic. Can. Psychiatr. Assoc. J. 22 (7), 371–380.

Goldstein, G., Suzuki, J.Y., 2015. The analyst's authenticity: "If you see something, say something. J. Clin. Psychol. 71 (5), 451–456.

Graves, T.A., Tabri, N., Thompson-Brenner, H., Franko, D.L., Eddy, K.T., Bourion-Bedes, S., et al., 2017. A meta-analysis of the relation between therapeutic alliance and treatment outcomes in eating disorders. Int. J. Eat. Disord. 50 (4), 323–340.

Haour, F., 2005. Mechanisms of the placebo effect and of conditioning. Neuroimmunomodulation 12 (4), 195–200.

Hara, K.M., Aviram, A., Constantino, M.J., Westra, H.A., Antony, M.M., 2017. Therapist empathy, homework compliance, and outcome in cognitive behavioral therapy for generalized anxiety disorder: partitioning within-and between-therapist effects. Cogn. Behav. Ther. 46 (5), 375–390.

Holmes, R.D., Tiwari, A.K., Kennedy, J.L., 2016. Mechanisms of the placebo effect in pain and psychiatric disorders. Pharmacogenomics 16 (6), 491–500.

Koole, S.L., Tschacher, W., 2016. Synchrony in psychotherapy: a review and an integrative framework for the therapeutic alliance. Front. Psychol. doi:10.3389/fpsyg.2016.00862.

McClintock, A.S., Anderson, T., Patterson, C.L., Wing, E.H., 2018. Early psychotherapeutic empathy, alliance, and client outcome: preliminary evidence of indirect effects. J. Clin. Psychol. 74 (6), 839–848.

Miller, W.R., Moyers, T.B., 2015. The forest and the trees: relational and specific factors in addiction treatment. Addiction 110 (3), 401–413.

Moyers, T.B., Houck, J., Rice, S.L., Longabaugh, R., Miller, W.R., 2016. Therapist empathy, combined behavioral intervention, and alcohol outcomes in the COMBINE research project. J. Consult. Clin. Psychol. 84 (3), 221–229.

Neacsiu, A.D., Smith, M., Fang, C.M., 2017. Challenging assumptions from emotion dysregulation psychological treatments. J. Affect. Disord. 219, 72–79.

Nienhuis, J.B., Owen, J., Valentine, J.C., Black, S.W., Halford, T.C., Parazak, S.E., et al., 2018. Therapeutic alliance, empathy, and genuineness in individual adult psychotherapy: a meta-analytic review. Psychother. Res. 28 (4), 593–605.

Palpacuer, C., Gallet, L., Drapier, D., Reymann, J.M., Falissard, B., Naudet, F., 2017. Specific and non-specific effects of psychotherapeutic interventions for depression: results from a meta-analysis of 84 studies. J. Psychiatr. Res. 87, 95–104.

Pihlaja, S., Sternberg, J.H., Joutsenniemi, K., Mehik, H., Ritola, V., Joffe, G., 2017. Therapeutic alliance in guided internet therapy programs for depression and anxiety disorders—a systematic review. Internet Interv. doi:10.1016/j.invent.2017.11.005.

Priebe, S., Dimic, S., Wildgrube, C., Jankovic, J., Cushing, A., McCabe, R., 2011. Good communication in psychiatry—a conceptual review. Eur. Psychiatry 26 (7), 403–407.

Rutherford, B.R., Roose, S.P., 2013. A model of placebo response in antidepressant clinical trials. Am. J. Psychother. 170 (7), 723–733.

Shatttock, L., Berry, K., Degnan, A, Edge, D., 2018. Therapeutic alliance in psychological therapy for people with schizophrenia and related psychosis: a systematic review. Clin. Psychol. Psychother. 25 (1), 60–65.

Sloan, E., Hall, K., Moulding, R., Bryce, S., Mildred, H., Staiger, P.K., 2017. Emotion regulation as a transdiagnostic treatment construct across anxiety, depression, substance abuse, eating and borderline personality disorders: a systematic review. Clin. Psychol. Rev. 57, 141–163.

Spencer, J., Goode, J., Penix, E.A., Trusty, W., Swift, J.K., 2019. Developing a collaborative relationship with clients during the initial sessions of psychotherapy. Psychotherapy (Chic) 56 (1), 7–10.

Sue, S., 1998. In search of cultural competence in psychotherapy and counseling. Am. Psychol. 53 (4), 440–448.

Tiger, L., 1979. Optimism: The Biology of Hope. Simon & Schuster, New York.

Tschacher, W., Junghan, U.M., Pfammatter, M., 2014. Towards a taxonomy of common factors in psychotherapy-results from an expert survey. Clin. Psychol. Psychother. 21 (1), 82–96.

Wampold, B.E., 2012. Humanism as a common factor in psychotherapy. Psychotherapy (Chicago) 49 (4), 445–449.

Wehmann, E., Kohnen, M., Harter, M., Liebherz, S., 2020. Therapeutic alliance in technology-based interventions for the treatment of depression: systematic review. J. Med. Internet Res. doi:10.2196/17195.

Yager, J., Feinstein, R.E., 2017. Tools for practical psychotherapy: a transtheoretical collection (or interventions which have, at least, worked for us). J. Psychiatr. Pract. 23 (1), 60–77.

Chapter 27

Conclusion

Fifteen forms of psychotherapy representing distinct major variants have been presented alphabetically to reduce any potential bias associated with the order of presentation:

- Acceptance and Commitment Therapy
- Behavioral Therapy
- Cognitive Therapy
- Compassion-Focused Therapy
- Emotion-Focused Therapy
- Existential Psychotherapy
- Gestalt Therapy
- Interpersonal Psychotherapy
- Mindfulness-Based Therapy
- Narrative Therapy
- Person-Centered Therapy
- Positive Psychotherapy
- Problem-Solving Therapy
- Psychoanalytic Therapy
- Rational-Emotive Therapy

Nonspecific psychotherapy factors including the placebo effect have also been covered.

For each of the sixteen intervention types a concise overview provides a solid sense of what is involved. Other than for the nonspecific factors each psychotherapeutic modality is typically hypothesized to work by remedying psychopathology, often initially starting with depression and then expanded to cover other forms of mental illness. In the third section, we will explore the feasibility of this approach, but indicate here that there are major conceptual and practical problems associated with this rationale. In contrast, all fifteen major forms of psychotherapy covered, plus nonspecific factors, do advance the states and processes for mental health consisting of:

- Activity
- Psychological Defense Mechanisms
- Social Connectedness
- Regulation (including over emotions)

States and Processes for Mental Health. DOI: 10.1016/C2020-0-00574-8

- Human-Specific Cognition
- Self-Acceptance
- Adaptability

For each form of psychotherapy at least two, and typically more, of these states and processes is directly and robustly advanced. Furthermore, the others can be advanced but of lesser probability, indirectly, or conditionally with the latter scenario highly intuitive when it arises. For example, behavioral therapy improves social activity and social connectedness when social activity is focused on, but is unlikely to when this form of activity is not addressed. Additionally, nonspecific factors including the placebo effect solidly enhance each of the states and processes characterizing mental health, with interactive effects often amplifying this outcome. The mode of delivery, such as individual, group, or Internet, does not matter, with the possible exception of the Internet mode reducing some of the social connectedness benefits due to the lack of therapeutic alliance inputs. However, given the human ability to anthropomorphism it is feasible that clients might form an alliance with an Internet-based delivery mode.

Of note, there appears to be a transtherapy influence of all forms and subtypes of psychotherapy on emotion regulation. This variant of regulation plays a key role in how the states and processes for mental health foster positive affectivity over negative affectivity (positive emotions exceeding negative emotions), by directly reducing negative emotions thereby favoring positive emotions. Psychological defense mechanisms likewise ensure positive affectivity over negative affectivity, by reducing negative emotions and bolstering positive emotions ongoing. Enhanced behavioral activation and reduced behavioral inhibition from solid activity, covered in the Activity chapter in the first section and the Behavioral therapy chapter of this section, also have a major impact in this regard with behavioral activation somewhat equivalent to positive affectivity, and behavioral inhibition linked to negative affectivity. As reviewed, in a world and universe ruled by entropy (order to disorder) the pursuit of happiness related to ongoing gains is misguided and futile, and if anything, it is the happiness of pursuit derived from the adaptive value of dissociative absorption in constructive activities. Hence, positive affectivity over negative affectivity, but not "happiness," follows from the states and processes for mental health, with powerful contributions from regulation, psychological defense mechanisms, and activity. Emotion regulation on its own translates into positive affectivity exceeding negative affectivity, and in an ongoing and sustainable fashion.

Conducting theoretical research over many years, I have learned that the fit is crucial. A theory must fit with both research evidence and clinical experience, and related to these is the feel: when a concept generated feels like trying to fit a square peg into a round hole, or even a round peg into a square hole where it will slot in but feels insecure, the theory is highly questionable and needs to be scrapped or massively revised. In the current instance of determining whether or not, and to what extent, major forms of psychotherapy and nonspecific factors enhance the states and processes for mental health, the fit is very smooth and emerged readily, although with the research emphasis on establishing efficacy and not so much mechanisms of action, I frequently had to rely on my theoretical background. The feel is one of round pegs into round holes and square pegs into square holes, with the understanding that for a given form of psychotherapy there is variation in the probability, directness, and conditionality of it advancing a particular state and process for mental health, an occurrence that could not be otherwise due to the particular emphasis of the psychotherapy type and how it is directed for a particular client.

Highly promising for the hypothesis are two outcomes. First, nonspecific factors including the placebo effect advance all of the states and processes for mental health, providing a solid explanation of how these mysterious factors actually operate to produce the psychotherapy benefits they are widely known to achieve. Second, how emotion regulation comprises a transtherapy influence, demonstrating that one of the states and processes is strongly impacted by all psychotherapy types (and nonspecific factors). Based on these two outcomes and how each form of psychotherapy and also nonspecific factors fit so well with the central hypothesis, it does appear that psychotherapy works by advancing the states and processes for mental health, a theme that we will further explore in the third section. An advantage of this approach is clearly defining when psychotherapy is required and gauging the effectiveness: if functioning in regards to one or more of the states and processes characterizing mental health is impaired, then psychotherapy is required (or some other mental health intervention), and the success of psychotherapy is evidenced by a shift from impaired to robust functioning on the states and processes for mental health.

Section III

The way forward with psychotherapy

Chapter 28

Problems with the discrete psychotherapy approach

The current approach to psychotherapy involves discrete forms that are hypothesized to work by remedying psychopathology. Positive psychotherapy might seem to be an exception, but the notion of mental illness arising from a lack of balance in key areas of life with restoration of balance resolving psychopathology does capture a similar theme. What positive psychology and psychotherapy does reveal is how the focus is almost entirely on negativity and psychopathology, but addresses this with yet another discrete form of psychotherapy. The purpose of this chapter is to demonstrate the problems that arise from this discrete psychotherapy approach focused on remedying psychopathology to improve mental health. They take the form of sheer numbers, research bias, fads and fades, and core rationale.

Sheer numbers

In the late 1800s and early 1900s, the only form of psychotherapy appears to have been psychoanalysis. Then with the rise of behaviorism behavioral therapy began in the early 1900s, initially focused on classical and operant conditioning. Person-centered therapy arose with Carl Rogers in the 1940s, followed by rational-emotive therapy created by Albert Ellis in the 1950s. From the 1960s on, there has been what might best be described as an explosion of psychotherapy variants. The 15 forms covered in Section 2 represent major types, but there are many more, with the sheer numbers overwhelming. Those that I encountered in researching this book (listed alphabetically) include:

- Abreaction Therapy
- Acceptance & Commitment Therapy
- Adventure Therapy
- Affect-Focused Body Psychotherapy
- Attachment Therapy
- Attack Therapy
- Behavioral Therapy
- Bibliotherapy
- Biodynamic Therapy

States and Processes for Mental Health. DOI: 10.1016/C2020-0-00574-8

- Body Therapy
- Cognitive Therapy
- Coherence Therapy
- Collaborative Therapy
- Concentrative Movement Therapy
- Compassion-Focused Therapy
- Contemplative Psychotherapy
- Contextual Therapy
- Core Process Psychotherapy
- Ecological Counselling
- Emotion-Focused Therapy
- Existential Psychotherapy
- Expressive Therapy
- Feminist Therapy
- Future-Oriented Therapy
- Gestalt Therapy
- Holistic Psychotherapy
- Human Givens Therapy
- Integral Psychotherapy
- Integrative Psychotherapy
- Interpersonal Psychotherapy
- Logic-Based Therapy
- Mentalization-Based Therapy
- Mindfulness-Based Therapy
- Mode Deactivation Therapy
- Morita Therapy
- Motivational Enhancement Therapy
- Multicultural Therapy
- Multimodal Therapy
- Narrative Therapy
- Nouthetic Counselling
- Object Relations Psychotherapy
- Pastoral Counselling
- Person-Centered Therapy
- Positive Psychotherapy
- Primal Therapy
- Problem-Solving Therapy
- Provocative Therapy
- Psychoanalytic Psychotherapy
- Rational-Emotive Therapy
- Reality Therapy
- Regression Therapy
- Relational-Cultural Therapy
- Self-System Therapy

- Social Rhythm Therapy
- Systemic Therapy
- Transpersonal Therapy
- Transactional Analysis
- Wilderness Therapy

The sheer number of these psychotherapy variants is incredible, and is an underestimate due to three processes: First, the generation of subtypes consistent with how people produce their own variants, much as with major versions of religion fragmenting into numerous subtypes. Second, how combinations of distinct forms and even subtypes have transpired. Currently, virtually every type has been combined with mindfulness for example, and many with cognitive therapy. Then of course there is cognitive mindfulness therapy. Third, the many variants specific to the mode of delivery, such as forms of couple, family, and Internet-based psychotherapies. Taking into account the distinct types, subtypes, and combinations, even omitting those specific to the delivery mode, there are hundreds of psychotherapy variants currently. Project ahead 50 to 100 years and the numbers will easily exceed a 1000!

While such an extreme diversity of psychotherapy types might seem positive in that it offers choice, the problems vastly outweigh this potential plus. Consumers face a bewildering array of options that will be difficult to navigate, particularly when a person is in distress and requires psychotherapy, as opposed to extensive homework to sort out the options and select the most optimal for their circumstance. Students of psychotherapy even now are overwhelmed by the diversity of options, but this reaction is subdued to what future aspiring psychotherapists will face. Schools of psychotherapy are unlikely to have the resources to teach more than a small fraction of the options, and selecting which ones will pose a problem that yokes into efficacy research covered next. The last but never least given how we live in a world based on money, is payers of psychotherapy struggling to determine which forms of psychotherapy to fund, that now and then will largely be decided by the competition of efficacy research. Based on these negatives associated with the sheer number of psychotherapy types now and certainly in the future, the discrete model is highly problematic.

Research bias

Given that psychotherapists have to earn a living, payment is required for psychotherapy. Throughout most of the world where psychotherapy is available, these payments are by insurance companies or governments. These payers typically want to see evidence of efficacy before funding a given form of psychotherapy. From what I understand, my own situation of the Ontario government funding psychotherapy at the discretion of the psychiatrist is a unique one that might well not persist. In researching this book, several fascinating things emerged: one being how there is a competition and even a race of sorts to establish efficacy necessary to secure funding for the psychotherapy type, which of course puts the given form of psychotherapy on the map so to speak. Taking a closer look, I noted that first, much of psychotherapy research is oriented to establishing efficacy, and second, most of this research is conducted by the originator of the psychotherapy type, students, and practitioners trained in the approach. This brings into play the very intriguing topic of research bias.

Whenever a product is involved, such as psychotherapy, the basic assumption needs to be that research will be biased when conducted by those with a vested interest in the outcome. In the mental health area, we encountered this with Selective Serotonin Reuptake Inhibitors (SSRIs) where published studies over-reported the number yielding a positive outcome and also efficacy over effectiveness, the former term referring to performance under ideal and controlled circumstances, as opposed to effectiveness under real-world conditions, such as most clients having a combination of conditions and not just pure depression (Kirsch et al., 2008; Turner et al., 2008, 2012). Bias took many forms as with pharmaceutical companies not publishing negative result studies or combining several into one research paper, while ensuring that positive result ones were published in the most prominent journal feasible. The positive outcome studies for SSRIs were overwhelming conducted by researchers receiving funding from the pharmaceutical industry (Kirsch et al., 2008; Turner et al., 2008, 2012).

Research bias even applies to early stage research that progresses to product development, with approximately 80% of results including those from top-tier labs published in top journals being false (Begley and Ellis, 2012; Prinz et al., 2011). Investigators working for Bayer conducted an analysis of research and development on early stage in-house projects (target identification and target validation) derived from external labs for their three main strategic research fields of oncology, women's health, and cardiovascular disease (Prinz et al., 2011). Amazingly they found that only 21% (14/67) of projects were characterized by published data being in line with in-house findings. Of the 14 projects only 1 perfectly reproduced the data, while 12 could be adapted, and 1 was not applicable. For two-thirds of the projects (43/67) inconsistencies between published results and in-house data were so great that the projects were scrapped (Prinz et al., 2011). Investigators at Amgen confirmed this outcome examining 53 "landmark" publications (papers in top journals from reputable labs) over the prior decade that they relied on to identify new targets for cancer drug development, finding that only 6 (11%) could be confirmed; a full 47/53 or 89% failed (Begley and Ellis, 2012). Relevant to these results, a client of mine working for a government regulating body was told by her highly experienced manager when she started, "Even though you will be shocked, 80% of research results we look at are false!" She doubted it but soon learned he was spot on. Massive research bias is systemic and not the exception!

In contrast to these more overt sources of bias, largely unconscious ones transpire as with the originator of a form of psychotherapy truly believing in the value, and somehow influencing outcomes through the passion of their belief. The probability of this occurrence is enhanced based on how psychotherapy research is typically conducted by those with a vested interest, and how neither the psychotherapists involved nor research participants can be blinded: clearly the psychotherapists know what form of psychotherapy they are providing and the client is at least somewhat aware of its nature. At times during the book I have mentioned entropy, a physics concept that rules our world and the universe, whereby order naturally progresses to disorder—our bodies decline with age and do not spontaneously improve over time, for example. With entropy, the natural state of things is for them not to work, but the assumption with research is often that it should work. Appreciating entropy and the proclivity for bias demands that we be very careful before concluding that a research outcome yields a true result. In the competition and race to establish efficacy for a given form of psychotherapy, this rigorous perspective is rarely adhered to.

The structure of psychotherapy research that needs to be applied to yield true outcomes is characterized by objectivity and independence. Both of these criteria demand that those providing psychotherapy to research participants not have any vested interest in the outcome. This requires that experienced therapists be trained in the technique but not practice it regularly, an occurrence I have almost never seen. Additionally, the researchers must be objective and independent enough to use measurement instruments that do not have any inherent bias in favor of the intervention type, and most importantly publish all negative result studies. When I looked over efficacy studies for a particular form of psychotherapy that were conducted by the originator and students, I cannot recall a truly negative outcome, and in a world and universe ruled by entropy this is next to impossible! Registering studies might seem promising, but rarely do those looking into a particular form of psychotherapy seek out registered psychotherapy trials not reported in any journal. In the Introduction to Section 2, efficacy research was mentioned with the ideal study format consisting of: a large number of participants that are representative of the respective population, investigators not vested in the outcome (independent and objective), and random assignment to four conditions—psychotherapy type being investigated, another well-validated form of psychotherapy such as cognitive, active placebo condition consisting of some activity that at least at face value seems psychologically relevant, and wait list. If the tested psychotherapy modality compares equally or better to the established form of psychotherapy, and both are superior to the active placebo and wait list groups, then the outcome can be considered valid, although replication of this result is best. How often have you as a reader encountered this level of rigor?

Another problem associated with the research bias issue is how certain forms of psychotherapy lend themselves to manualized approaches while others do not. I have noted a fascinating pattern whereby the presence and extent of manualized approaches seemingly correlates positively with efficacy outcomes: the more manualized the form of psychotherapy is the greater the efficacy research support. Ones that have resisted the manual approach, such as gestalt and existential psychotherapy, do not acquire much support. Indeed, efforts are underway with many forms of psychotherapy to put them in a manual format, with the goal of building solid efficacy research support. However, just because a form of psychotherapy is scripted in a manual does not mean that it is any more effective, and flexibly responding to a client's needs at a given moment is very adaptive and beneficial. Furthermore, while standardization derived from manuals might assist with research, it often does not align with psychotherapy in real-world conditions. Based on discussions with psychotherapists and clients, it appears that in a real-world setting, many psychotherapists deviate from the manual in response to client needs, and hence nonmanual flexible approaches will yield valid effectiveness outcomes given that representative conditions are present. Skilled therapists that do not have a vested interest in a given form of psychotherapy but are training in its application can deliver it to research participants adhering to the principles and process of that form of psychotherapy without manuals. Overall then it can be said that there is a tremendous amount of bias, or at least the potential for it, in psychotherapy efficacy research that really needs to be addressed and rectified, and the bias is largely motivated by the need to establish validity to secure funding, both scenarios far from ideal but inherent in the discrete psychotherapy approach.

Fads and fades

Fads tend to characterize mental health interventions. Fads occur when the popularity substantially outstrips the evidence. For example, during the time when SSRIs were under patent protection they seemed to be the answer to everything, even for common less than ideal mood states in some instances. Then when the patent protection expired and pharmaceutical company money ceased to influence academic psychiatrists and others involved in promoting them, SSRIs lost their luster. This SSRI fad came with a cost, namely that psychotherapy was de-emphasized, a logical follow-up to the notion that SSRIs worked for everything so why bother with psychotherapy. Meanwhile, experienced clinicians applying both psychotherapy and pharmacotherapy noted that while these medications have a role, they are not a solution to everything, and the combination of psychotherapy and medication often works best. I believe that this is one of the major reasons why psychotherapy struggles for funding necessitating efficacy competition.

Psychotherapy is not immune from fads. Psychoanalysis dominated for decades during the first half of the 20th century, with the popularity outstripping evidence, particularly considering that objective psychotherapy research was not common then. Back in the 1940s, Carl Roger's Person-Centered Therapy was extremely popular and applied in many setting including political encounter groups, the success well beyond the limited empirical evidence. Albert Ellis's Rational Emotive Therapy was widespread in its application a decade later, and even though there was more emphasis at this point on research evidence, it was limited compared to how successful this form of psychotherapy was. Currently, mindfulness is applied to many forms of psychotherapy, and has been extended well beyond the psychotherapy realm. Furthermore, mindfulness is one form of meditation, and likely does not work any better than concentrative variants, although we really do not hear much about this other type despite its application in Eastern culture for hundreds of years—think of the repeated chant "Om" to indicate the primordial vibration from creation as a common process in concentrative meditation. Why has mindfulness swept the market and the concentrative form not, despite the latter being linked to creation? The answer is that mindfulness has reached the popularity of a fad, heavily promoted whereas the concentrative variety lost out. Van Dam et al. (2018) point to how mindfulness has really become a fad based on both researcher and media involvement, with research glossing over variations.

Applied to popular culture fads can be fun and mostly harmless, although I wonder how many women suffered from impossibly high stiletto heel shoes in their day, or young men during the 1970s when platform shoes for men were the fad. Placing mental health and fashion in the same category, based on the predilection for fads, is not complimenting mental health interventions, and distances it from science. Can you image if Einstein's relativity theory was in for a few years as a fad and then out. Hence, if we are to end the fad aspect we have to align interventions for mental illness with science. In this regard, a crucial change will be to shift from discrete to continuous approaches: in my opinion and based on research presented in Mental Illness Defined: Continuums, Regulation and Defense (Bowins, 2016), mental illness manifestations are continuous, whereas the Diagnostic and Statistical Manual (DSM) in the latest version (DSM-5) maintains that there are numerous discrete entities, such as Major Depression and Minor Depression (American Psychiatric Association, 2013), that even at face value seem dubious. There is no truly solid scientific evidence for these discrete entities, with most of the data derived from studies comparing one hypothesized type to another and finding that different features apply, such as "generalized anxiety" distinguished by worry. However, a closer insightful look reveals that many of the features that supposedly distinguish conditions are actually continuous, such as worry in anxiety generally, depression, and stress (Olatunji et al., 2010), and panic attacks arising from severe anxiety as an emergent property, being present in all "types" of anxiety (Bowins, 2016).

I have proposed the Continuum Principle: natural phenomena tend to occur on a continuum, and any instance of hypothesized discreteness requires unassailable proof (Bowins, 2015). Supporting this principle is research from varying disciplines that have also reached the conclusion that psychological events are structured continuously. Alfred Kinsey in his studies of human sexuality captures this occurrence perfectly: in Sexual Behavior in the Human Male (Kinsey et al., 1948), he states, "The living world is a continuum in each and every one of its aspects," and adds in Sexual Behavior in the Human Female (Kinsey et al., 1953), "It is a characteristic of the human mind that tries to dichotomize in its classification of phenomena." Studying brain development in youth (United States National Institutes of Health Magnetic Resonance Imaging Study of Normal Brain Development), Hudziak et al. (2014) comment that their research group has uncovered many sources of behavioral genetic evidence in support of a dimensional model of mental illness. They further indicate that a categorical (discrete) depiction of psychopathology fails to capture the true nature of behavior and its underlying biology, and that emotions and behaviors exist on a continuum, rather than in discrete categories. Since natural occurrences tend to be continuous aligning with trait variation and natural selection, the intuitive probability of a fully discrete model of mental illness being accurate is extremely low. However, it does align with a proclivity to favor discreteness to simplify information processing demands and marketing needs, given that discrete entities are perceived to be easier to market. Psychotherapy repeats the pattern of numerous discrete entities instead of an integrated and continuous approach. I strongly believe that we need to get away from fads and distortions that satisfy our own psychological needs and that of special interests like pharmaceutical companies, and bring mental health into the science realm which at a very basic level entails a shift from discrete entities to a continuous model.

One might wonder why fads apply to mental health interventions, as well as diagnosis? The answer has several components, one being promotion instead of true outcomes. Much as with medications psychotherapy is a product and products require marketing and promotion to succeed. Biased research to establish efficacy plays a key role in this process, standing in contrast to a truly independent and objective quest for true outcomes (see Research Bias in this chapter). Additionally, there is the intense personal effort that originators of psychotherapy types apply to establish it in mainstream practice. Several of these intriguing individuals are relentless promoters through research, courses, talks, media coverage, and more, with their impressive efforts playing a key role in the success of the particular form of psychotherapy, but what happens when this effort declines?

Fades is the downside of fads! A very striking occurrence I noted in doing the research for this book, is how once the originator of a psychotherapy type fades, and at most a generation or two of students, the form of psychotherapy also tends to fade and usually very quickly. For example, Carl Rogers created person-centered therapy during the 1940s and extended it into many realms. He died in the 1980s and currently this once very popular form of psychotherapy is rarely practiced outside of techniques applied to eclectic psychotherapy. Albert Ellis originated rational-emotive therapy a decade after Carl Rogers, and despite its recognition and quite widespread success, it is not typically practiced as a discrete approach any longer. Demonstrating tremendous vitality, Les Greenburg relentlessly promotes emotion-focused therapy, but what does history predict will happen after he no longer can do so and a generation or two of students pass? It has been said that the only thing we learn from history is that we learn nothing from history, but what we might learn is that the success of a particular form of psychotherapy is directly related to its promotion, and when the fad fades so does the psychotherapy form even if it has robust aspects.

Core rationale

We have already seen how the sheer number of psychotherapy types, research bias, and fads and fades, create seemingly insurmountable problems for the discrete approach to psychotherapy, but what about the core rationale? Each form of psychotherapy is believed to work by remedying psychopathology. Implicit in this rationale is the notion that psychopathology constitutes a problem, or if not why try and remedy it? Two fundamental flaws exist with the core rationale both related to generalizability and the targeting of psychotherapy for these psychopathology problems. First, problems are specific entities that require specific solutions. If your car is not working, there is a specific problem necessitating a particular intervention. Likewise, if a physical health problem arises such as diabetes or heart disease, the intervention is specific to it. In the case of mental illness, numerous psychotherapeutic interventions are directed at one problem such as depression. We covered 15 major forms of psychotherapy, and I listed many others each with a different focus. Then there are the subtypes and combinations. It does not logically follow that for a given problem (a type of psychopathology) so many diverse approaches could actually work. This scenario is analogous to the mechanic fixing a piston problem by targeting the cylinder, spark plugs, valves, crankshaft, sump, connecting rod, cooling system, lubrication system, oxidizer-air inlet system, and even reflecting the diversity of psychotherapy approaches, working on the exhaust system, axle, and other parts tied into the engine. Similarly, to manage diabetes an internist targeting all aspects of carbohydrate metabolism, related systems dealing with fat and protein metabolism, and also extending interventions to broader but linked biological systems. There are just too many psychotherapeutic interventions for specific psychopathology problems. Even worse for the core rationale, nonspecific factors are effective for many forms of mental illness, extending the generalization problem with diverse forms of psychotherapy for a particular problem to an absurd level.

The second problem related to generalizability and the targeting of psychotherapy is how virtually every form of psychotherapy is targeted beyond the initial problem. In many or most instances, the initial problem is depression, but very shortly the psychotherapeutic intervention is applied to several other types of mental illness. Take for example compassion-focused therapy that began with the new millennium and has already been extended to a diverse range of psychopathology that appears to be growing yearly. This generalization to many forms of psychopathology is the norm, not the exception. When it comes to specific treatment strategies, in contrast, such as exposure and response prevention for obsessive-compulsive behavior, this generalization is much less likely. If psychotherapy works by remedying psychopathology how can a given focus benefit so many diverse conditions? Furthermore, this applies to virtually all forms of psychotherapy and also nonspecific factors. It is analogous to a piston repair remedying damage to other engine parts, or an intervention for carbohydrate metabolism correcting problems with diverse aspects of metabolism, and even less probable all intervention types doing so. If a given psychotherapeutic modality actually works by remedying psychopathology, then it does not logically follow that it will be beneficial for a diverse array of mental illness problems, and totally unrealistic that this scenario applies to all forms of psychotherapy and also nonspecific factors.

Hence, the way that so many diverse forms of psychotherapy, as specific solutions, work for a given type of mental illness, and how virtually all forms are extended to a wide range of psychopathology, makes the core rationale—psychotherapy works by remedying psychopathology—untenable. Applied to other domains such as mechanics and internal medicine, this scenario is ludicrous. Excessive generalization in terms of too many forms of psychotherapy directed as distinct solutions to a particular problem and each form targeted at multiple types of psychopathology, plus the role of nonspecific factors in both scenarios, really necessitates a conceptual shift in how we understand psychotherapy.

Summary note

Major advances often follow from conceptual shifts and this change is really necessary for psychotherapy if it to align with science and remain viable. The sheer number of psychotherapy variants currently being applied is overwhelming, with the numbers almost certain to increase with time. This will present an impossible scenario for consumers, students and providers, educators, and payers. Currently, in the efficacy competition with all the other forms of psychotherapy to gain funding, substantial research bias exists, at least if we contrast what is transpiring to a fully independent and objective research model. Psychotherapy is a product and all such entities are highly vulnerable to research bias that distances them from science that is at the core oriented to true outcomes. The way that mental illness interventions frequently represent fads, in part based on research bias, further distances psychotherapy from science. Fads are fine (I suppose) for popular culture, but for mental health? The downside of fads is fades, and this unfolds with forms of treatment that have become fads largely through intense promotion fading once the originator and a generation or two of students fades.

Solid science that captures true outcomes such as the double helix model of DNA, and relativity and quantum theories for physics, do not work via fads and fades. I strongly suggest that we attempt to put psychotherapy on the same stable foundation, which brings us to the core rationale of psychotherapy. The underlying concept is that psychotherapy works by remedying psychopathology which entails specific problems and specific solutions for them. Meanwhile, excessive generalization with first, too many forms of psychotherapy and nonspecific factors as solutions to a particular problem, and second, most forms targeted at multiple types of psychopathology, makes the core rational untenable and frankly unscientific. The way forward requires a tenable core rationale that replaces the discrete psychotherapy model with an integrated and continuous system, research oriented to true outcomes, and the fading of fads. In addition, this new approach really needs to explain the powerful role of nonspecific factors in a fashion that aligns them with specific forms of psychotherapy.

References

American Psychiatric Association, 2013. Diagnostic & Statistical Manual 5. American Psychiatric Publishing Inc, Washington, DC.

Begley, C., Ellis, M., 2012. Drug development: raise standards for preclinical cancer research. Nature 483 (7391), 531 -531.

Bowins, B.E., 2015. Depression: discrete or continuous? Psychopathology 48 (2), 69–78.

Bowins, B.E., 2016. Mental Illness Defined: Continuums, Regulation, and Defense. Routledge, New York, London.

Hudziak, J.J., Albaugh, M.D., Ducharme, S., Karama, S., Spottswood, M., Crehan, E., et al., 2014. Cortical thickening maturation and duration of music training: health-promoting activities shape brain development. J. Am. Acad. Child. Adolesc. Psychiatry 53 (11), 1153–1161.

Kinsey, A.C., Pomeroy, W.B., Martin, C.E., 1948. Sexual Behavior in the Human Male. W.B. Saunders, Philadelphia.

Kinsey, A.C., Pomeroy, W.B., Martin, C.E., Gebhard, P.H., 1953. Sexual Behavior in the Human Female. W.B. Saunders, Philadelphia.

Kirsch, I., Deacon, B., Huedo-Medina, T., Scoboria, A., Moore, T., Johnson, B., 2008. Initial severity and antidepressant benefits: a meta-analysis of data submitted to the Food and Drug Administration. PLoS Med. doi:10.1371/journal.pmed.0050045.

Olatunji, B.O., Broman-Fulks, J.J., Bergman, S.M., Green, B.A., Zlomke, K.R., 2010. A taxometric investigation of the latent structure of worry: dimensionality and associations with depression, anxiety, and stress. Behav. Ther. 41 (2), 212–228.

Prinz, F., Schlange, T., Asadullah, K., 2011. Believe it or not: how much can we rely on published data on potential drug targets? Nat. Rev. Drug Discov. 10 (9), 712–717.

Turner, E., Matthews, A., Linardatos, E., Tell, R., Rosenthal, R., 2008. Selective publication of antidepressant trials and its influence on apparent efficacy. New England J. Med. 358, 252-260.

Turner, E., Knoepflmacher, D., Shapley, L., 2012. Publication bias in antidepressant trials: an analysis of efficacy comparing the literature to the US food and drug administration database. PLoS Med. 9 (3). doi:10.1371/journal.pmed.0050045.

Van Dam, N.T., Van Vugt, M.K., Vago, D.R., Schmalzl, L., Saron, C.D., Olendzki, A., et al., 2018. Mind the hype: a critical evaluation and prescriptive agenda for research on mindfulness and meditation. Perspect. Psychol. Sci. 13 (1), 36–61.

Chapter 29

Advancing psychotherapy effectiveness

In the first chapter of this section we covered how the current discrete model of psychotherapy has insurmountable problems derived from sheer numbers, research bias related to the competition for efficacy outcomes, fads (popularity substantially outstripping evidence) and fades, and the core rational. An additional problem is the puzzling and intriguing way that nonspecific factors, such as the therapeutic alliance, hope, and the placebo effect, also produce a benefit. How can this be given the core rationale that specific forms of psychotherapy work by remedying psychopathology? The answer is that it almost certainly cannot. Most psychotherapists live with this conceptual tension knowing that the nonspecific factors are at work but do not really align with the notion of specific forms of psychotherapy. The resolution of this mystery resides in how both specific factors (forms of psychotherapy) and nonspecific factors advance the states and processes for mental health. The Nonspecific factors chapter demonstrates how robust the nonspecific factors actually are in this regard. The ease at which specific and nonspecific factors are brought into alignment supports the position that psychotherapy actually does work by advancing the states and processes for mental health—activity, psychological defense mechanisms, social connectedness, regulation, human-specific cognition, self-acceptance, and adaptability—with each of these, and in particular activity, psychological defense mechanisms, and regulation, ensuring that positive affectivity exceeds negative affectivity. Indeed, I believe that for any model of psychotherapy to be viable it must address and resolve the role of nonspecific factors. As demonstrated by the resolution of the specific and nonspecific factors issue, moving away from the discrete psychotherapy model to an integrated focus on advancing the states and processes for mental health is crucial.

Psychologically we tend to gravitate to the negative, an occurrence embedded in the current rationale of psychotherapy directly remedying psychopathology. A much more positive approach is advancing the core states and processes for mental health, with improvements in psychopathology naturally ensuing: both formal and informal mental illness manifestations are resolved and good mental health is in place when activity, psychological defense mechanisms, social connectedness, regulation, human-specific cognition, self-acceptance, and adaptability are robust. This proposal entails applying strategies designed

States and Processes for Mental Health. DOI: 10.1016/C2020-0-00574-8

to advance these core states and processes for mental health, with a clear focus on each. This outcome can be achieved by strategies not linked to any particular form of psychotherapy (general) including nonspecific factors, and also by applying principles and approaches from existing forms of psychotherapy. Additionally, future research can investigate the less dominant forms of psychotherapy to determine if these yield solid strategies.

In the process of advancing the states and processes for mental health, the general strategies and those specific to a given form of psychotherapy resolve deficits underlying various forms of mental illness. Some strategies constitute transdiagnostic (across diagnoses) and transtherapy (across therapies) interventions such as behavioral activation, emotion regulation enhancement, and cognitive reframing (Boswell, 2013; Boswell et al., 2013; Farchione et al., 2017; Kaplan et al., 2018; Neacsiu et al., 2015; Sloan et al., 2017). Behavioral activation is a key component of the Activity state and process for mental health (see the Activity chapter). It has been identified as a transdiagnostic strategy for depression across a wide range of settings and clinical populations, that is designed to enhance positive reinforcement for adaptive healthy behavior and reduce behavioral avoidance (Farchione et al., 2017). Emotion regulation is a crucial component of the regulation state and process for mental health (see the Regulation chapter). Transdiagnostic interventions emphasize emotion regulation, such as the Unified Protocol applicable to disorders with an emotion dysregulation aspect (Boswell, 2013; Boswell et al., 2013). Emotion dysregulation impacts many aspects of functioning including identity (Neacsiu et al., 2015). Sloan et al. (2017) cite emotion regulation as a transdiagnostic treatment construct across anxiety, depression, substance abuse, eating disorders, and borderline personality disorder, and this impact has been noted for each of the specific forms of psychotherapy covered in Section 2 (transtherapy). Indeed, emotion regulation does seem to be advanced by all forms of psychotherapy.

Maintaining positive cognitions is an integral component of the psychological defense state and process for mental health (see the Psychological defense mechanism chapter). Cognitive reframing from negative to positive is a major transdiagnostic approach that can be applied to a range of psychopathology (Kaplan et al., 2018). The integrated and continuous approach proposed here is transdiagnostic in that the states and processes for mental health span diagnoses, and the strategies for advancing these states and processes apply to various forms of mental illness. It is also transtherapy because strategies from specific forms of psychotherapy enhance the states and processes for mental health. Ultimately, the reason for why transdiagnostic and transtherapy approaches work, is that they enhance these core states and processes! It might be suggested that the transtherapy and transdiagnostic strategies emphasized in current research, such as behavioral activation, emotion regulation, and cognitive reframing, are sufficient to account for how psychotherapy works, but first, they cannot explain improvements in all mental illness manifestations, and second, they act by advancing the states and processes for mental health, highlighting the importance of this approach.

Given that strategies from various forms of psychotherapy are to be applied, those indicated do not require a manualized approach, with flexibility paramount. We will now explore each of the states and processes for mental health, applying both general strategies and those specific to a given form of psychotherapy, presenting the most robust options, to see how this might look. Note that for each strategy derived from the major forms of psychotherapy only a brief summary has been provided here, and those seeking more detailed information and examples can explore the relevant form of psychotherapy in Section 2.

Activity

A general way as a psychotherapist to advance activity for clients is to suggest, guide, and support the application of various forms of activity. In Activity for Mental Health (Bowins, 2020), I demonstrate how physical, social, nature, cognitive, art/hobby, and music forms of activity are very helpful for mental health, and provide the reasons for why this occurs. At the very core, human hunting and gathering evolution ensured that we had to be active, in contrast to our tree-based higher primate relatives (Pontzer, 2017; Raichlen and Alexander, 2017). Hence, by becoming active in various ways mental health is furthered and in a very natural fashion. Diverse activities also foster balance in life adding to the mental health benefit. The absorption in positive foci that occurs with activity disconnects people from negativity and fosters positivity from the rewards. Another way to enhance activity is to be aware of and apply behavioral activation and behavioral inhibition (see the Activity chapter): depression involves low behavioral activation and high behavioral inhibition, while several other forms of mental illness including anxiety have high behavioral inhibition (Akiskal and Pinto, 1999; Bowins, 2008; Eckblad and Chapman, 1986; Jamison et al., 1980; Koukopoulos et al., 2003). Both high behavioral inhibition and low behavioral activation result in inhibited and withdrawn states, usually worse with depression due to the combination. Hypomania, on the other hand, involves high behavioral activation and low behavioral inhibition enabling it to counter or override depression and anxiety, without the dysfunction of mania (Akiskal and Pinto, 1999; Bowins, 2008; Meyer et al., 1999). By encouraging clients to be very active and not inhibited beyond safety concerns, high behavioral activation and low behavioral inhibition is instilled, clearly moving them away from depression and anxiety. An added benefit derives from how behavioral activation is linked to positive affectivity, while behavioral inhibition aligns with negative affectivity. Hence, by advancing the former and reducing the latter, positive affectivity will exceed negative affectivity (positive over negative emotions), and as has been mentioned this is a key way that the states and processes for mental health induce this emotion outcome in a sustainable way.

The principles and approaches of certain forms of psychotherapy, covered in Section 2, robustly advance activity and can be readily applied. **Acceptance and Commitment Therapy** has a unique focus that is ideally suited to enhancing activity: acceptance of adversity, including anxiety, that is a blocking activity due to experiential avoidance, and committing to a course of action to achieve valued goals. Having a client accept that some adversity such as anxiety is tolerable and refrain from avoiding it in the moment, and then committing to actions to achieve their valued goals are very straightforward psychotherapy strategies to apply, and certainly do not require a manual. Valued activities (goals) are noted, fears and anxiety blocking attempts to engage identified, the rationale for accepting the adversity explained with encouragement to persevere, and then supporting committed actions to achieve the goal/s. Activity of diverse forms can readily be advanced from the main principles and strategies of acceptance and commitment therapy.

Behavioral Therapy powerfully enhances activity as the name suggests. The focus is on behavior with thoughts not directly addressed. From my experience a major advantage of applying it is that the approach circumvents how people, and even many therapists, first attempt to instill thoughts, emotions, and motivation conducive to activity, often with the outcome that fear and the amplified version, anxiety, persists and inhibits the person from acting. Behavioral therapy is highly beneficial by getting the client to act first and experience the cognitive, emotional, and motivational benefits afterwards derived from the reinforcement achieved. This reversal of the normal sequence is very significant as it has a powerful impact on mental health. Activities are always positive in some way to the person ensuring that there will be reinforcement. The graded way that fear-inducing challenges are approached instills confidence and motivation with progressive successes. Behavioral therapy ensures that behavioral activation is high and behavioral inhibition low, with the added benefit of positive affectivity > negative affectivity in a sustainable fashion.

Positive Psychotherapy advances activity via the straightforward emphasis on engagement and achievement providing reinforcement, in turn motivating further activity. The theme of leading a meaningful life is realized from activity in positive spheres. Additionally, the extensive journaling work enhances mental activity. **Problem-Solving Therapy** also fosters activity from the very active approach to issues involving the sequential steps of problem identification, clarification, generating realistic solutions, selecting the best option, developing an action plan, implementing it, and monitoring the outcome. Activity of various types is implicit in this process and the approach can be readily applied when there is a problem blocking activity.

The strategies advancing activity inherent in acceptance and commitment therapy, behavioral therapy, positive psychotherapy, and problem-solving therapy are highly compatible with one another. Acceptance and commitment therapy encourages the acceptance of adversity and commitment to a course of action to achieve valued (read reinforcing) goals. Behavioral therapy encourages activity to secure reinforcement without waiting for the right motivation. Positive psychotherapy emphasizes engagement and achievement yielding reinforcement. Problem-solving therapy applies sequential steps to resolve problems blocking activity and foster engagement in constructive actions. Combined with the general ways not tied into any particular form of psychotherapy, activity can be very strongly advanced.

Psychological defense mechanisms

In the chapter with this name we went over the two psychological defense mechanism templates of positive cognitive distortions and dissociation, with classical Freudian defenses subsumed under the former, although some have solid elements of dissociation. Positive cognitive distortions can be advanced in therapy simply by having the client place positive spins on occurrences. Depression and anxiety are characterized by negative distortions (Beck, 1991; Bowins, 2004). Shifting to positive distortions bolsters this defense countering depression and anxiety. As covered in the Psychological defense mechanism chapter, the term distortion is applied because reality is elusive being difficult to fully capture, and with emotions there is either positive, negative, or both: positive and negative coexist and do not cancel to neutral. The nonspecific psychotherapy factor of hope robustly advances positive cognitive distortions, and certainly when circumstances are challenging as they often are for those entering psychotherapy. Hence, providing clients with hope is a powerful general way to enhance psychological defense mechanisms.

Regarding classical Freudian defenses, they appear to naturally shift from immature to mature defenses with longer term psychotherapy, and certainly of a psychodynamic form (Perry, 2001; Perry and Bond, 2004; Van Wijk-Herbrink et al., 2011; Vlastelica et al., 2005). A technique I have applied for those demonstrating immature defenses is to first address the psychological defenses the person is applying, but usually unaware of. Second, explain and demonstrate the use of mature defenses that actually can be consciously controlled. This intervention does seem to assist in the progression from immature to mature defenses, at least when the person is somewhat psychologically minded. For example, acting out feelings shifted to channeling the negative energy into constructive actions and pursuits (sublimation), such as journaling feelings.

Adaptive dissociation takes the form of absorption in positive foci and compartmentalization. Absorption involves immersion in a constructive pursuit removing a person from negativity, which aligns with sublimation. Everyone is familiar with this defense, such as absorbing oneself in a good book, watching an interesting YouTube video, or hobby pursuit. Applying it consciously takes very little effort and does distance a person psychologically and emotionally from negative thoughts, feelings, and experiences. Compartmentalization, consisting of separating sources of stress into distinct psychological compartments, becomes easier with practice, and is a key way to contain and manage adversity helping to ensure that problems in one area do not spill over and contaminate functioning in other spheres of life. Psychotherapists can advance absorption and compartmentalization, what I refer to as adaptive dissociation (Bowins, 2012), by explaining these strategies and guiding a client in the use of them.

Several forms of psychotherapy provide strategies that can powerfully advance psychological defense mechanisms. **Acceptance and Commitment Therapy** enhances adaptive dissociation through cognitive defusion, which means stepping back from thoughts favoring experiential avoidance to obtain a more objective perspective. Psychotherapist can encourage people to step back from an entrenched perspective by imagining it in another person, or similar distancing strategies. **Behavior Therapy** fosters absorption in positive rewarding pursuits enhancing adaptive dissociation. **Cognitive Therapy** is primarily oriented to shifting negative thoughts and themes underlying them to positive cognitions, thereby clearly advancing the positive cognitive distortion psychological defense mechanism template. At the core this entails identifying negative thoughts and underlying schema, and then reframing them in a positive way. A manual is not required, and it can be applied whenever negative perspectives emerge. **Compassion-Focused Therapy** shifts a person from thoughts that are critical of oneself and others (negative distortions) to self-supportive thoughts and understanding perspectives regarding others (positive distortions), by applying compassion-oriented reasoning, behavior, imagery, and feelings. The focus on compassion then advances the positive cognitive distortion defense. Absorption in compassionate cognitions and behavior distances a person from negativity, thereby enhancing adaptive dissociation. **Emotion-Focused Therapy** fosters positive cognitive distortions by providing corrective emotional experiences: altering negative emotional responses not adaptive to circumstances and the escalation of these, to more positive emotional reactions appropriate to circumstances. Focusing on how adaptive or maladaptive a client's emotional response is will assist in this process.

When elements of experience are dissociated and not fused, as seems to occur with trauma (Bowins, 2010), strategies that assist in the fusion are very helpful. **Gestalt Therapy** appears to achieve this through full experiential awareness and clear expression of relevant thoughts and emotions, transforming incomplete gestalts into complete ones. Grieving is likely occurring with this strategy, and healthy grieving is capable of fusing dissociated elements of trauma (Bowins, 2010). Hence, encouraging and supporting traumatized clients in grieving losses associated with the traumatic event resolves the dissociation that although adaptive in the moment of trauma, is negative in the longer run. Another way of framing this is restoring more adaptive dissociation.

Mindfulness-Based Therapy, and almost certainly any form of meditation, probably works via dissociative absorption (see the Psychological defense mechanism chapter). In the process of experiencing the present moment without distraction or focusing on an object as with concentrative meditation, absorption in a positive focus is transpiring helping to distance the individual from negativity. By not reacting to negative intrusions this psychological distancing is furthered. **Narrative Therapy** advances adaptive dissociation via externalization, consisting of the client distancing themselves from the problem, as opposed to the person being the problem. This dissociation of the problem from the person fosters a sense of psychological control. The generation of coherent, dominant, and positive self-narratives powerfully enhances positive cognitive distortions, and is quite an easy strategy to apply, often being experienced as uplifting to the client. To build a positive story it is helpful to have the person first journal positive aspects of their life, as these components form the basis of the positive storylines.

As the name strongly implies, **Positive Psychotherapy** very much advances positive cognitive distortions. Negative distortions are replaced by positive ones through strategies such as gratitude journaling, designing a beautiful day, and self-esteem journaling, and the encouragement of hope, engagement, achievement, and balance. This intense positive focus also facilitates absorption in positivity adaptively dissociating the person from negativity. **Problem-Solving Therapy** fosters compartmentalization by breaking down seemingly insurmountable problems when experienced as a whole, into manageable components, an approach that is widely applied to challenging issues and not just in this form of psychotherapy. Last but certainly not least when it comes to psychological defense mechanisms, **Psychoanalytic Therapy** advances this important state and process characterizing mental health, with shifts from immature to mature defenses transpiring with at least a longer term therapy (Perry, 2001; Perry and Bond, 2004; Van Wijk-Herbrink et al., 2011; Vlastelica et al., 2005). A technique that can be applied is assessing defense mechanism functioning, a process that does not have to be based on tests. However, it does require knowledge of classical defense mechanisms, as well as recognition of them from client–therapist interactions and what the client discusses regarding relationships outside of therapy. Strategies can be taken to counter immature defenses and foster mature ones. For example, if a client is projecting their own negative states such as anger, accusing the therapist of being angry at them for being late, a transference interpretation can help the person see where the anger originates and take ownership. When applied properly with a high index of belief that it is occurring, transference interpretation is very powerful in helping clients become more self-aware, including of psychological defenses. A therapist can then foster mature defenses such as positive anticipation of problems, as with lateness and timing issues addressed through proactive planning.

Psychological defense mechanism functioning can then be robustly advanced by both general strategies and those derived from major forms of psychotherapy. Eleven major forms of psychotherapy—acceptance and commitment therapy, behavior therapy, cognitive therapy, compassion-focused therapy, emotion-focused therapy, gestalt therapy, mindfulness-based therapy, narrative therapy, positive psychotherapy, problem-solving therapy, and psychoanalysis—offer strategies to enhance positive cognitive distortions, adaptive dissociation in terms of absorption and even compartmentalization, and also classical Freudian defenses.

Social connectedness

During at least 95% of human evolution we were connected to others in hunting–gathering groups, but in industrial society people are often quite isolated. Psychotherapists can generally bolster social connectedness by encouraging clients to become more socially active, attempt to form relationships, and bond with others. How this might look can vary, as with just picking up the phone and calling old friends or relatives, interacting more with coworkers, trying to find a romantic partner, or getting involved in community social activities. Anxiety is commonly present resulting in avoidance of social scenarios. In such instances the client must face their fear and approach rather than avoid, often overcoming early life attachment issues. As a nonspecific factor, the quality of the therapeutic relationship is a template for social connectedness, and in itself can provide a sense of being emotionally bonded to another person. Therapist empathy plays a key role in the therapeutic alliance and contributes to trust, openness, caring, compassion, support, understanding, consistency, high engagement, positive regard and affirmation, relevant feedback, and collaboration, further advancing social connectedness.

Various forms of psychotherapy enhance social connectedness, often conditionally upon this being focused on, thereby offering helpful strategies. When social involvement is an area subject to experiential avoidance, **Acceptance and Commitment Therapy** works by having the client accept the anxiety and commit to social actions designed to foster a connection. **Behavioral Therapy** will advance social activity when targeted as something positive to the client, although perhaps feared. Social activity in itself does not guarantee a sense of being connected to others, but it is a prerequisite: without social activity, it is difficult to truly feel connected. By increasing social behavior in a graded way to overcome the anxiety, behavioral therapy can create the right scenario for social connectedness. **Cognitive Therapy** addresses negative cognitions blocking social activity and connectedness when this is an issue. By reframing thoughts that distance a person from others to ones that support engagement, social connectedness is advanced. This positive reframing aligns with the Masi et al. (2011) metaanalysis mentioned in the Social connectedness chapter, finding that for social isolation the most effective intervention is reframing negative cognitions hindering social interactions.

Compassion-Focused Therapy offers a unique approach to enhancing social connectedness via prosocial behavior, derived from understanding and compassion toward oneself and others. Harsh attitudes directed at others create a social distancing and when directed at the self reduces confidence limiting prosocial behavior. Compassion overcomes both sources of social isolation fostering connectedness. According to **Gestalt Therapy**, problems with social interactions occur due to contact boundary issues, involving impaired identification of what arises from the self and others. Alienation transpires due to the person seeing their own faults in others and reacting negatively. By assisting clients in clarifying their own limitations and that of others interacted with, the person will take ownership of their own role and not react negatively to other people, setting the stage for social connectedness. As might be expected from the title, **Interpersonal Psychotherapy** offers robust ways to advance social connectedness. Improving social skills definitely increases the likelihood of a person forming solid relationships with others. Resolving role disputes restores the bond that previously was present. Managing complicated bereavement and role transitions enables a person to progress to new relationships.

Social connectedness can then be advanced generally by encouraging clients to be more socially active and form relationships, with the therapeutic alliance a solid template and an instance of social connectedness in and of itself. Empathy plays a key role in the therapeutic alliance and fosters many prosocial behaviors further enhancing social connectedness. Several major forms of psychotherapy offer strategies that strongly advance social connectedness, often contingent upon this being a concern and focus. Advancing a sense of belonging aligns with human evolution and how this long history has instilled a need for relationships.

Regulation

Maintaining emotions, thoughts, and behavior within healthy limits is crucial to mental health. A general way to foster regulation in psychotherapy is to have clients become aware of when negative emotions, thoughts, and behavior are too extreme. With this understanding actions can be taken to regulate the issue of concern, such as inhibiting negative behaviors that are excessive. Emotion regulation can be advanced by discussing emotion information processing, identifying the type of cognitive activating appraisal that triggers key emotions: loss-sadness, threat or danger-fear, violation or damage-anger, gain-happiness, for instance. Also, how thought processes amplify these emotions (the amplification effect) shifting sadness to depression and fear to anxiety. This straightforward information provides clients with the capacity to understand why certain emotions arise, and survey circumstances both external and internal to discern the source. I have found that clients readily process this information and can apply it to limit negative emotions. For instance, "I'm feeling angry so I must be perceiving a violation of sorts." Identifying the source and working with it, such as adjusting the perspective if not accurate or managing the source if realistic, enables the emotion to be regulated.

Emotion regulation appears to transpire with all forms of psychotherapy operating across all types of psychopathology, as covered in the Behavioral therapy chapter (Sloan et al., 2017). This benefit likely transpires due to how psychotherapy enhances the psychobiology of emotion regulation, including prefrontal cortex activity providing top-down regulation of excessive limbic system activity (Stein, 2008). Other nonspecific factors also regulate emotions including therapist influences, with empathy crucial, and interpersonal synchrony (see the Nonspecific factors chapter). In addition to these transtherapy aspects, some forms of psychotherapy offer approaches to regulate emotions and other aspects of psychological functioning. **Acceptance and Commitment Therapy** assists in regulating disturbing emotions by having a client accept the emotion and not engage in actions to avoid it, the result being that the negative emotion loses its power to motivate and influence. People naturally attempt to eliminate adverse emotions, which in many ways reinforces the power of these emotions, but by seeing that they can be safely lived with emotion regulation is advanced. This form of psychotherapy also facilitates regulation of dysfunctional behaviors, such as excessive food consumption in the context of eating disorders.

Behavioral Therapy enhances regulation via absorption in positive pursuits that shift a person away from the negative focus. Frequently, negative emotions and thoughts mutually reinforce one another with negative thoughts increasing negative emotions, creating an emotional climate for further negative thoughts, and so on. Absorption in positive activity cancels this negative scenario, and helps establish mutual reinforcement between positive emotions and thoughts, although behavioral therapy does not directly focus on emotions and thoughts. **Cognitive Therapy** powerfully advances emotion regulation by targeting the negative thoughts triggering negative emotions, and replacing these thoughts with positive ones yielding positive emotions. The mutually reinforcing cycles of negative thoughts and negative emotions are then countered, and positive cycles fostered. There is substantial evidence that cognitive therapy and related approaches actually comprise cognitive regulatory therapies, providing top-down neural regulation of excessive limbic system activity (Bowins, 2013; Stein, 2008). Cognitive therapy applied to psychotic-level thoughts is effective in normalizing these extreme cognitive distortions. Having the person attempt to provide evidence for the psychotic belief, and going over how there must be clear evidence casts doubt on their hypothesis. Generating alternative explanations dilutes the belief, and testing the explanations instills a rational process further regulating the psychotic-level cognitive distortion.

Compassion-Focused Therapy counters the way that self-criticisms and harsh perspectives toward others generates excessive negative emotions, such as shame, guilt, sadness, anxiety, and anger, that are difficult to regulate. The compassionate approach to oneself and others sooths negative emotions and fosters positive feelings. **Emotion-Focused Therapy** has a powerful impact on emotion regulation as would be expected with this title. This transpires by having a client understand emotional responses relative to circumstances, why maladaptive emotional responses are occurring, how there can be detrimental emotional responses to emotions, and providing a corrective emotional experience. For psychotherapists not trained in this highly manualized modality, simply a focus on emotion information processing and applying this as a guide to how adaptive or maladaptive the client's emotional responses are, can assist in providing a corrective emotional experience with an outcome of adaptive emotional reactions to circumstances.

Existential Psychotherapy robustly regulates negative emotions, and certainly anxiety, arising from the core conflicts we all experience pertaining to death, aloneness, meaninglessness, and freedom and responsibility. Addressing and not avoiding the conflict between these themes and what we would prefer, reduces negative emotions. Meaningful and authentic life changes further regulate negative emotions associated with the core conflicts, by creating favorable outcomes increasing positive emotions. **Gestalt Therapy** enhances emotion regulation by fostering full experiential awareness of emotions and thoughts in the moment via active expression, as opposed to discussing them in a detached way such as part of the past, enabling a client to integrate the experience into a meaningful whole. This process settles adverse emotions. **Mindfulness-Based Therapy** appears to bolster various components of regulation including emotion regulation, self-regulation, and self-control, likely in my opinion via absorption in the peaceful aspects of present moment and not responding to negativity. In addition to mindfulness, other forms of meditation also advance regulation via absorption (Bowins, 2012). There is substantial evidence of top-down regulation presented in the Mindfulness-based psychotherapy chapter.

Narrative Therapy is able to bolster emotion regulation by shifting negative and limited self-narratives generating excessive negative emotions, to positive and coherent narratives about oneself favoring positive emotions. The technique of deconstruction, whereby overly complex negative scenarios are transformed into manageable ones, also advances regulation due to how overwhelming scenarios trigger negative emotions that are difficult to regulate, but when the scenario is limited and manageable these emotions are reduced. By shifting immature psychological defenses to mature ones, emotion regulation is advanced by **Psychoanalytic Therapy**: immature defenses are inadequate for regulating emotions whereas mature ones such as sublimation, positive anticipation, suppression, altruism, and humor are excellent for managing negative emotions. As mentioned earlier, this shift occurs with longer term psychotherapy and certainly of a psychoanalytic nature, but likely with others, and mature psychological defenses can be taught and consciously applied. **Rationale-Emotive Therapy** enhances emotion regulation based on how irrational inflexible beliefs generate no shortage of negative outcomes and emotions that are challenging to regulate, whereas very direct efforts to get clients to relinquish these beliefs and adopt rationale and flexible beliefs yield positive outcomes and emotions.

Regulation and most prominently emotion regulation can be advanced by general psychotherapy strategies. Awareness of when negative emotions, thoughts, and behavior are excessive and consciously taking steps to limit the expression comprise very basic strategies to advance regulation. Emotion regulation can be enhanced by focusing on emotion information processing. It is also advanced by therapist empathy and interpersonal synchrony. A diverse range of approaches derived from many of the major forms of psychotherapy also foster regulation. Of great significance, there is evidence that emotion regulation is a transtherapy benefit occurring regardless of the type of psychotherapy, that likely operates via enhanced top-down neural regulation of excessive limbic system activity.

Human-specific cognition

This crucial aspect of mental health including basic cognition (largely executive functions), social cognition, and motivation (see the Human-specific cognition chapter for a complete description) is the most challenging to enhance through psychotherapy, or likely any means. For each component, general strategies not linked to particular forms of psychotherapy can potentially be helpful, but the impact is not certain. Executive functions might be improved by commercial programs such as Lumosity which a therapist can recommend, although the evidence is not conclusive and a person really has to engage. Also, recall that when a commercial product is involved research bias enters the picture if the researchers have a vested interest, so any supporting research must be looked at critically unless conducted by fully independent and objective researchers. A simpler way to improve some executive functions is have a client practice the task. The feasibility of this is best for memory which beyond the school years many people do not use, and memory has largely been outsourced to computer devices. I have had clients complain of poor memory, and later report that their memory is better after practice.

Social cognition lends itself more to improvement from general psychotherapy strategies. Consistent with our social nature many clients are concerned about their social functioning, having trouble deciphering the intent of others, and understanding how they contribute to social outcomes. Psychotherapy generally can assist in this understanding through discussions regarding various interactions and also the client–therapist relationship. The psychotherapeutic relationship is unique in that a person can gain supportive feedback about their role and how they approach interactions.

Motivation can be enhanced by the therapist applying a cost-benefit analysis and motivational interviewing. Even though it often occurs unconsciously, people tend to weigh the pluses and minuses of a given option, and are motivated when benefits > costs. Having clients elevate this to a conscious level, even writing out the advantages and disadvantages can increase motivation when there is a clear net gain from a given option. Motivational interviewing relies on cognitive dissonance and other strategies to increase motivation, the former consisting of pointing out the inconsistency between a negative behavior and values/goals. For instance, "You indicated how you value education but have not progressed to college or university." Since the person cannot alter the latter part, motivation for attending is increased. The supportive therapeutic relationship as a nonspecific factor can also enhance motivation. Through these various strategies not linked to any one form of psychotherapy, executive functions, social cognition, and motivation can be improved.

Some of the major forms of psychotherapy improve human-specific cognition, and the strategies can be applied to advance this crucial state and process for mental health. **Behavioral Therapy** advances motivation via reinforcement: behavior leading to outcomes that are positive to a person is engaged in regardless of thoughts and feelings, and the reward instills motivation. Frequently, anxiety inhibits actions and the person never acquires the reward resulting in limited motivation. **Emotion-Focused Therapy** improves social cognition by assisting in the understanding of emotions, and the role they play in interactions. The client is also likely to advance in their capacity to accurately read emotions in others and respond appropriately. As mentioned in the Emotion-focused therapy chapter, this form of psychotherapy is overly complex, but the approach of having clients understand the information value of emotions, and learn to work with this understanding does not require a manualized approach, more just an emphasis on emotions and the therapist being familiar with emotion information processing. **Interpersonal Therapy** also improves social cognition when there are deficits. By deciphering how the client relates to others and reacts, and from these actions how others respond to them, the person gains a unique insight into their social behavior thereby advancing social cognition, with this applied to relationships. The technique of role playing can be very effective for altering how a client interacts with others. Exploring role disputes can also enhance social understanding and hence social cognition.

Mindfulness-Based Therapy benefits the executive functions of attention, inhibition, and cognitive flexibility, although research results are somewhat mixed. There is an intuitive logic to meditation improving attention given that a person learns to control what is consciously attended to. This action also entails inhibiting competing thought streams in some instances, and flexibly shifting the focus. **Narrative Therapy** can improve motivation by replacing limiting negative self-narratives that demotivate with positive inspiring ones. It is very straightforward to have clients generate positive stories about themselves building on positive features. In a related fashion, **Positive Psychotherapy** enhances motivation via the positive focus, with the ongoing journaling (gratitude and self-esteem) work instilling this as a pattern. **Problem-Solving Therapy** can improve executive functioning from the very cognitive nature of the approach: a client has to identify problems, clarify them, generate realistic solutions, select the best option, develop an action plan, implement it, and monitor the outcome. Several executive functions are activated in this process, such as attention, set shifting (cognitive flexibility) by generating various solutions, inhibition pertaining to nonviable options, planning in regards to actions, and monitoring by evaluating outcomes. It actually has the potential to significantly ramp up executive functioning, and is almost certainly the most promising psychotherapy option for improving this crucial aspect of human-specific cognition that is typically very difficult to change.

Hence, despite being challenging to advance compared to the other states and processes for mental health, basic cognition (largely executive functions), social cognition, and motivation do respond to psychotherapy interventions not tied to a particular modality, and also from select major forms—executive functions with problem-solving therapy, and perhaps mindfulness; social cognition from emotion-focused therapy and interpersonal therapy; motivation with behavioral therapy, narrative therapy, and positive psychotherapy.

Self-acceptance

Self-concept (self-perspectives) and self-esteem (self-evaluations) are the basis of self-acceptance. Both self-concept and self-esteem can be enhanced from psychotherapy by the nonspecific factor of a solid therapeutic alliance fostered by robust empathy, given that perspectives and evaluations of oneself are linked to social input. Positive engagement does help people improve how they view themselves. Beyond this basic level, providing positive feedback to the client can be very helpful, instead of just focusing on dysfunctional behavior and thoughts. A therapist can point out the person's strengths and build on these for progress. For example, "The way you describe your work experiences indicate that you are conscientious." Of course, the comments need to capture real strengths of the client and not be contrived.

Self-acceptance is robustly advanced by several of the major forms of psychotherapy covered, and the strategies can be readily applied. By having a person accept some adversity and still progress to achieve valued goals, positive outcomes will ensue from **Acceptance and Commitment Therapy** improving self-perspectives and self-evaluation. The commitment to action helps ensure that this transpires, increasing the likelihood that self-acceptance will be enhanced. **Behavioral Therapy** fosters diverse activities that are positive to the person and reinforcing. Success with activities of interest that were previously avoided or inhibited should further self-concept and self-esteem, and hence self-acceptance. By reframing negative self-referential thoughts and any underlying schema to positive thoughts about oneself, **Cognitive Therapy** can strongly advance self-perspectives. Outside of a manualized format a psychotherapist can readily apply this approach by listening for negative self-perspectives, drawing attention to them, and assisting the person in reframing them in a positive fashion. Encouraging the person to practice this on their own, and ask for examples the next session, always helps ensure that the process is continued outside of sessions.

Compassion-Focused Therapy strongly advances self-acceptance because self-compassionate perspectives bolster the core of one's being, leading to improved self-concept and self-esteem. Many people who seek psychotherapy are very self-critical, eroding the core foundation supporting their self-concept and self-evaluations. The compassionate approach from the therapist provides a solid template for how to be self-compassionate. **Existential**

Psychotherapy helps people become more self-aware of how core conflicts pertaining to death, aloneness, meaninglessness, and freedom and responsibility, generate anxiety in all of us. The client is also made aware of how some anxiety from these sources is unavoidable, and by managing the conflicts a person can identify what makes for an authentic and meaningful life for them. The changes that transpire improve self-perspective and self-evaluation. Since everyone, including the psychotherapist, has these concerns discussions are easy to engage in, and definitely do not require any advanced knowledge of philosophy.

There are at least two ways that the strategies of **Gestalt Therapy** improve self-acceptance. A key one is the emphasis on full self-awareness, with a focus on blending foreground and background features of self-perspective: people are caught up in a focus on negative foreground features with the more positive background aspects faded. By having a person refocus on the background to their life a balanced and more positive picture emerges, advancing self-concept and self-esteem. The strategy of identifying and removing blocks to personal growth and self-actualization also advances self-acceptance. **Narrative Therapy** clearly enhances self-acceptance by generating positive self-narratives that are coherent and balanced, thereby bolstering the foundation supporting self-perspectives and self-evaluations. **Person-Centered Therapy** robustly advances self-acceptance, based on how the client is to discover themselves, identify inconsistencies between the actual and ideal self, devise solutions to achieve congruency, and recruit their resources to achieve it. This approach is very empowering improving self-concept and self-esteem. **Positive Psychotherapy** enhances self-acceptance, with self-esteem journaling listing what a person has done well at, comprising a specific strategy to achieve this outcome. The engagement and achievement focus yields real gains supporting improved self-acceptance. **Problem-Solving Therapy** empowers a client by breaking problems down into manageable components, devising solutions, and then implementing them. This empowerment combined with improved outcomes enhances self-concept and self-esteem.

Both general psychotherapy strategies and those derived from major forms of psychotherapy robustly advance self-concept, self-esteem, and from these, self-acceptance. The nonspecific factor of a solid therapeutic alliance fostered by empathy bolsters self-acceptance due to the importance of social input. Focusing on a client's realistic strengths instead of limitations is an easy way for therapists to improve self-acceptance. Ten of the fifteen major forms of psychotherapy offer robust approaches to improving self-concept and self-esteem that are readily applied without a manual. Furthermore, several of these approaches overlap assisting in the ease of application. For example, enhanced self-awareness transpires fostering positive changes in thoughts and behaviors, and compatible positive self-referential perspectives are instilled, such as from cognitive therapy, compassion-focused therapy, gestalt therapy, narrative therapy, and positive psychotherapy.

Adaptability

Flexibly adapting to ever-changing circumstances is key to mental health. Generally, this can be advanced in psychotherapy by examining how a client perceives behavior in relation to circumstances. I have noted that many clients think in terms of good-bad, right-wrong, and the like, applying absolutes. Shifting their perspective to what is adaptive for the given circumstances can be quite enlightening, paving the way for more adaptive behavior. Encouraging the person to think of behavior relative to circumstances ongoing instills this approach as a pattern. The general way that nonspecific factors appear to foster neural plasticity (see the Nonspecific factors chapter) enables them to enhance adaptability.

Adaptability is advanced by strategies drawn from different major forms of psychotherapy. **Acceptance and Commitment Therapy** does so by having the client flexibly adjust behavior in the service of valued goals. Behavioral flexibility, labeled psychological flexibility, is encouraged to achieve these goals despite adversity. Cognitive flexibility itself is enhanced by producing broad and balanced perspectives to minimize avoidance responses. **Cognitive Therapy** also advances psychological flexibility and so adaptability, largely by the reframing of negative perspectives including specific thoughts and underlying beliefs. Adhering to unreasonably negative thoughts typically results in maladaptive outcomes, whereas flexibly shifting perspectives to see the positive side fosters behavior that aligns with circumstances. When relationships are a focus, **Interpersonal Psychotherapy** produces more adaptive behavior by resolving role disputes, fostering smoother role transitions, and improving social skills. Role issues often involve inflexible thoughts and actions, such as a man expecting his wife to do all the housework like his mother, and by adjusting expectations for this role transition, adaptive alterations in behavior ensue. If interpersonal skill deficits are a concern, improving these skills will provide for a more extensive range of social behaviors increasing the probability of adaptive outcomes.

Mindfulness-Based Therapy improves adaptability by instilling greater cognitive flexibility, likely due to improved control over attention, inhibiting negative thought streams, and shifting to a focus on the peaceful present. By altering negative and limiting self-stories to positive ones that are coherent and balanced, **Narrative Therapy** advances adaptability: limited and negative self-narratives often occur with repetitive maladaptive behavior, such as "I can never win," whereas positive and more comprehensive narratives favor actions adaptive to circumstances, with an example being, "I can win when the task matches my skill set." Psychotherapists can readily assist a client in producing narratives that favor adaptive behavior. "Innovative moments" in story generation appear to shift rigid self-narratives into more flexible and adaptive stories.

Even the title, **Problem-Solving Therapy** suggests that it can promote adaptive behavior. Problems that bring people into psychotherapy commonly involve inflexible repetitive approaches that do not fit with circumstances. Solutions derived from the problem-solving steps—problem identification, clarification, generating realistic solutions, selecting the best option, developing an action plan, implementing it, and monitoring the outcome—will fit behavior to circumstances enhancing adaptability. **Rationale-Emotive Therapy** is ideally suited to improving adaptability given its focus on irrational negative beliefs that are not consistent with the demands of reality. Assertively addressing these irrational beliefs in therapy, and having the client develop rational beliefs fitting with reality greatly advances flexibility and adaptability.

Psychotherapy generally can advance adaptability if the therapist looks at how the client perceives behavior in relation to circumstances. The common emphasis on absolutes such as good-bad and right-wrong favors inflexible and maladaptive actions. Encouraging, guiding, and supporting the client in processing behavior in relation to circumstances will produce much more adaptive behavior. Neural plasticity appears to increase as a nonspecific psychotherapy influence, thereby fostering adaptive thoughts and actions. Several major forms of psychotherapy provide strategies to advance psychological flexibility, producing a shift from inflexible maladaptive perspectives and actions to flexible and adaptive behavior aligning with circumstances.

Bringing it all together in psychotherapy

General psychotherapy strategies and those from major forms of psychotherapy robustly advance the states and processes for mental health—activity, psychological defense mechanisms, social connectedness, regulation, human-specific cognition, self-acceptance, and adaptability. Nonspecific factors operate across all variants of psychotherapy to achieve this outcome. Moving ahead with psychotherapy the best option is to focus on the states and processes for mental health, and apply therapeutic strategies that advance them. This novel psychotherapy focus might seem overwhelming, but is actually quite straightforward when not applying manual approaches from major (or minor) forms of psychotherapy. In my experience, every form of psychotherapy can be readily applied without a manual based on the core principles and processes. This approach is more flexible enabling interventions that work at a given time to be applied. For example, if practicing cognitive therapy in a manual form and a powerful transference issue arises, the therapist cannot easily venture there, but certainly can to the benefit of the client if flexibly applying strategies from various forms of psychotherapy. Indeed, this flexible approach is more adaptive aligning with one of the states and processes for mental health—adaptability. Learning the various strategies presented above is likely easier than mastering a highly manualized form of psychotherapy, and of course with experience a psychotherapist can adopt more strategies ensuring that their interest factor remains high.

The approach to psychotherapy that I am proposing might on the surface appear to be a variant of eclectic psychotherapy, and while it does incorporate strategies both general to psychotherapy and specific to major forms of psychotherapy, it is very different. Eclectic psychotherapy, which I am very familiar with, applies various strategies to remedy psychopathology, based on the client's presentation at a given time. The focus is on psychopathology and remedying it. The approach advocated here is to focus on advancing the states and processes for mental health, with improvements to mental illness naturally following. A key benefit of this approach is the seamless merging of nonspecific factors operating across all forms of psychotherapy and those specific to a form of psychotherapy: both work by advancing the states and processes for mental health. From this outcome, the incomprehensible way that nonspecific factors operate within the discrete psychotherapy model focused on remedying psychopathology becomes highly comprehensible. Essentially, the distinction between nonspecific and specific factors is dissolved, as both work in the same fashion! An additional benefit is being able to define when psychotherapy is required—when one or more of the states and processes for mental health are compromised—and gauging its effectiveness based on improvements in these states and processes.

To achieve this major conceptual and practical shift in psychotherapy, both general strategies and those derived from major forms of psychotherapy are to be applied. Future research can examine more minor forms of psychotherapy to reveal additional robust strategies for advancing one or more of the states and processes for mental health. As mentioned at the start of the book, it might be the case that there are other states and processes for mental health that can be identified, but I strongly caution against diffusing them to the point of being meaningless, either due to a researcher trying to create their own variant as has occurred with forms of psychotherapy, or as a way of weakening this approach to support the discrete model. The states and processes for mental health were carefully considered and researched, and do seem to cover the mental health spectrum. Some researchers will be tempted to add a happiness theme, but in its true context happiness as an emotional reaction to gain is impossible to sustain in a world and universe ruled by entropy (order to disorder), and as such is misguided. Instead of the pursuit of happiness, the happiness of pursuit as a form of adaptive dissociative absorption (a major form of psychological defense mechanism) is viable. Whereas "happiness" does not qualify as a state and process for mental health, positive affectivity over negative affectivity does, and this follows from the other states and processes with a heavy contribution from regulation, psychological defense mechanisms, and activity, the latter derived from how high behavioral activation and low behavioral inhibition entail elevated positive affectivity and reduced negative affectivity. Emotion regulation is noteworthy in that it appears to be advanced by all forms of psychotherapy (transtherapy) and nonspecific factors including the placebo effect, highlighting the crucial role that regulation plays in mental health and how natural healing processes attempt to restore it. Emotion regulation ensures that positive affectivity exceeds negative affectivity in a sustainable fashion, by directly reducing negative emotions, thereby shifting the balance in favor of positive emotions.

A major advantage of this integrated approach to psychotherapy is that it dispenses with the problems that arise from the discrete psychotherapy model—sheer number of psychotherapy types, research bias arising from the competition to establish efficacy for funding purposes, the way that psychotherapy has fads that then fade when the originator and students fade, and weaknesses in the core rationale (see the Problems with the discrete psychotherapy approach chapter). Psychotherapy training will focus on robust strategies to advance the states and processes for mental health, drawing significantly from existing forms of psychotherapy which will help perpetuate them in a more sustainable way than the current fads and fades manner. Students will develop a highly flexible and targeted way to deliver psychotherapy, and payers will not have to make decisions on the basis of what is often biased efficacy data. Perhaps most important, consumers will benefit from an integrated approach oriented to advancing the states and processes crucial to their mental health. Although a manualized format is not likely to aid in delivering psychotherapy as described and will probably reduce the flexibility of its delivery, a condensed assessment form to evaluate a client's functioning on the seven states and processes for mental health will be of benefit: impairments to activity, psychological defense mechanisms, social connectedness, regulation, human-specific cognition, self-acceptance, and adaptability, produces formal and informal mental illness necessitating psychotherapy, while robust functioning on these core states and processes characterizes mental health, hence a clear way of assessing them will be helpful. The way forward usually involves major theoretical shifts, and in the case of psychotherapy this entails transitioning from a focus on remedying psychopathology to advancing the states and processes for mental health, a shift that resolves the major problems with the current discrete psychotherapy approach, dissolves the distinction between specific and nonspecific factors, and provides an integrated and continuous model of psychotherapy.

References

Akiskal, H.S., Pinto, O., 1999. The evolving bipolar spectrum: prototypes I, II, III, and IV. Psychiatric Clin. North Am. 22, 517–534.

Beck, A., 1991. Cognitive therapy: a 30-year retrospective. Am. Psychol. 46 (4), 368–375.

Boswell, J.F., 2013. Intervention strategies and clinical process in transdiagnostic cognitive-behavioral therapy. Psychotherapy (Chicago) 50 (3), 381–386.

Boswell, J.F., Farchione, T.J., Sauer-Zavala, S., Murray, H.W., Fortune, M.R., Barlow, D.H., 2013. Anxiety sensitivity and interoceptive exposure: a transdiagnostic construct and change strategy. Behav. Ther. 44 (3), 417–431.

Bowins, B.E., 2004. Psychological defense mechanisms: a new perspective. Am. J. Psychoanal. 64, 1–26.

Bowins, B., 2008. Hypomania: a depressive inhibition override defense mechanism. J. Affect. Disord. 109, 221–232.

Bowins, B.E., 2010. Repetitive maladaptive behavior: beyond repetition compulsion. Am. J. Psychoanal. 70, 282–298.

Bowins, B.E., 2012. Therapeutic dissociation: compartmentalization & absorption. Couns. Psychol. Q. 25 (1), 307–317.

Bowins, B.E., 2013. Cognitive Regulatory Control Therapies. Am. J. Psychother. 67 (3), 215–236.

Bowins, B., 2020. Activity for Mental Health. Academic Press, Cambridge, MA.

Eckblad, M., Chapman, L.J., 1986. Development and validation of a scale for hypomanic personality. J. Abnorm. Psychol. 95, 214–222.

Farchione, T.J., Boswell, J.F., Wilner, J.G., 2017. Behavioral activation strategies for major depression in transdiagnostic cognitive-behavioral therapy: an evidence-based case study. Psychotherapy (Chicago) 54 (3), 225–230.

Jamison, K., Gerner, R., Hammen, C., Padesky, C., 1980. Clouds and silver linings: positive experiences associated with primary affective disorders. Am. J. Psychiatry 137, 198–202.

Kaplan, D.M., Palitsky, R., Carey, A.L., Crane, T.E., Havens, C.M., Medrano, M.R., et al., 2018. Maladaptive repetitive thought as a transdiagnostic phenomenon and treatment target: an integrative review. J. Clin. Psychol. 74 (7), 1126–1136.

Koukopoulos, A., Sani, G., Koukopoulos, A.E., Minnai, G.P., Girardi, P., Pani, L., et al., 2003. Duration and stability of the rapid-cycling course: a long-term personal follow-up of 109 patients. J. Affect. Disord. 73, 75–85.

Masi, C.M., Chen, H.Y., Hawkley, L.C., Cacioppo, J.T., 2011. A meta-analysis of interventions to reduce loneliness. Pers. Soc. Psychol. Rev. 15 (3), 216–266.

Meyer, B., Johnson, S.L., Carver, C.S., 1999. Exploring behavioral activation and inhibition sensitivities among college students at risk for bipolar spectrum symptomatology. J. Psychopathol. Behav. Assess. 21, 275–292.

Neacsiu, A.D., Herr, N.R., Fang, C.M., Rodriguez, M.A., Rosenthal, M.Z., 2015. Identity disturbance and problems with emotion regulation are related constructs across diagnoses. J. Clin. Psychol. 71 (4), 346–361.

Perry, C., 2001. A pilot study of defenses in adults with personality disorders entering psychotherapy. J. Nerv. Ment. Dis. 189, 651–660.

Perry, J.C., Bond, M., 2004. Long-term changes in defense styles with psychodynamic psychotherapy for depressive, anxiety, and personality disorders. Am. J. Psychiatry 161 (9), 1665–1671.

Pontzer, H., 2017. The crown joules: energetics, ecology, and evolution in humans and other primates. Evol. Anthropol. 26 (1), 12–24.

Raichlen, D.A., Alexander, G.E., 2017. Adaptive capacity: an evolutionary neuroscience model linking exercise, cognition, and brain health. Trends Neurosci. 40 (7), 408–421.

Sloan, E., Hall, K., Moulding, R., Bryce, S., Mildred, H., Staiger, P.K., 2017. Emotion regulation as a transdiagnostic treatment construct across anxiety, depression, substance abuse, eating and borderline personality disorders: a systematic review. Clin. Psychol. Rev. 57, 141–163.

Stein, D.J., 2008. Emotional regulation: implications for the psychobiology of psychotherapy. CNS Spectr. 13 (3), 195–198.

Van Wijk-Herbrink, M., Andrea, H., Verheul, R., 2011. Cognitive coping and defense styles in patients with personality disorders. J. Pers. Disord 25 (5), 634–644.

Vlastelica, M., Jurcevic, S., Zemunik, T., 2005. Changes of defense mechanisms and personality profile during group analytic treatment. Coll. Anthropol. 29 (2), 551–558.

Concluding word

An unfortunate occurrence I have noted in the mental health field is seemingly intense resistance to change. For instance, how the Diagnostic and Statistical Manual of Mental Disorders persists with a discrete model that even at face value is questionable, as with minor and major forms of depression, and bipolar depression somehow different than unipolar depression. Psychotherapy, likewise, is stuck in a resistance to change rut repeating the perspective that the mechanism of action consists of remedying psychopathology via numerous discrete forms of psychotherapy, to indirectly improve mental health. To perpetuate this notion insurmountable problems with the model are not considered: too many forms of psychotherapy each with its special sauce applied to a given problem, the way that many forms are extended to multiple mental health issues, and the impossibility of understanding how nonspecific factors operate within this discrete psychotherapy model.

The way forward involves being aware of our propensity to focus on the negative, in this instance psychopathology, and appreciate that psychotherapy actually works by directly advancing the states and processes for mental health: activity, psychological defense mechanisms, social connectedness, regulation, human-specific cognition, self-acceptance, and adaptability, with positive affectivity over negative affectivity following from them if it is to be sustainable. The theoretical and empirical proof of concept provided supports this assertion for 15 major forms of psychotherapy, and nonspecific factors. The model proposed represents a transdiagnostic and trans-therapy approach, based on the application of both general strategies and those specific to various forms of psychotherapy, to directly advance each of the states and processes for mental health. An advantage of this model is its capacity to distinguish mental illness from mental health: impairments to one or more of the states and processes characterizing mental health produce formal and informal mental illness, and mental health transpires with robust functioning on these parameters. Consumers, students and providers, educators, and payers will benefit now, and certainly in the future when the number of psychotherapy types will be completely overwhelming. Furthermore, instead of the fad and fade scenario playing out over history with psychotherapy types, the components of each that robustly advance mental health will be preserved. In addition to these very practical considerations, the new model conceptually aligns nonspecific and specific psychotherapy factors.

While change is always challenging, it is worthwhile given that the prevalent approach to psychotherapy has insurmountable practical and conceptual problems. The game changing model presented here resolves these concerns and advances psychotherapy effectiveness by focusing on states and processes for mental health.

Index

FSC
www.fsc.org
MIX
Papier | Fördert
gute Waldnutzung
FSC® C083411

Kolibri 360 GmbH
Ferdinand-Jühlke-Straße 7
99095 Erfurt, Deutschland
produktsicherheit@kolibri360.de